DR.

Natural Cures for Health Disasters

KNOWLEDGE HOUSE PUBLISHERS
Buffalo Grove, Illinois

Copyright, 2005 Knowledge House Publishers

All rights reserved. No part of this book may be reproduced without the expressed written consent of the publisher. Note: copyright infringement is a fraudulent practice and is punishable according to Federal laws by severe penalties.

Revised edition, originally *Lifesaving Cures*

Printed in the United States of America on recycled paper.

ISBN: 1-931078-11-4

Disclaimer: This book is not intended as a substitute for medical diagnosis or treatment. Anyone who has a serious disease should consult a physician before initiating any change in treatment or before beginning any new treatment.

To order this or additional Knowledge House books call 1-866-626-5888. or order via the web at: www.knowledgehousepublishers.com

To get an order form send a SASE to:
Knowledge House Publishers
105 Townline Rd., Unit 116
Vernon Hills, IL 60061

Contents

	Introduction	5
Chapter 1	**It Will Happen**	17
Chapter 2	**Natural Cures**	25
Chapter 3	**Nutrient Dense Foods**	85
Chapter 4	**Wilderness Foods**	107
Chapter 5	**Illnesses**	115
	Appendices	359
	Bibliography	374
	Index	376

Introduction

The objective of this book is simple. It is to describe the most effective and easy ways to cure disease. Plus, it is to provide the quickest methods to do so. It is to elucidate the safest natural remedies for a wide range of illnesses. It is to demonstrate which substances can be relied upon to improve the odds of survival in the 21st century. It is to prepare the individual for the decades ahead. There will be a time which will herald health crises of mammoth proportions. Then, disability, disease, and death beyond human imagination will far exceed the capacity of modern medicine alone to resolve. Thus, it is critical that the individual become capable of self-care through natural cures, which are non-toxic, easy to use, and lifesaving.

Few people know how to take care of themselves in the event of a collapse of personal health, let alone a national crisis. Yet, the need for self-help in the health field is greater now than ever before in modern history. This book helps prepare the individual for the potential health consequences of breakdowns in infrastructure in Western countries as well as disease/epidemics. When health disasters strike, the individual must have available natural substances that work quickly, safely, and reliably, that is for reversing common illnesses and injuries.

The need for such remedies is vast. Billions of humans suffer pain, agony, and distress from potentially curable conditions. Yet the greatest hope for cure lies in the remedies of nature. The use of safe/natural remedies to cure disease is based upon the principles of the Hippocratic Oath, which every physician testifies to upon graduating. This oath is above all "do no harm." In other words, it is superior to do nothing than to in the attempt to cure cause greater damage. In modern medicine such an event—actual harm inflicted upon a patient by the doctor or hospital—is routine. This is why natural medicines are so essential. The fact is the medicine of Hippocrates, the supposed father of medicine, was based exclusively on food and herbs.

The health of Americans is declining, largely because of the devastation of the immune system. This is the result of modern living. Bizarre germs are on the attack, and the immune system of many individuals fails to successfully combat them.

Regarding loss of productivity cold and flu viruses wreak the greatest devastation. What's more, epidemics of food poisoning afflict tens of millions yearly, while killing hundreds and permanently disabling thousands. Powerful viruses, many of them stealth in nature, infect the internal organs at will, causing untold misery and/or permanent damage. Hepatitis viruses are also a significant cause of such disruption. The fact is in North America there is a vast hepatitis epidemic, particularly of hepatitis C, with millions of people afflicted with this disease. No one knows for certain how this pandemic occurred. Ticks infest human beings with rodent-derived germs, which are impossible to eradicate with medications. People are led to believe they are well immunized. Yet, whooping cough and diphtheria are returning. Antibiotics were supposed to protect humanity. Yet, there are thousands of bizarre mutant germs which are immune to antibiotics. In particular, drug-resistant staph, strep, salmonella, enterococcus, pneumococcus, mycobacteria, candida, shigella, clostridium, and E. coli are causing frightening and often lethal epidemics. Infectious diseases are no longer seasonal. They disrupt human lives on a monthly, weekly, and, in some instances, daily basis.

Natural disasters are also increasing the risks, and not just in disaster zones. Epidemics which start in distant regions can spread rapidly, afflicting humanity globally. Mass transport has made this a reality. The year of 1998 heralded the greatest disasters of this generation. Over 50,000 people were killed and tens of millions injured and/or displaced by monster disasters. Hurricanes Georges and Mitch, devastating tornadoes in the southwestern USA, massive earthquakes in Afghanistan, Japan, and Columbia, volcanic eruptions in Mexico, the great Yangtze flood, typhoons and tempests in the South Seas, and disastrous forest fires all over the world have destroyed the lives of people, as well as the infrastructure, including the ecosystems. Yet, the greatest damage to humanity is forthcoming. Surely, the great Indian Ocean tsunami, the 2004 Florida hurricanes, as well as the Bam, Iran, earthquake, have proven that.

As a result of these monstrous disasters untold thousands, rather, millions, more will likely suffer from potentially fatal illnesses. Disaster zones, especially flood zones, breed disease. The decimation in the aftermath of natural disasters will likely be even greater than the original disaster. In 2004 this certainly proved true in the aftermath of hurricanes, which left hundreds of thousands of people vulnerable. The vulnerability is largely for mold contamination, which can lead to lethal diseases. The fact is during 2004 through 2005 tens of thousands of Southerners, particularly Floridians, developed a wide range of bizarre symptoms, which are likely due to mold poisoning: wheezing, asthma attacks, chest congestion, spots on the lungs, nose bleeds, night sweats, sinus disorders, pain in the face, stiff neck, stuffy sinuses, and numerous others. As a result of these devastating disasters there is no way to estimate the long term effects, but they will be monumental.

The financial toll is beyond count. The *Chicago Tribune* reported in November 1998 that natural disasters in that year wrought some 90 billion dollars in damage. The editors note that this is more damage than all the disasters of the prior decade, perhaps as much as two prior decades, combined. The massive snowstorms of 1999 were another promise of more disastrous events and expenses to come. This makes it clear that the 21st century will only be worse. This has already been proven in 1999 by the massive Turkish earthquake, the mammoth mile-wide Oklahoma tornado, the Bam, Iran, earthquake, the 2004 multiple hurricanes of the Deep South and the 2004 Indian Ocean tsunami, disasters the likes of which have never been seen in modern history.

In one year, 1998, there were a greater number of severe natural catastrophes than those occurring in the entire decade from 1988 through 1998. What can be expected in the 21st century? Assuredly, at a minimum the same level of destruction is likely. Yet, there will be events in the 21st century delivering destruction of even greater magnitude, a level of human suffering far beyond the 1998 experience. In fact, the degree of destruction, deluge, disease, and despair likely to strike in the 21st century will surely be unfathomable. The 2004 Indian Ocean tsunami has proven that. The fact is unless abated the negative effects of human meddling will inevitably destroy the planet and the human race.

Certain individuals, including so-called experts, might regard this as "doomsday advice." Yet, these are the same individuals who failed to predict, advise, or warn about the potential for disasters, such as Hurricane Mitch, which destroyed Nicaragua and Honduras. The destruction of an entire country is unprecedented in modern history. None of these "experts" predicted it. Nor do these individuals warn the public about the disasters of modern medicine: antibiotic resistance, super-germs, mutant viruses, toxic drug reactions, the toxicity and futility of chemotherapy, the excessive use of radiotherapy, the toxicity of margarine, the destructive/toxic actions of depleted uranium, which is destroying the health of innocent civilians, as well as military personnel, and the toxic effects of genetically engineered food. These are the truly great American disasters. Consider this: In North America drug therapy alone causes nearly a half million deaths yearly.

They have complicity with such deaths. Governments authorize policies which cause vast destruction, particularly to the environment. When they mandate such destruction, how could it be expected that they would protect the people? Consider the government sponsoring of vaccines, invasions of sovereign nations, and the bombing of the innocent with so-called depleted plutonium. These are criminal acts, which only cause despair. Then, they would supposedly protect the people? The fact is the government will not offer truly valuable preventive advice, nor will they find the much-needed cures. Nor did they or would they prepare the populace for toxic chemical or radiation disasters such as those which occurred in Bhopal, Three Mile Island, and Chernobyl, as well as the fallout of depleted plutonium. Neither do they warn of the disastrous effects of daily exposure to poisonous chemicals such as pesticides, herbicides, fungicides, chlorinated hydrocarbons, and similar carcinogenic substances. One wonders what the motives are of those who warn the public not to listen to valuable or lifesaving advice. What would be the motive of covering up or distorting the truth? Is it anything other than greed?

Think about it. It doesn't require a major disaster for the individual to be forced to rely on natural medicines. After all, doctors no longer make house calls and being stranded is a reality despite modern technology. For instance, entire cities, in fact, entire states, may be isolated merely by a snowstorm or perhaps a flood. Hundreds, even thousands, of lives may be left at risk. Sudden storms, particularly ice storms, may disrupt electricity, cutting off power to thousands of individuals for as long as three weeks. Incredibly, in such events thousands of individuals will suffer from cold exposure. Furthermore, as a result of poor quality food and water hundreds will contract infections. Imagine what would happen if a national power outage or some other disruption affecting food/water purity occurred; millions could develop significant infections.

The same can occur with great snowstorms, where people may be unable to reach physicians or hospitals. Such storms may cause the stranding of potentially millions of travelers. Due to the stress and disruption the risks for infections, particularly the flu, increase. Yet, it was the 2004 Indian Ocean tsunami which proved to be the disaster of all disasters. Here, the morning after Christmas in numerous regions throughout the Indian Ocean all infrastructure was destroyed. The fact is in many regions all that humankind had built was washed into the sea. For the survivors it was each individual on his/her own: with their own hearts and souls, with their own creator.

The world is increasingly stricken with massive disasters: earthquakes, tidal waves, deluges, blizzards, epidemics, tsunamis, volcanic eruptions, and toxic contamination. Monstrous earthquakes have struck Turkey, Iran, China, Japan, and Taiwan. In 2004 in southern Iran as the result of a devastating earthquake an entire city was destroyed. Typhoons pummel southeast Asia. Hurricanes destroy the southern states. As a result, epidemics loom. None of this happens by chance.

Everyone has his/her own disaster story to tell. Think about how much more secure such individuals would feel if they developed a working knowledge of natural/home remedies and, more importantly, if they had such remedies on hand. If it is merely stress, disrupted schedules, and a lack of sleep that are the sole consequences, the individual will recover and life will quickly return to normal; the natural cures would be used to relieve aggravation and stress. However, if such a circumstance is combined with a health disaster, whether it be a horrible bout of the flu, a cold, an earache (which is particularly disastrous when flying, causing perhaps further delay), severe pain, or perhaps something worse, it could be devastating. What a disaster this would be, unless a person is prepared. Armed with a thorough knowledge of natural cures, the individual would be prepared and could handle virtually any crisis more efficiently. These are remedies that can be packed in any luggage, backpack, or purse. Many fit easily in a pocket. In such circumstances is there anything else that the populace could rely upon?

Natural cures may be useful for preventing catastrophes that could cost life or limb or which could result in pain or misery. Here, the objective is to provide alternatives which are unavailable in modern medicine. The fact is regarding disaster-related injuries and chronic illnesses medicine is largely impotent. Other than antibiotics, painkillers, and first aid what else does medicine offer?

True, medicine has a critical role. Yet, regarding self care for disasters, as well as many chronic diseases, there are few if any options. Here modern medicine is impotent. Regarding massive or global disasters these options are also essential. However, the paramount need is for the use of natural cures for everyday illnesses. This is because these are an enormous cause of disability. What's more, there is no way that modern medicine will be able to handle the health consequences of massive disasters due to radiation releases, germ epidemics, the release of biogerms, chemtrails, or toxic chemical exposure. Here, the individual must assume the responsibility for survival. The fact is rather than curing them through their ill-conceived policies the power-monopolists are causing vast disorders. Consider the Gulf War Syndrome: is it anything other than government-issue?

To be optimally prepared people should comprehend options which are safe and most effective. This book provides precisely that information. As a result of its thorough study the individual will learn the following to assist in preparing for the precarious future:

- the most effective self-remedies for infections, *when antibiotics fail*
- the most valuable cures for healing wounds
- the most powerful substances for gaining strength and energy
- foods which offer the greatest fuel and energy power
- foods which offer the greatest nutrient density for the money
- the most effective home remedies for halting or preventing epidemics
- the most useful painkilling self-remedies
- the safest self-remedies for children and the elderly
- natural cures which do not severely interact with prescription medications
- the top natural cures for reversing radiation poisoning
- the top natural cures for reversing toxic chemical damage
- the best natural cures for combating burns
- the most effective natural cures for inactivating venomous wounds
- the top self-remedies for reversing poisoning by prescription medication and other potentially toxic substances, that is antidotes for poisons that are safe to administer in the field
- the most effective self-remedies for sunburn and exposure to the elements
- the best self-remedies for combating the stress and pressure that occur during difficulties/catastrophes or as a result of injury
- the most chemical-free and natural sources of supplements available

A knowledge of natural remedies is essential for guaranteeing the best odds for survival. Certainly, relying upon the typical nonprescription items is virtually useless. In fact, their use may prove dangerous. If there is a health disaster, the worst thing to do is to potentiate it. The dispensation of prescription medications by the general public is totally ill-advised. No one should consume these drugs unless under a physician's care. Nonprescription drugs are equally precarious. In fact, basic drugs, such as aspirin, acetaminophen, and ibuprofen, result in thousands of deaths yearly, even through "normal" use. So, if non-prescription medicines, such as aspirin, digestive aids, antiinflammatory agents, and topical antibiotics, offer little hope and if such prescriptions are too risky to self-consume, what remains? It is only the natural cures which contain the power and safety that only nature itself can produce. They alone are the agents which can be relied upon for survival and cure.

Objections have been raised that no research has been done with the natural cures. It may even be suggested that they may not always be safe. Yet, if care is taken and if only the most natural unadulterated products are used, such products would be far safer to consume than nonprescription drugs. For instance, wild food and herbs have been used for centuries with great success, and research verifies this. These wilderness foods/herbs are completely safe for human consumption. In contrast, biologically or chemically altered products present unknown variables and significant problems. Chemically or genetically altered products have no record of safety. In fact, according to recent research their safety is dubious.

All the survival remedies described in this book are safe, effective, and easy to use. Even children can be taught to use these lifesaving substances. Health disasters create panic, but preparedness can avert further calamities and perhaps needless deaths. Study this information; master it. It could prove lifesaving.

Everyone deserves to know about simple life-enhancing emergency procedures. The public must know as much as possible about safe and easy-to-access remedies, which may be used for health improvement as well as emergencies. The federal government is attempting to restrict free speech, essentially violating the constitution, by blocking the dissemination of valuable information in the field of natural healing. This blockade is largely instigated by special interest groups which profit by restricting such information. This is especially true of the pharmaceutical cartel. This cartel is notorious for its attempts to restrict freedom of choice.

Government proposes to be the agent for protecting the public. Yet, it gives the public no audience for informed choice. The information blockade is to the detriment of the general public. While the sale of natural/herbal products is allowed, valuable, as well as scientific, information about such products is restricted and/or prohibited. What is the reasoning behind the policy to allow a product to be sold and yet disallow information? In fact, it is a costly and dangerous method. Information would allow the individual to make an intelligent choice. It would further the proper use of a product. It would aid in the determination of what is helpful or harmful.

The fact is it is the lack of information that is dangerous. This is the opposite of the government view. It was David Kessler, M.D., then acting FDA Commissioner, who expressed on national TV the government's position, saying, essentially, 'trust us (i.e. you mindless idiots), we will make the decisions for you.' In other words, he was demanding, 'do not take your health into your own hands.' Yet, it was Kessler who was dismissed from the FDA for misappropriating government funds.

North Americans have for too long relied upon doctors for preventive medicine. Physicians are poorly trained in this regard. This book is the opposite of the medical attitude: that is aggressive crisis care. Nature too can be relied upon for emergencies, even for life-threatening diseases. With natural medicine lives can be saved, even in disasters. These are lives that would otherwise be lost, since medicine offers no reliable solutions. Now, the individual will know, nutritionally and herbally, precisely what to do—and what to take—during a disaster. Deadly diseases are now disarmed, all through natural cures. With the following information people will be able to care for themselves in case access to doctors is restricted or impossible.

Chapter 1
It Will Happen

There will be epidemics of mammoth proportions in the 21st century. The world's leading scientists share this viewpoint. It was Dr. J. Lederberg, Nobel Prize winner and current President of Rockefeller University, who said that the threat of a massive epidemic sweeping the Western world is "real...and looming." Virtually no one will be completely prepared. Lederberg states that there is no way that the government will be prepared and that the hospitals are ill-equipped and will be "absolutely swamped."

The epidemics of the 21st century will involve a wide range of germs and a massive number of people. Virtually every country will be affected. No one will be fully prepared. Yet, a thorough knowledge of self-remedies and natural cures will place the informed in an elite, perhaps enviable, position.

Regarding the issue of massive epidemics there should be great concern. Concern is protective, because it creates action. In contrast, inaction, the bane of modern humanity, is deadly. Don't be reticent. You yourself might be one of the unfortunate statistics if you fail to develop a knowledge of what can be done to protect yourself, your loved ones, and perhaps a total stranger.

AIDS is a global epidemic. So is hepatitis. Fungal infections are the bugaboo of Western societies, and infections by an extensive range of fungi, including Candida albicans, are widespread. Drug-resistant microbes—strep, staph, E. coli, salmonella, enterococcus, pseudomonas, clostridium, and numerous others—are decimating the population, yearly afflicting tens of millions of individuals. The *JAMA* (*Journal of American Medical Association*) noted in 1997 that antibiotic-resistant germs kill on a yearly basis a minimum of 250,000 hospitalized patients alone. These are largely pharmaceutically induced deaths. This fails to include the number of people who die from such infections in their homes or in care centers, for instance, hospices and nursing homes. Nor does it include deaths from allergic or toxic reactions to antibiotics. A reasonable total is some 400,000 deaths, all from germs that are modern aberrations, freaks of nature, and which are drug-created. Thus, epidemics, many of which are man-made, already exist. However, as the 21st century progresses these epidemics will worsen. Thus, it is crucial to be prepared so you can protect yourself. If you become the victim, you can't even help yourself, let alone anyone else. What's more, if you fall ill, there will be no one to come to your aid.

Can the consequences of epidemics of such a massive scale that tens of millions of individuals will become infected be imagined? Microbiologists insist such a scenario is inevitable. They claim it is a natural cycle of human civilization. Yet, epidemics already exist, especially in America. This is largely because chronic infections by mutant germs afflict tens of millions of Americans. It is also because of man-made germs, which have escaped from biological laboratories or have been purposely disseminated into the public.

In 1999 a bizarre flu-like illness struck millions, the flu shot seemingly offering little if any protection. Instead of lasting the typical week or so, symptoms persisted as long as six weeks, severely weakening infected individuals.

In late 2003, suddenly, a bizarre flu-like illness struck American children. Some 60 children died. In a number of these children the vaccine appeared to increase the vulnerability to sickness and likely contributed to the deaths. Thereafter, studies performed by a number of investigators, including Susan Dolan of Denver Children's Hospital, documented the virtual uselessness, rather, danger, of giving such vaccines to children.

As mentioned previously the toxicity of flu shots is well reported. As a result of such injections numerous individuals developed serious side effects, including paralysis, heart disorders, and brain damage. What's more, a recent study conducted at the NIH (National Institutes of Health) concluded that for the elderly the flu shot was of no benefit.

Regarding the flu there is great hype. Much of this hype is generated by the pharmaceutical cartel in order to promote its wares. This is despite the fact that there are no medical cures for this condition. Rather, evidence points to medical therapies, notably mass vaccination, as the cause of epidemics. For example, the 1918 pandemic, which killed globally some 80 million people, originated in the vaccinated: the heavily vaccinated soldiers, who, fully infected, returned home after the war.

Modern viruses are stealth in nature. This means they are bizarre, and mutated. It means they can escape immune surveillance. Thus, they are incredibly dangerous. It is not a matter of if they will strike—they are already here, attacking and disabling us.

Judy Kay Gray, M.S., research scientist, describes a frightening scenario: "Global warming is the incubator for the newest wave of infectious diseases; warmth breeds germs. The melting of the icebergs is releasing vast numbers of germs frozen in time for thousands of years. Along with the mutations of virulent germs already in existence the human race is being exposed to killer pathogens previously not encountered by the current generation. This enormous germ burden will inundate the global population, which has no immunity to these freakish germs. As a result disease, disability, and death will reach a level never before previously experienced." Yet, if a thorough knowledge of natural cures is acquired, no such catastrophe need occur. This is because viruses are readily destroyed by natural substances.

The new millennium will be fraught with uncountable disasters, both naturally and humanly induced, causing an unprecedented degree of strife and suffering. The fact is such human despair is currently happening, for instance, disease outbreaks in Honduras and Nicaragua, the tropical diseases infesting the Chinese as a result of the Yangtze flood or the more recent incomprehensible disaster, the Indian Ocean tsunami. What's more, in the Western world unrelated to the powers of nature there is a yearly catastrophe, since tens of thousands of Westerners suffer from chronic infections due to antibiotic-resistant germs. Other tens of thousands abruptly die from such germs, fully a man-made catastrophe. Likewise, hundreds of thousands of others suffer the consequences of insect-borne diseases such as Lyme disease and mosquito-borne encephalitis.

There was particular concern about the global consequences of the great 1999 through 2005 natural disasters. The enormous numbers of individuals displaced by natural disasters validated this prediction. Displacement consequently results in disease. The masses are crowded virtually upon each other with nowhere to live, eat, breathe, sleep, or hide. In this setting of strife, stress, and poor nutrition, communicable diseases spread rapidly. In other words, the germs spread like a wildfire. As a result, rampant epidemics strike humanity, and the loss of lives is countless. For instance, in China in 1998 a world record flood occurred along the Yangtze River, displacing over 20 million people. What's more, the flood occurred, from the point of view of the spread of infectious disease, at the worst possible time: the summer, which aids in the breeding of germs. Local disease outbreaks become international epidemics.

The Chinese population, as well as the animals of China, harbor a wide variety of novel germs, notably influenza viruses, corona viruses (the supposed cause of SARS), and parasites. These germs are notorious for causing epidemics. Recall the

Swine Flu concerns of the 1970s, as well as the more current Hong Kong and bird flu syndromes. Mexico/Central America is another hot zone for the spread of infection. In Central America Hurricane Mitch forced tens of thousands from their homes, immediately resulting in outbreaks of dengue fever, malaria, influenza, cholera, and fungal infections. In March 1999, an encephalitis epidemic struck Malaysia, leading to over 120 deaths. Most of the deaths occurred in pork farmers/processors, and, in fact, the virus was proven to be transmitted from swine to humans. No medicine could be found to halt the infection. In an attempt to control the epidemic the Malaysian government resorted to the slaughter of tens of thousands of pigs. The point is that if this virus had invaded the population at large potentially thousands of humans would have been killed. The Malaysian experience proves that such catastrophes are highly likely to occur in the future.

Throughout the United States floods have accelerated the growth of bizarre fungi and molds capable of decimating health. Potentially millions of individuals are developing illnesses from these highly toxic molds. In the Ohio and Mississippi River valleys hundreds of thousands of individuals are sickened by the highly poisonous mold chemicals known as mycotoxins: many die and the cause is not even known.

Today, further catastrophes have been wrought. In 2004 hurricanes of unbelievable fury struck the American South, devastating much of Florida as well as Alabama. Millions of people have been displaced, many losing their homes. The death toll is unknown. However, the infrastructure has been devastated, which greatly increases human vulnerability. This will surely accentuate the spread of a wide range of infections. The residents of such regions are at great risk for mold and fungal infections. This is largely due to the trapping of moisture inside homes and buildings, which causes mold to flourish. Exposure to such mold greatly damages the immune system. These molds produce mycotoxins, which are exceptionally dangerous and can cause life-threatening diseases. The amount of mycotoxin on the head of a pin is sufficient to kill an individual. In particular, the flu will spread like wildfire in such an environment, since mold greatly weakens the immune system. Yet, regarding water damage and water-borne diseases none can compare to the disaster of the century: the Indian Ocean tsunami. Here, every conceivable water-related disease will occur: cholera, typhoid fever, dengue, malaria, dysentery, intestinal worm infection, leptosporosis, E. coli, shigella, and dozens of others. Mold will be less of an issue than the aforementioned, since the hot sun helps reduce mold counts. However, in flood-damaged buildings standing water can lead to fulminant mold growth, which can cause potentially fatal diseases. In such a scenario due to rotting corpses and the potential of rat infestation even plague could develop. This would be devastating, sparking the outbreak of a potentially catastrophic global epidemic. A greater issue is parasitic and bacterial infections, which in the aftermath will be fulminant.

Even so, the majority of illnesses are unrelated to acts of nature. They happen to individuals in daily life. An example of this is the disaster of a health care worker who contracts AIDS or hepatitis or perhaps some unknown infection from human contaminants. Other examples include the crisis of a surgical patient who develops a bizarre drug-resistant infection, which is more dangerous than the original procedure, and the individual whose organs are attacked by a virus or bacteria after receiving tainted blood. There is also the individual who contracts a disastrous internal infection from merely eating commercial, but tainted, food. Or, a person has a reaction to a drug, which leads to a weakened immune system, and, then, infection. These are the disasters of everyday life that account for a greater degree of disability, pain, and anguish than any other factor.

Medical mishaps increase the risks for global epidemics as well as local crises. The overuse of antibiotics in hospitals leads to thousands of outbreaks of infections, which are virtually impossible to halt, even with the most potent of all medicines. Tens of thousands, in fact, millions, of deaths have been attributed to these drug-induced outbreaks. Research labs carelessly release test germs, which may gain a foothold in the environment, leading to potentially bizarre diseases. The current West Nile outbreak is an example of this. Genetic engineering leads to the introduction of unknown proteins, as well as bizarre mutated germs, in food and vegetation, which will cause new illnesses and severe allergic reactions.

This was recently proven by the association of vitamin E with an increase in disease risk. The fact is the majority of vitamin E is derived from soy, which is genetically engineered. Thus, the creation of a natural non-genetically engineered vitamin E source is mandatory. In what is acclaimed as "science for the future of humankind" genes from chicken, bacteria, and fish are added, that is spliced, to vegetable or fruit genes. This fabrication would never develop in nature.

The potential damage in humans from such fabrications has never been carefully assessed. Yet, with nearly 50% of all modern food containing genetically engineered components, soon, the effects of this "experiment" will surface. Far from being scientific or altruistic, this is a global commercial movement, which has exclusively financial motivations. It is to the detriment of the human race, as well as the world's precious array of animals and plants, to alter the gene pool in an invasive, unnatural way.

Already, nearly half of all deaths globally are attributable to infections. Even with cancer, the majority of deaths are due to infectious complications, such as pneumonia, blood poisoning, kidney infections, etc., rather than any direct effects of the tumors. Hostile germs and drug-resistant bacteria are currently the cause of unmitigated global crises. Invasive medical procedures, as well as potent medications, are responsible for additional damage and disease, particularly in the Western world. Since there is already chaos, any breakdown in the status quo and/or infrastructure, as has prominently occurred in the aftermath of recent disasters: the destruction of the city of Baghdad, the Indian Ocean tsunami, and the massive Floridian hurricanes, will accentuate the danger. The result will be an increased incidence of life-threatening illnesses, that is global health crises.

In the 21st century Westerners will be at a high risk for natural and man-made disasters. Aging infrastructure, human error, and natural catastrophes all contribute to this risk. Sabotage, while admittedly a risk, is comparatively insignificant. The following is a list of potential dangers to acknowledge and prepare for:

- chemical and radioactive pollution
- lack of potable water
- inadequate clean, safe, and nutritious food
- rampant infections from highly invasive germs
- inadequate protection from the elements, i.e. an excess of heat or cold with no means of mitigating it (power outages, disaster-induced loss of shelter, etc.)
- lack of sewage disposal and garbage disposal
- violent tendencies of individuals, especially those who are totally unprepared for disasters, technology breakdowns, etc.
- angry hostile individuals who take out their stress on others
- repeated disasters, which destroy existing infrastructure such as homes, hospitals, and medical centers as well as roads, telephone systems, and electrical structures

Chapter 2
Natural Cures

If options are compromised and a person is forced to abandon everything, never go without home remedies. It is these remedies that make the difference between survival and disaster. This book aids in the selection of items which are easy to use and readily available. Lack of toxicity is crucial in these scenarios, and, thus, virtually all the remedies described herein are non-toxic. In other words, they cannot kill anyone or damage the internal organs. In fact, they can only help. In other words, they will help the person get well and will preserve health and even save lives.

Aloe vera

Since 3000 B.C. aloe vera has been used as an emergency medicine. Aloe is versatile, because it speeds the healing of wounds, plus it kills germs. However, its main use in wound healing is for sunburn. It induces healing, prevents scarring, and helps cool the body. Thus, it is useful to apply in the event of heat exhaustion and sunburn. Aloe, directly from the plant, is also useful for virtually all types of skin irritations. What's more, research performed in Chicago indicates that aloe may offer another anti-burn action: frostbite. Dr. M. Robson, a surgeon, discovered that aloe taken directly from the plant and added to a skin cream fully cured frostbite, an amazing finding preventing amputation in serious frostbite cases. Other uses for aloe include healing of chemical burns, steam burns, cold sores, canker sores, swollen/sore gums, open wounds, and skin cancer. It is the ideal agent for use on damaged or irritated skin. It is also useful in the treatment of skin cancer. This is especially true when combined with oil of wild oregano (i. e. Oreganol P73).

Bee propolis

Bee propolis is the bees' natural antibiotic. Bees collect a substance from the buds of trees resembling a type of resin. They convert this resin to propolis. A flavonoid-rich substance, propolis exhibits both antiinflammatory and antiseptic properties. It is also an anti-toxin, helping to reverse or protect against toxic chemical and/or radiation exposure. The fact is propolis is one of the most powerful natural medicines known.

Propolis is defined in Webster's dictionary as "bee glue." Despite its valuable germ-killing properties bees use it primarily as a glue for cementing their hives. Yet, it serves a dual function, because it is a germ-resistant coating. It is so powerful that it fully keeps the hive sterile. Plus, it is so rich in protective substances, that is antioxidants, that it reduces all other antioxidants into insignificance. The fact is it is the most powerful natural antioxidant known.

Bees use propolis to prevent germ infestation in the hive by carefully coating the entire surface, internally as well as externally, with this precious substance. The power of propolis in this respect is evident to anyone who sees an abandoned hive. The hive remains intact for years or, perhaps, decades without visible decay.

Bees also use propolis to coat foreign objects, which gain entry to their hives. Astonishingly, a mouse was once found in a bee hive. After stinging it to death, the bees coated it with propolis. Incredibly, the propolis coating preserved the mouse virtually intact, mummifying it. In other words, it halted all microbial actions. Obviously, propolis is a natural preservative. The reliance upon it also explains why thousands of bees can live in tight quarters without the risk of devastating epidemics.

Propolis is one of nature's most unique antibiotics, offering germ-killing powers against virtually any organism, including viruses, bacteria, fungi, and parasites. In contrast to prescription antibiotics germs are unable to develop resistance to it. Furthermore, it is safe to self-administer during a crisis, both topically and internally.

Propolis is non-toxic, that is as long as it is pure and free of pollutants. The problem is that propolis may contain lead. The lead is not exclusively from pollution. The fact is it is from the man-made hives which are often painted with lead-based paint. When the propolis, which the bees glue to the hives, is scraped off, paint is also removed. Propolis is so sticky that once it is contaminated there is no way to remove the paint. Thus, when the propolis is processed, lead and other chemicals from the paint are perilously intermixed. When buying propolis, be sure it is assayed and proven lead-free. Ask the manufacturer for such an analysis, that is for any propolis which is to be taken internally.

The importance of guaranteed lead-free sources is aptly illustrated by the following case history:

CASE HISTORY:
A 45-year-old woman aggressively used bee propolis for a severe gum infection. Buying a standard brand of propolis tincture, she consumed as much as one-half ounce per day. Within a week, she developed visual changes, fatigue, nausea, and blinding headaches. A complete blood count was performed. Tests revealed an abnormality known as basophillic stippling, which is a classic marker for lead poisoning. Thus, this patient developed acute lead poisoning from contaminated propolis. After halting the propolis, the symptoms eventually diminished.

Propolis is highly effective against herpes viruses. In particular, it is an aggressive cure for cold sores as well as shingles. It is also effective against genital herpes. Used topically, it rapidly eliminates pain and swelling. The potency of propolis is increased greatly by the addition of essential oils. Such oils are also antiviral. A combination of propolis and essential oils is now available, called PropaHeal. This is the preferred treatment for any herpetic lesions, even the genital type. The oil helps purge the herpes virus from the internal organs, blood, and nervous system. The power of PropaHeal is demonstrated by the following:

CASE HISTORY:
Ms. J. suffers from frequent cold sores. These sores break out suddenly, particularly as a result of stress. Interestingly, Ms. J. relates her vulnerability to herpes to the high number of vaccines she received, particularly the numerous polio shots as well as oral polio exposures (i. e. the tainted sugar cube). Soon after the vaccinations she broke out in numerous oral herpetic lesions and since that outbreak she has been plagued with these lesions. Recently, a massive cold sore suddenly developed. Her upper lip was so swollen it was almost turned inside out. Typically, such a lesion would last for weeks. PropaHeal was applied. Immediately, she felt relief. She was shocked to see that the swelling diminished rapidly. Within thirty minutes virtually all pain, swelling, and redness were eliminated. This was the first time ever that she gained such rapid results.

Even more compelling is the case of the physician who was exposed to a highly dangerous form of herpes during his clinical rounds:

CASE HISTORY:
Mr. K. is a busy physician, who treats post-surgical patients. One such patient had recently undergone numerous operations and was exposed to blood products. He was severely ill. After staying at the patient's bedside for a prolonged period he noticed an itching, irritating sensation about his mouth. Within a few hours lesions

developed at the corner of this mouth, and then within 24 hours a massive and painful cold sore broke out in the middle of his lower lip. There were also cold sore-like lesions on the corners of the mouth. PropaHeal was applied and also taken internally. Previously, he had tried numerous other herbal medicines. Immediately, he gained relief, and within 24 hours the lesions were reversed. In his case it took numerous applications due to the virulence of the hospital-acquired strain.

Black seed (Nigella seed)

It was the Prophet Muhammad who brilliantly proclaimed that Nigella seed could potentially cure nearly any disease. This seed is a native of the Mediterranean and African regions and has been used as food and medicine for thousands of years. Found in the Pharaohs' tombs, it was renowned in numerous ancient Mediterranean civilizations for its health-giving properties. The Greeks and Romans regarded it as one of their top medicinal herbs. Dioscorides (1st century A.D.) gave dozens of uses for it. Nigella, he claimed, eradicated headaches, sinus problems, toothaches, menstrual disorders, and intestinal parasites. Today, its antiparasitic actions are perhaps most renowned. African/Asian herbalists use it to purge the bowel of worms, especially in children. It is also relied upon for reversing gas, stomachache, bloating, and intestinal cramps. In India it is taken extensively to enhance breast milk formation and is perhaps the most effective herb known for this purpose. I have personally found it effective for curtailing the devastating symptoms of the flu. Its antiseptic value is demonstrated by the following:

CASE HISTORY:
Ms. A. was travelling in her car on a long trip. She had developed flu-like symptoms, and black seed (as Black Seed-plus) was the only natural medicine she had available. She took several capsules every 10 to 15 minutes, and within four hours all the symptoms of flu disappeared.

Modern research confirms black seed's significant therapeutic properties. Egyptian physicians determined that it reversed asthma better than common medications. Other studies point to the spice's immune-boosting powers. Apparently, it is one of the most powerful immune-enhancing agents known.

Nigella seed is exceptionally pungent. This is what accounts for its medicinal properties. It is very rich in natural oils, which nourish and soothe the body. The highly aromatic components warm the tissues, stimulate digestion, and activate metabolism. Thus, it is a tonic valuable for nearly all ailments. It is available commercially as Black Seed-plus (North American Herb & Spice).

Bromelain

Enzymes are the most powerful living force of the body. They are the body's workhorses, performing thousands of essential functions.

Bromelain is an extremely useful enzyme, and it was selected for its versatility and potency. It is a protein digesting enzyme extracted from the green stems of pineapples, not the fruit. It is a potent antiinflammatory agent, plus it has germ-killing properties.

Bromelain is one of the most reliable tissue healing agents known. It aids in the healing of any injury. It does so by stimulating circulation, in other words, it increases blood flow. It also helps eliminate swelling and inflammation.

Only uncoated bromelain, the type found in capsules, is reliable as a supplement. The best bromelain is certified by assay to digest protein in an activity against milk protein, i.e. milk clotting units (MCU), or against gelatin, i.e. gelatin dissolving units (GDU). Never purchase enteric coated or hard tablet bromelain. These tablets are ineffective compared to the uncoated variety. The process of hard coating requires heat which destroys the enzymes.

A typical dosage for combating trauma is 2 to 4 capsules taken on an empty stomach several times daily. A high grade product measures a minimum of 400,000 MCU, that is Milk Clotting Units, or 2000 GDU (Gelatin Dissolving Units) per 1000 mg. Continue this dosage until improvement is noted. Then, reduce the amount to 1 or 2 capsules twice daily. Papain, the protein digesting enzyme from papayas, works synergistically with bromelain. This enzyme is measured both in Milk Clotting Units and Proteolytic Units. Ideally, a top quality product should contain both enzymes. The papain should measure a minimum of 1000 MCU or 25,000 Proteolytic Units per 1000 mg.

Don't expect pineapples to provide enough bromelain to exert a physiological effect. The enzyme is concentrated in the green stems, not the fruit, although fresh pineapple contains a greater amount than the canned. Papaya fruit contains a considerable amount of papain, however, the highest concentration is found in the seeds. The greener a papaya is the richer it is in enzymes.

Infla-eez is a formula containing only the highest potency bromelain/papain. Fully meeting the aforementioned it is a powerful antiinflammatory agent, fully capable of reversing swelling, infection, and pain. This formula is rich in enzymes as well as antiinflammatory flavonoids. Infla-eez can be ordered from finer health food stores or by calling 1-800-243-5242.

Wild bush greens

Wild bush greens are one of the most versatile of all emergency remedies. This is due to the ability of such greens to bind toxic chemicals, removing them from the body. Such wild greens, when converted into a wild chemical-free extract, help the body detoxify pesticides and herbicides. They also aid in the expulsion of chlorinated hydrocarbons, including dioxins.

Research proves that the wild greens, if raw and unpolluted, can save lives in the event of any type of disaster, especially toxic chemical and radiation exposure. Such an extract can also be taken on a daily basis as a preventive.

Another benefit with these greens is that they are, essentially, pure protein. The type of protein this contains is complete and is digested into a usable form. Essentially, it is a vegetable steak. Thus, the wild greens serve as a source of daily, as well as emergency, nourishment. However, its greatest utility is in the event of chemical poisoning, heavy metal exposure, cyanide poisoning, toxic smoke exposure, etc. In the event of such poisoning this greens extract must be used aggressively. Improvement is usually rapid.

The wild bush greens are available as the original type, GreensFlush (formerly Gene's Wild Greens). This is the original raw greens extract made from fully wild greens, which grow in the far northern wilderness. This is safe to take in large quantities, because it is essentially a food rather than a medicine. If necessary, the GreensFlush taken with Nutri-Sense (see page 70) can sustain life for a prolonged time.

Cilantro/coriander oil

This is one of the most fascinating of all herbal oils. It was again the Prophet Muhammad who apparently stated that with the exception of cancer, the cilantro/coriander plant could, if taken regularly, cure virtually any disease. Both cilantro and coriander are fine tonics for the gut. They stimulate digestion and aid in elimination. They are excellent warming agents, meaning they help increase metabolic rate. Today, herbalists use cilantro/coriander for reversing nausea, diarrhea in children, intestinal cramps, stomachache, and hemorrhoids. It is also used for nerve disorders, including migraines, neuralgia, liver disorders, heart disease, and stress syndromes. The latest research edifies its importance for liver function, particularly coriander oil. This spice oil greatly enhances the liver's ability to metabolize cholesterol, aiding in bile synthesis and reducing blood cholesterol levels. This may explain why individuals who regularly consume this spice have a reduced incidence of liver problems as well as heart disease.

The best cilantro/coriander comes from the Mediterranean, where it grows wild. Here, the cilantro is derived from the green shoots of the coriander plant. The cilantro typically used in recipes, that is the fresh type, isn't from the coriander tops. The tops are used in cooking, especially Mexican fare.

The medicinal cilantro/coriander is entirely different than the Mexican type. This is a true Mediterranean type, which to a degree grows wild. North American Herb & Spice Co. provides an oil of cilantro made from the seeds of the cilantro/coriander plant. Thus, it is a true oil of cilantro, that is the type used since ancient times as a medicine. Incidentally, this is an exotic food additive and may be used to enliven virtually any recipe, especially meat and poultry dishes. For the latter it acts as a mild antiseptic as well as a preservative. It is ideal for adding to marinades.

Cinnamon

This is one of the most ancient of all spices. Historically, it was used both as a medicine and flavoring. Blair's *Biblical Herbal* describes how cinnamon was more valued in ancient Rome than gold. Then, it was relied upon to aid digestion and to cure diarrhea. It was also known as an effective germicide.

According to Lee Broadhurst, Ph.D., herbal researcher, cinnamon exhibits significant anti-diabetic actions. However, to achieve an anti-diabetic effect significant amounts must be consumed, like a teaspoon or two daily.

Cinnamon is a top spice for survival, plus it is easy to store and virtually impervious to spoilage. Do not use commercial or aromatherapy grade cinnamon oil, which is made from the leaves instead of the edible bark. Use instead the regular commercial spice, or, preferably, freshly ground cinnamon sticks (which may be processed in a coffee grinder). Or, take edible cinnamon oil. This type of oil is made only from the unprocessed natural cinnamon bark, the same type used for the spice. Avoid aromatherapy-grade cinnamon oils. These are usually produced from the leaves and/or root bark, both of which are unfit for human consumption. According to research published by Jean Valnet, a French medical doctor and famous essential oil researcher, edible oil of cinnamon is capable of killing most germs. In a concentration of less than one percent, cinnamon oil sterilized septic water.

Cinnamon has been extensively reported for its value in diabetes. Apparently, this spice acts as an insulin-like agent. Certainly, for diabetics and hypoglycemics adding cinnamon to the diet is productive. This is because this spice helps regulate the digestion and metabolism of carbohydrates. However, concentrates of cinnamon and other blood sugar-regulating spices are an option. Oregulin, which contains extracts of cinnamon, fenugreek, and wild cumin, is a potent blood sugar regulator. Clinical trials demonstrate that this formula helps lower blood sugar levels by some 40%. Incredibly, Oregulin also causes weight loss in a natural and physiological manner. This is because it eliminates the physiological disruptions related to impaired carbohydrate metabolism.

Cranberries

The main value of cranberries is in the prevention or reversal of urinary tract infections. Thus, they should be utilized primarily by individuals vulnerable to these infections. They are an excellent tonic for the kidneys.

Researchers have thoroughly proven that cranberry juice, as well as the extract in capsules, is highly beneficial in preventing bacteria from attacking the urinary tract. It does so by blocking the ability of the germs to attach to the mucous membranes of these organs. Thus, the microbes are simply flushed out before they can infect the tissues. Only a few berries possess this action, and they all belong to the cranberry family. The active components within these berries are called tannins, also known as proanthocyanidins.

Cranberry Juice

Commercial cranberry juice is not a lifesaving food. It is high in sugar and/or corn syrup. Cranberry concentrate is the ideal type to utilize. It can be readily reconstituted simply by adding water and is free of sugar and additives.

Cranberry is a tart berry, and this is why it is so useful as a health aid. The sour taste is due to a group of compounds known as organic acids. These acids include gallic, in which it is most rich, and malic acid. These organic acids are actually types of flavonoids. A recent article published in *Life Science* by Dr. T. Wilson shows that cranberry extract is highly beneficial to the heart and circulation. Plus, because of the anti-germ effects of the cranberry acids, it is highly useful in the prevention and treatment of urinary tract disorders, including bladder, prostate, and kidney infections.

A wild cranberry supplement is available. Known as CranFlush this is the ideal cranberry supplement for reversing urinary conditions. CranFlush rapidly eliminates all germs from the urinary tract. It is also useful for prostate disorders. CranFlush has been found to be effective for a wide range of common complaints, including bladder infections, kidney infections, sluggish kidneys, and kidney stones. CranFlush is made exclusively from wild remote cranberries, which are hand-picked. This is a cold-sterilized extract. Thus, it is the only true raw wild cranberry extract available.

Cumin

While it is one of the most relied upon of all herbs in antiquity, cumin is little known in America. Yet, if ancient tradition is correct, it is another spice worth its weight in gold. This is because this highly pungent spice is a potent natural medicine. Unfortunately, today, it is only used in veterinary medicine. Yet, its utility for humans is immense, especially for disorders of the gut.

Most Americans realize how pungent and aromatic oil of cumin is, especially Mexican food lovers. Yet, that is why it is such a valuable substance. Its aroma is due to its high content of special substances known as aldehydes. Specifically, cumin is rich in cuminaldhehyde, and that is what gives it its medicinal power.

Cumin has been used medicinally for thousands of years and was a favorite natural remedy of the ancients; it is mentioned at least twice in the Bible. Mathias notes in *Economic Botany* that this spice has been used as food and medicine since "earliest written records." Apparently, the ancients administered it primarily for digestive and circulatory disorders as well as for headaches. Now it is known that cumin and, particularly, oil of cumin, is one of the most powerful of all antioxidants. When researchers matched oil of cumin against a variety of antioxidants, it showed supremacy over all of them. Cumin oil greatly enhanced the ability of the body to fight toxicity by increasing the synthesis of a critical enzyme called glutathione peroxidase as well as glutathione-S-transferase. One study found that as a result of enhanced glutathione activity the ability of organs to remove toxic compounds was increased by up to 700%. This oil is difficult to find and the wild cumin oil is available only from North American Herb & Spice. It is also a component of Oregacyn capsules.

As mentioned previously since antiquity cumin has been respected as a digestive aid. Now we know that this effect is due to its valuable actions on the digestive organs, particularly the liver and pancreas. One study found that oil of cumin increased the liver's output of bile, which is critical for the digestion of fat, by as much as 300%. That is an enormous increase. Another study found that cumin preserves and enhances the function of the pancreas.

Cumin also possesses significant antiseptic properties. In particular, it was found to be highly effective in destroying the larvae and eggs of parasites. Yet, it is one of the few natural substances possessing potent actions against a wide range of microbes, including worms, protozoans, amoebas, bacteria, and fungi. Furthermore, of all spices tested cumin was one of the few capable of preventing one of the most pervasive of all health issues: food spoilage. The crude essential oil of cumin thoroughly halted the production of dangerous compounds secreted into food by mold/fungi known as mycotoxins. What's more, as reported in the *Journal of Food Science* cumin is an aggressive antifungal agent, which completely inhibited fungal growth, even in tiny amounts. Lastly, it is an anti-toxin, meaning it aids the body in the removal of toxic chemicals.

Oil of cumin is extremely pungent, so start by using a small amount, like 2 or 3 drops twice daily. Ideally, add it to tomato/V-8 juice or fatty foods. Then, increase the amount to as much as 20 drops twice daily. Fill a gelatin capsule with the oil for easy administration. Stools tend to become a normal rich dark color, which is an excellent effect and is due to improved bile flow. Because of its dramatic actions in purging the liver of bile, this is one of the most valuable antidotes to poisonous chemicals known.

A special type of oil of cumin made from wild cumin is available. This is in a base of black cumin seed, that is nigella seed, oil. Known as oil of cumin this is the most potent cumin seed oil available. Oil of cumin is derived from the steam extraction of wild cumin seeds. The black cumin seed oil is derived by cold-pressing the wild seeds. The potency is due to the fact that it is wild. ORAC antioxidant testing shows that next to wild oregano oil cumin seed oil is the most potent herbal antioxidant known.

LivaClenz is made exclusively of edible spice oils containing cumin oil as an active ingredient. It is designed specifically for assisting liver function as well as for detoxification. It contains the oils of a variety of mountain-grown spices, including cumin, fennel, rosemary, coriander, and oregano. All these oils have been proven in scientific research to aid in bile production. As a general tonic and preventive agent take 5 drops twice daily. For reversal of mass exposure to toxic chemicals take 20 or more drops three times daily. Both oil of cumin and LivaClenz are useful in assisting liver function. Note: the scientifically based emulsion of edible spice oils with extra virgin olive oil was invented by North American Herb & Spice Co. This is the ideal means for the consumption of dietary spice oils.

Fennel

Fennel is the herb which Grecian marathon runners traditionally consumed. This is because it gave them physical strength and endurance. It has a history as a medicine as ancient as human society itself.

Today, primitives depend upon fennel for treating a number of diseases. In the Middle East it is respected as a dependable tonic for virtually any digestive problem, especially gas and bloating. The ancient Greeks deemed it invaluable for improving vision and increasing life span. It was also used to stimulate weight loss and is apparently very effective for this purpose. This may be explained partially by the fact that fennel, particularly its essential oil, is an aggressive diuretic, speeding the elimination of excess fluid. Fennel is also an excellent aid to liver function. Researchers determined that oil of fennel dramatically increased the output of bile, more than doubling it. In the Mediterranean it is utilized as a gallbladder/liver tonic. It is also respected as a breast tonic. In fact, researchers have proven that oil of fennel dramatically increases breast milk synthesis. It may also aid in normalizing the girth of the breast in the event of malformation.

Fennel contains a variety of substances offering natural hormone-like actions. This explains its prolonged use by societies as an aid to female health. Thus, it has been used for menstrual difficulties, bloating, ovarian disorders, and hot flashes. It is far safer as a menopausal aid than synthetic or commercial estrogens.

Care must be taken in the consumption of fennel oil. It is safe, as long as it is derived from the edible seed. The finest fennel comes from its native regions, for instance, the Middle East. In contrast, European, American, or South American fennel oils are of inferior quality. Such oils should never be taken internally. An edible wild Middle Eastern oil of fennel of the highest quality is available from North American Herb & Spice. Be sure that the oil is certified edible before consuming it.

Folic acid

One of the most important of all vitamins, folic acid is critical for the function of every cell in the body. In particular, it is required by the body's DNA repair systems. In other words, when DNA—the genetic material—is damaged (i.e. broken), a process which afflicts each individual daily, folic acid stimulates the repair. The critical importance of this nutrient is exemplified by the recent reversal of the government posture regarding its daily requirement. The RDA (now known as the RDI) has been nearly tripled, from 150 to 400 mcg per day.

For nearly 50 years the medical profession and U.S. government underestimated the value of this vitamin, even discouraging individuals from consuming large amounts. This was to the detriment of the population. Physicians simply discouraged the consumption of large amounts of this vitamin, that is over 800 micrograms (twice the RDA). They were in error. In fact, their anti-folic acid stance caused significant harm. For instance, tens of thousands of birth defects, ranging from spina bifida and cerebral palsy to cleft palate, could have been prevented through the daily intake of one or more milligrams of folic acid.

A recent study proves the degree of error perpetrated by the U.S. government and the medical profession, as well as the pharmaceutical houses, regarding folate intake. Dr. R. A. Jacobs, publishing in the *Journal of Nutrition*, found that in order to halt or prevent DNA damage, the minimum daily intake should be approximately 500 mcg, that is over three times the "old" RDA. When Jacobs gave this amount of folic acid to volunteers, their DNA repair returned to normal. Yet, recent reports indicate that for optimal protection even larger amounts may be needed, as much as 5 mg daily.

The minimum of 5 milligrams seems to be the magic dose. A study by Dr. Michel Leeka of Free University Hospital in the Netherlands found that this amount helped completely reverse the damage due to folic acid deficiency. Folic acid deficiency has been associated with a wide range of diseases, including heart disease, cancer, hardening of the arteries, malabsorption syndrome, irritable bowel, and birth defects. The fact is virtually all of these diseases could be prevented—perhaps cured—by the regular intake of large amounts of this vitamin.

What is perhaps even more absurd is the fact that cancer patients have been prohibited from taking folic acid. The presumption is that this vitamin somehow stimulates the growth of cancer cells. This is utterly false, as is proven by the latest research, which clearly shows that cancer is caused by a deficiency of this nutrient. The vitamin is needed for the growth of normal healthy cells, including white blood cells, which protect the body from cellular degeneration. It is required for the synthesis of DNA, the genetic material which governs the repair of cellular structures and the growth of healthy tissue.

The DNA within human bodies is being assaulted on a vast scale, especially in the chemically-polluted Western world. Westerners suffer virtual epidemics of diseases directly related to folic acid deficiency. Thus, for such individuals folic acid supplementation is a must.

Garlic

A detailed knowledge of the health benefits of garlic will always prove handy. This is because it is one of the safest and most versatile of all medicinal herbs. Researchers have proven that garlic is enormously valuable for combating a wide range of illnesses. It is one of those rare substances that is a universal tonic. This means it provides a certain degree of protection for virtually any illness.

Researchers have discovered that garlic is a natural germicide, capable of killing virtually any microbe. Bacteria, parasites, viruses, and fungi all succumb under its powers. It was even found capable of killing the notoriously difficult-to-eradicate skin fungi, the type that causes athlete's foot. Thus, garlic is universally valuable as a home remedy. It is versatile, available, and inexpensive. It offers anti-toxin, anti-bacterial, anti-viral, anti-fungal, anti-parasitic, and anti-venom powers. It boosts immunity, increases blood flow, stimulates digestion, purges the liver, and strengthens the heart. All these actions have been thoroughly documented by modern science.

Here is a simple tip that everyone can apply in the event of a crisis. If medical care is unavailable and a serious infection develops, for instance, in a wound or on the skin, what could be procured virtually anywhere on this Earth that would sterilize the wound, eliminate the pain, or neutralize the venom? Garlic can be purchased anywhere. Simply crush a few dozen cloves of garlic to remove a few teaspoons of juice. Add the juice to a body or face cream. Apply this mixture to wounds, abrasions, lacerations, burns, venomous bites, or any other infected or inflamed lesions. Note: a significant stinging sensation may occur. Also, some people find garlic offensive, while others may be allergic to it. In these instances the Oreganol P73 (oil of wild oregano) is the preferred antiseptic. Even so, a high quality garlic formula has recently become available. Known as Garlex it is an oil of garlic supplement, made from cold-pressed mountain-grown garlic cloves. This is the ideal form of garlic for germicidal purposes. Garlex is well tolerated and as a germ killer is far more potent than the typical garlic pills. The cloves used for pressing this garlic oil are unique. They are yellow in color, a representation of their rich content of sulfur and other minerals. This explains the luscious taste of this supplement.

Glutathione

Glutathione is perhaps the most important protein/enzyme compound of the human body. It is the primary molecular tool for protecting the body against the assaults of living: poisons, aging, stress, and poor diet. It is the number one substance for detoxifying chemicals such as heavy metals, radiation, hydrocarbons, pesticides/herbicides, food additives, and other noxious compounds.

There are dozens of types of glutathione molecules in the body. Glutathione peroxidase, its enzyme form, is the most potent type. This enzyme is protected by certain nutrients, notably riboflavin, vitamin C, and vitamin E. Thus, these vitamins are crucial for maintaining glutathione at the highest biological activity in order to maintain the detoxification of poisons.

Glutathione is a relatively simple molecule, so it can be readily produced by the body. However, it is also quickly depleted, especially if the individual is under a great deal of stress, suffering from a chronic disease, or is exposed regularly to toxic chemicals.

In the vitamin/mineral kingdom the most important glutathione boosters are vitamin E, selenium, riboflavin, and vitamin C. Herbs/spices that boost glutathione levels include cumin, oregano, rosemary, and sage. Such herbs are far more aggressive in boosting glutathione levels than mere vitamins. Other herbs, such as silymarin or turmeric, are helpful, however, the aforementioned are the most aggressive and powerful. For instance, one study found that cumin oil alone increased tissue glutathione levels by nearly 700%, while rosemary boosted it by some 400%.

Taking glutathione-boosting vitamins along with the herbs/spices dramatically improves the operations of the internal glutathione factories, giving the individual ideal health as well as the best chances for combating a deadly disease or toxic crisis. Two supplements which dramatically boost glutathione levels are the LivaClenz, Oregacyn Liver, and the oil of wild cumin.

Honey, unprocessed

This is the ideal substance for combating crisis and illness, because it is both food and medicine. Honey is perhaps humanity's original medicinal food, being utilized for at least 60,000 years. All ancient civilizations relied upon it for nourishment as well as for combating disease.

Honey is a predigested food. This means it is readily digested by virtually anyone. Cane sugar or molasses requires energy to digest; honey requires none. The fact is it helps produce energy. Contrary to popular belief, crude raw honey is well tolerated by infants and is entirely safe for their consumption.

Certain medical doctors prohibit the consumption of honey in infants. In fact, the medical profession has made this policy prevalent in the United States and Canada, but it is not a prevalent attitude in all Westernized countries such as those in Europe or Asia. The honey condemnation arises from the same medical profession which taught mothers to place infants face down for sleeping, a policy which led to the death of countless thousands of infants from sudden death syndrome. Using fear tactics instead of science, today's physicians prohibit the consumption of a totally natural food, which could only aid infant health.

There is no increased risk for illness or botulism in infants who are fed raw honey. The fact is it is harmless. Rather, the consumption of this natural antiseptic food protects infants from such diseases. The fact is when this substance is placed on wounds infected by the botulism organism, it sterilizes them. Raw honey has been consumed by the primitives and their children for thousands of years. It never has and never will cause botulism. Infants and children are fed all manner of poisons: drugs, antibiotics, sugar water, soda pop, candy, sugary cereals, sweetened and dyed fluid replacements, and deep-fried foods, not to speak of the toxic food additives found in virtually all processed foods. Yet, ill effects are rarely if ever considered. One dose of chicken nuggets, bologna, or a can of soda pop should be a source of far greater concern for causing ill health than a spoonful of crude raw honey, which mothers in the United States and Canada have stringently avoided for their children for decades on the basis that it could somehow cause fatal disease. What a loss it has been and, how ludicrous is such thinking.

Raw honey kills germs. A study performed in England found that as a result of honey applications, wounds infected by a variety of germs were sterilized within a few days. The *Journal of Pediatrics* found that honey, even the commercial variety, worked better than the typical pediatric remedies in halting infantile diarrhea. However, the more crude, that is unprocessed, a honey is the more effective it is as a topical antiseptic. Currently, British surgeons use it on burns with great success. They note that the honey sterilizes the wounds and halts scarring. Here are just a few of the immense uses of honey against disease:

- for halting diarrhea and intestinal cramps
- for preventing infection and scarring in burns
- for firming up sloppy stools (especially in infants)
- for healing wounds and killing germs in wounds
- for application to abrasions, cuts, and sores
- for easing constipation
- for halting coughs and lung congestion
- for aiding in the growth of natural/healthy intestinal bacteria

Guaranteed raw honey made by bees which are never fed sugar is difficult to find. Usually, such honeys are produced only overseas, particularly in the Mediterranean. A variety of Mediterranean honeys have recently become available. These include wild oregano honey, wild thistle honey, and wild Mediterranean mountain honey. To order these non-sugar fed bee honeys call 1-800-243-5242. These types of wild honey help naturally boost the immune system.

Kelp

A rich source of iodine and other trace minerals kelp is one of the most nutrient dense of all food supplements. It is the best naturally occurring source of iodine, which is sorely needed for the function of the glands, particularly the thyroid gland.

Kelp's most critical use is to regenerate the thyroid gland. It greatly balances it, often singlehandedly bringing its function to normal. Tens of millions of Americans, particularly women, suffer from abnormally functioning thyroid glands. Whether the thyroid gland is overactive or underactive, kelp is highly effective, because it normalizes thyroid function. Yet, this is only true of high grade kelp from deep (relatively unpolluted) ocean water.

Kelp's actions on the thyroid gland also explains its enormous value for disasters. Radiation poisons the thyroid gland. This is the first internal organ to be damaged as a result of radiation exposure. Radioactive iodine is rapidly absorbed into the body, and the thyroid gland vigorously traps all iodine molecules, so if it is exposed to the radioactive type, it doesn't differentiate. Thus, it unwittingly destroys itself. The secret to preventing this is to bombard the thyroid with as much natural iodine as possible to block the entry of the poisonous type. This is utterly crucial. Doing so will prevent cancer and save lives, especially if a nuclear power plant explodes or if some similar radiation disaster occurs. Other forms of iodine should be consumed such as potassium iodide. If a nuclear disaster occurs, overload the body with iodine in the form of kelp, potassium iodide, iodized salt, and crude unbleached sea salt. This one step may save your life.

Warning: There are many inferior types of kelp. They are inferior, because they are harvested from pollution zones. Researchers have discovered that commercial kelp tablets are contaminated with heavy metals. Kelp possesses great affinity for trapping minerals, and it fails to differentiate. It has a particular affinity for arsenic. For instance, several cases of arsenic poisoning have occurred in kelp users. Kelp harvested from remote regions is free of industrial pollutants and is devoid of measurable levels of arsenic or other heavy metals. Thyroset by North American Herb & Spice is one such brand. It is assayed and proven to be free of toxic chemicals, arsenic, or heavy metals. Before buying kelp be sure to investigate the source. Demand an analysis or procure verbal verification from the maker that it is arsenic/chemical free. Such a pure type of kelp will be a great aid to health, since it is one of the richest sources of nutrients known. The Thyroset is guaranteed free of any such contaminants. High grade kelp is also an active ingredient of NukeProtect.

Lactobacillus

There is no question that Lactobacillus bacteria, that is the healthy flora, are of value for crisis situations. However, their greatest value is in the prevention or treatment of digestive disorders, particularly diarrhea as well as constipation.

Definitive proof of the power of lactobacillus came from the University of Nebraska Medical Center. Here, researchers discovered that it was powerful enough to reduce antibiotic-induced diarrhea by 300%, a highly significant finding. Previously, the researchers determined that regular consumption of these healthy bacteria speeded recovery from viral gastroenteritis. Thus, lactobacillus is of particular value for children, who are the primary victims of viral diarrhea. What's more, when taken regularly it apparently helps prevent the diarrhea typically contracted when traveling abroad. This may be why residents of the tropics and the Mediterranean, where food/water sanitation is inferior to that in the Western world, regularly consume lactobacillus-rich foods on a daily/weekly basis. I have seen individuals in these regions eat or drink yogurt by the quart every day.

In the event of diarrhea a high quality lactobacillus supplement is an ideal defense. There are dozens of lactobacillus products on the market. However, use your money wisely. Check with the manufacturer to ensure that the potency is guaranteed and/or that research has been performed on the product. For excellent protection against harmful germs take such a product on a daily basis and increase the consumption of Lactobacillus-rich fermented foods.

One of the most well investigated healthy bacteria supplements is Health-Bac. This is a high grade natural bacteria supplement, primarily a combination of Lactobacillus acidophilus and bifidus. It does not require refrigeration, so it is the ideal type for use in traveling. One problem with commercial natural bacteria formulas is that the results are not sustaining due to failure to implant. According to studies in Europe the strain of healthy bacteria in Health-Bac vigorously implants into the colon. This is the ideal type for reversing the toxicity of antibiotics. The Health-Bac is available at finer health food stores, or to order call 1-800-243-5242.

Lavender oil

Lavender oil is an immense asset for reversing disease and injury, especially in a crisis. It is one of those unique substances that possesses a broad range of activities. This aromatic flower oil has been a requirement for making life more pleasant for thousands of years. In ancient times the sweet smelling lavender was respected more for its medicinal properties than its scent, while today the opposite is true. Thus, modern society is largely ignoring this oil's greatest attribute: its health-giving properties.

During biblical times extracts of lavender were used for wound healing. In ancient Persia and Greece lavender was applied as a germ killer. In Medieval times it was famous as an antidote for psychological and neurological disorders. During the 18th century it was part of a world-renowned formula for beautifying skin and assailing skin ailments. Recent research proves that oil of lavender is an invaluable agent for repairing damaged skin. What's more, it has also been proven to aid in the treatment and prevention of a variety of lung diseases. A. Bissas notes in her article, *Lavender—The Essential Oil,* that, currently, lavender is successfully used for combating insomnia, tension, water retention, bad breath, sinus congestion, dandruff, and sluggish circulation. This is not mere folklore. Bissas' comments were recently echoed by the prestigious British journal, *The Lancet,* which described how fumes from lavender oil induced sleep equally as well as sleeping medications.

Lavender's sedative actions are broad spectrum. It is a reliable relaxing agent for virtually any condition associated with stress or tension, and that means practically all illnesses. Europeans currently use it for migraines. Dr. Jean Valnet, the famous French essential oil expert, used lavender oil for healing skin diseases as well as open wounds. Tisserand notes that it exerts a calming action on the heart and nerves as well as the digestive tract. He describes its European use for colic, nausea, vomiting, gas, and heartburn. A highly technical journal has reported that lavender is an anti-cancer agent. Writing in *Cancer Biotechnology Weekly* the authors provide data indicating that the oil works as well as chemotherapy drugs without side effects. Currently, lavender oil is being researched by a number of universities for its obvious anti-cancer powers against a wide range of conditions, including breast, intestinal, prostate, and ovarian cancers.

Virtually all the commercially available lavender oil is derived from farm-raised plants. What's more, there are dozens of varieties of the farm-raised species, which are mere hybrids used primarily for perfumery and floral purposes. Bissas notes that these types are "less potent and...inferior to the true lavender." Oil of Lavender by North American Herb & Spice Co. is the "true" lavender, plus it is guaranteed 100% wild, harvested from the deep Mediterranean. In fact, it is the only guaranteed wild high mountain lavender available. The lavender utilized grows wild in the mountains as high as 6000 feet above sea level and is free of chemicals, pesticides, and/or solvents. This is the original wild lavender described by the ancients as a potent natural medicine. It is a most rare and precious oil. This wild lavender oil (in olive oil) makes a highly invigorating rub; apply it vigorously anywhere on the body. Use a few drops of this wild oil internally as needed. Or, for even superior action regarding topical issues use the Oreganol cream, which contains wild lavender, St. John's wort, and myrtle oils, all in a propolis/honey base.

Myrtle oil

The leaves of the myrtle bush, a native of the Mediterranean, are the source of a unique and versatile essential oil. The leaves and flowers, which are highly aromatic, have been used both as food and medicine for thousands of years.

Myrtle aids the skin as well as the respiratory system. The ancient Greeks relied upon myrtle as a skin tonic for enhancing beauty and for healing damaged tissues. It was also used for curing bladder infections, wounds, and skin diseases.

Today, the primitives administer myrtle for a wide range of conditions. In North Africa it is relied upon as an anti-diabetic agent. In Turkey it is used to reverse chronic cough and for alleviating sinus distress. The Turks also use it for diabetes. Modern research documents that myrtle truly is a fighter of diabetes, finding that it helps protect the pancreas from chemical-induced damage. Hungarian researchers discovered that it also kills fungi, particularly the difficult-to-kill Candida albicans. Today, herbalists use myrtle for asthma, sinusitis, chronic cough, lung congestion, skin wounds, vaginitis, bladder infections, hemorrhoids, and sore throat. Rub it into the scalp to combat itching and dandruff. Regarding diabetes it is an active ingredient of the supplement, Oregulin.

Perhaps myrtle's greatest use is in the healing of skin. It is an invigorating tonic for normal skin as well as for aging skin. Yet, it is also invaluable for emergencies such as wounds, burns, abrasions, cuts, and scratches. It is specifically acknowledged for inducing the healing of damaged skin and mucous membranes. Apply it to virtually any skin wound or lesion. For instance, one woman reported that the oil "eradicated" on her face brown spots, which were due to sun damage. As mentioned previously myrtle is an active ingredient of Oreganol cream.

Myrtle is also an exotic oil, that is it is an aphrodisiac. The smell alone is stimulating. Applied topically to the appropriate areas, it regenerates even the most feeble of sexual functions for both men and women.

N-acetyl cysteine (NAC)

This amino acid is currently available in emergency rooms for the treatment of drug overdose. It is particularly valuable for reversing poisoning by acetaminophen, the active ingredient of Tylenol.

The reversal of drug toxicity is the main use of NAC. In this respect it helps prevent and reverse drug-induced liver damage and/or failure. However, it is also a proven aid for combating nuclear radiation. Thus, it is a versatile agent for aiding in the detoxification of harmful chemicals of all types. For an herbal therapy to achieve the same results LivaClenz is effective.

Olive oil

Extra virgin olive oil is useful both as a nutrient rich food and a potent medicine. It is easily stored and has a prolonged shelf life. When opened, it rarely spoils.

Recently, an article illustrating the novel properties of olive oil was published in the reputable journal, *Nutrition Reviews*. The authors discovered that olive oil's beneficial effects go far beyond its vegetable/healthy fat content. The oil contains a variety of powerful antioxidants known as polyphenols.

Apparently, it is these compounds which account for its therapeutic properties. While the researchers note that olive oil research is "in its infancy," the fact is this God-blessed substance has been relied upon as a survival food, as well as medicine, since the beginning of time. Olive oil provides fuel fats, which help nourish critical organs, including the brain, liver, and kidneys.

Olive oil may be preserved virtually indefinitely by adding certain herbs/spices. After opening, crumple and add fresh wild sage, oregano, cumin, and/or rosemary. Or, as an even more potent preservative add oil of sage, oregano, cumin, and/or rosemary. Simply add 5 to 10 drops of these oils per quart of oil. This will prevent oxidation of the oil after it is opened. One study determined that the oil's shelf life was increased nine-fold by simply adding antioxidant spices/herbs.

Oregano

For a crisis anything powerful enough to destroy sewage but harmless to the human body would be of great value. It was Jean Valnet, M.D., in *The Practice of Aromatherapy* who described how a researcher named Cavel stumbled upon it. Cavel searched the plant kingdom for germ-killing substances, deciding that essential oils were the most powerful. To evaluate them he used sewage water and fed it beef broth to stimulate growth. Various oils were added, one at a time, to determine antiseptic activity. Oil of oregano was among the most powerful, completely sterilizing the water in a 1% concentration. Other powerful antiseptics included oil of orange, lemongrass, cinnamon, and clove as well as lavender, cumin, and rosemary.

It took nearly six times the amount of synthetic germicides to equal the power of wild oregano oil. In fact, all of the aforementioned antiseptic oils were more powerful than the synthetic. Incredibly, wild oregano oil was 6.5 times more effective than garlic oil, the latter being notoriously respected as one of the most powerful natural germ killers. Thyme was also exceptionally potent, that is wild thyme (*Thymus vulgaris*). However, the latter is less commonly consumed as a food, so its internal use is less respected compared to highly edible substances such as oregano, cumin, rosemary, cinnamon, and lemongrass. Wild thyme from the edible species might be useful as a topical antiseptic, but it must be emulsified in olive oil. Note: wild thyme is entirely different than the commercially available Thymus species, which are unfit for human consumption.

Cavel's work is corroborated by modern research. In 1998 microbiologist Daniel Fung and colleagues at Kansas State University discovered that oregano impedes the growth of E. coli, preventing it from infecting the body. Siddiqui found (*Medical Science Research*, 1996) that oil of oregano was so powerful against viruses that it caused "disintegration", which was observed under the electron microscope. The respected Cornell University proved that oregano, even as a spice, killed all 30 organisms against which it was tested, including E. coli and salmonella. At Microbiotest Labs, as reported in *Antiviral Research,* a combination of three spice extracts, known as OregaBiotic, proved to be an exceptionally powerful virus killer. In a mere twenty minutes in tissue culture it killed all traces of the human cold virus.

These modern findings merely edify the historical record. It was Fleisher who thoroughly documented the fact that wild oregano is biblical Hyssop. The ancient Hebrew text contains the word *ezov,* which was erroneously translated as "hyssop." Furthermore, during the 12th century Maimonides of Islamic Spain made it evident that the hyssop of the Law is simply the wild oregano which grows in the mountains. Earl Smith, biblical researcher, notes that the burning bush of Moses could represent the wild oregano that grew on Mt. Sinai. This makes sense, since Moses unquestionably had to combat plague and pestilence during his prolonged and arduous tour. What's more, certainly, God's guidance is oriented for physical as well as spiritual benefits.

Oil of oregano is an edible oil made from wild mountain-grown oregano. To be edible the spice must be the *wild mountain-grown oregano* found in the hot climate of the Mediterranean. European, Spanish, and/or so called Mexican oregano types have not been subjected to the rigorous research as have the wild Mediterranean types. What's more, true original oregano species are not found in Europe, Morocco, Mexico, or Spain. There is a simple means to avoid the confusion. Look for the researched type, P73 wild oregano oil.

Mexican oregano isn't oregano. Rather, it is listed in botany books as an entirely different plant of the *Lippia* genus. It is rarely useful as a medicinal oregano and is also inferior as a spice.

Currently, there is a lack of continuity in the essential oil market. Plus, there is a deficiency of aggressive quality control. With regards to oregano oil Julia Lawless confirms this confusion in the *Encyclopedia of Essential Oils*, saying that the typical commercial oregano oil is not a true oregano but is either marjoram or Thymus. This is because the commercial oils have not been carefully screened to be sure they are edible. North American Herb & Spice originated the use of edible oil of oregano. The high quality of such edible oil is due to its source: the distant and high mountains of the Mediterranean. This is the real wild 100% Mediterranean oregano and is free of non-oregano plants like Spanish thyme or Mexican Lippia. With the North American brand oil quality control is exceptional and raw material sourcing rigorous. The wild oregano is picked by hand high in the Mediterranean mountains. One ton of the raw spice produces a mere 8 kilograms of oil. It is extracted only with steam.

Beware of oils made from cheap imitations which are not edible and/or which are made from Spanish thyme (*Thymus capitus*), Origanum vulgare (i.e. marjoram), or Mexican sage. Do not consume these types internally. It is the oil of wild oregano, made from the wild spice, which is truly safe. This is the Oreganol P73, commonly found in high quality health food stores.

Recently, there has developed a trend to genetically engineer virtually everything. Unfortunately, soon, spices, including oregano, will be genetically produced. Genetically engineered spices must be farm raised on commercially treated soils or in greenhouses. Furthermore, the seed is produced by cloning, in other words, it is genetically altered.

The purveyors of these genetically reconstituted spices are aggressively attempting to market their wares. They hope to "standardize" oregano and other spices by growing them in the laboratory. Genetically engineered spices/herbs are inferior to the wild types. These are not the types of antiquity, the Hyssop of the Bible, the wild oregano of the Law. Only the substances growing in the Fertile Crescent are of the correct biblical species. Only wild oregano is the basis of modern research elucidating medicinal powers. North American Herb & Spice did the research and supplies guaranteed wild oregano from the Fertile Crescent, hand picked in the mountains and valleys of the Mediterranean. Ask for wild oregano, because that is the highest in quality and safest for human consumption. Plus, the wild oregano is the type which has been utilized by societies since the beginning of human history and which is unaltered by human hands. Wild oil of oregano (Oreganol P73) may be purchased at finer health stores and pharmacies. Ask for the distinctive blue label with the black medicine dropper cap. For proven quality look for P73 on the bottle, which stands for proven by research.

In summary, the properties of the P73 oil of oregano proven by modern research include:

- destruction of all molds and fungi
- disintegration of RNA and DNA viruses, including herpes viruses
- inhibition of bacterial growth, including staph, strep, and E. coli

- destruction of the parasite, *Giardia lamblia*
- destruction of mold spores in the air
- halting of the growth and/or destruction of skin fungi
- increasing the output of bile
- reversing pain and inflammation
- improving the detoxification capacities of the liver

Note that virtually all of the research has been done using wild oregano from the deep Mediterranean, not Spanish oregano, Spanish thyme, Thymus capitus, or thymol. The types that are consumable either as oil or herb are the edible oreganos from the Mediterranean and Middle East. These are similar to the types used in the spice trade but are of a higher quality and purity. The point is simple: for internal consumption the spice must be edible, plus it should be the type upon which the majority of the significant research has been performed. It must be the type which has been utilized since antiquity and which is safe for internal consumption in any form.

There are three forms of wild oregano available: the oil, the crushed herb, and the juice. The oil is extracted from the high mountain spice, which grows up to 8000 feet above sea level. The juice is produced by a special process which yields the water soluble fractions from the spice. It is a natural source of oxygenated compounds and flavonoids. The crushed herb grows on mineral-rich mountain soil. In fact, this oregano often grows directly on rock. Thus, it is a dense source of naturally occurring minerals, particularly calcium, magnesium, phosphorus, iodine, and potassium. Known as OregaMax capsules, this is a village formula, consisting of wild oregano, Rhus coriaria (mountain sumac berry), garlic, and onion. OregaMax is the maximum strength crude herb. Interestingly, all of the aforementioned spices are natural antiseptics. North American Herb & Spice's oil of oregano (i.e. Oreganol P73) and OregaMax capsules are 100% wild and are *not* genetically engineered.

Pantothenic acid

This should be regarded as the "speed healing" vitamin. This is because this vitamin accelerates the healing of virtually any injury and is particularly reliable for aiding in the recovery from trauma. It accelerates the healing of a wide range of wounds/injuries, including post-surgical wounds, bed sores, broken bones, sprains, burns, stomach ulcers, and bruises.

Pantothenic acid, or vitamin B_5, is critical for the function of every internal organ. It plays a basic role in the metabolism of food and is also essential for the proper utilization of numerous other vitamins. It is required for the metabolism of protein, carbohydrate, and fatty acids, in other words, virtually every function within the body is dependent upon it. It is the key vitamin responsible for stimulating the synthesis of natural cortisone, which largely accounts for its wound healing actions. The vitamin also offers significant anti-stress powers. In fact, inability to cope with stress is one of the major symptoms of its deficiency. Top sources of naturally occurring pantothenic acid include royal jelly, organ meats, peanut butter, salmon, and eggs. It is notable that these foods are rarely consumed currently. Thus, pantothenic acid deficiency is endemic, that is the majority of Westerners suffer from the deficiency.

Red grape powder (Resvital, formerly Resvitanol)

Like spices, grapes and grape extracts have been relied upon medicinally from the beginning of time. They are mentioned with a hint of medicinal value in all of the holy books, particularly the Qur'an. Such grapes of antiquity were obviously of a type different than commercial American grapes.

Due to its alcohol content wine is contraindicated during a crisis. Nor is it a reliable cure for disease. Fortunately, there are other ways to achieve the health benefits of grapes without drinking wine. This is because there are other means to concentrate the healing attributes of grapes.

The powers in grapes are found primarily in a family of chemicals known as polyphenols (or merely phenols). Researchers at the University of Denmark determined that phenols found in the pure grape, notably the skin of red grapes, worked as well as wine in reversing circulatory damage and preventing cardiovascular disease. The researchers produced a concentrate from the grape skins, which are a residue of the wine industry. These grape skin/seed antioxidants are among the most potent agents for protecting the blood vessels and heart from toxic damage.

The medicinal properties of grapes are being heartily investigated by hundreds of researchers. Yet, the true power is found in the whole grape, the skin, seed as well as the vine and leaf. Red or purple grape extracts provide components which are highly protective against heart disease, cancer, and arthritis. A recent report published in the *Journal of Biological Chemistry* indicates that a grape compound, known as resveratrol, may be more effective than common drugs, such as aspirin, in reversing or preventing arthritis, heart disease, cancer, and even Alzheimer's disease. The compound completely blocked the toxic reaction which precipitates these diseases. What's more, researchers believe that this effect may explain why individuals living in regions where fresh grapes form a large part of the diet have a much reduced incidence of heart disease and cancer. The active ingredient of the grape extracts is a potent flavonoid called *resveratrol*.

Italian researchers discovered something even more profound regarding the chemistry of resveratrol. They determined that this unique chemical revitalizes nerve cells. In fact, resveratrol induced portions of the nerves to regenerate, in other words, the nerves started growing again, a feat formerly deemed impossible. A reasonable conclusion is that resveratrol is a major protector of the genes, in other words, it prevents chromosome damage.

Grape extracts offer another mechanism of action. Apparently, they are directly toxic to cancer cells. Researcher S.

Joshi found that when grape seed extract was placed in the test tube with various cancer cells, some of the cells died. H. Preuss of Georgetown University also made this determination, finding that an extract of grape seed inhibited the growth of human cancers, killing some cancer cells outright, while increasing the strength of normal cells. Other researchers have determined that the red grape components offer significant anti-pain and anti-inflammation powers. Imagine the benefits to the human body by naturally concentrating the medicinal components of grapes. Such a grape extract, as a natural antiinflammatory, anti-toxic, and anti-cancer agent, would have potentially lifesaving actions. It was Folts from the University of Wisconsin who proclaimed that a pill of *concentrated grape flavonoids,* not just one or two synthetic components, would be powerful preventive medicine for Americans. Fortunately, now such a product is available. Known as *Resvital* it is the only grape product available that provides all of the components from the grape without the sugar. A "village formula," it is made in a primitive fashion, which preserves its therapeutic essence. Picked while still sour the entire grape bunch is sun-ripened until fully dried. What is produced is a powder rich in minerals, flavonoids, and vitamins which are naturally concentrated in the vine, seed, skin, and leaves.

Resvital is made from pulverized wilderness red sour grapes. Thus, it is a truly unprocessed grape product, the only such product available made from not only the seeds and skin but also the vine and leaves. Did you know that many of the commercial grape products are processed with solvents? With Resvital all the benefits of the grape are gained without the chemicals.

Resvital is a dense source of flavonoids, vitamins, and trace minerals. It is one of the most mineral packed and nutrient dense substances ever analyzed. Analysis reveals that it is an excellent source of a wide range of minerals, notably calcium, magnesium, chromium, potassium, iron, and silica. Incredibly, it contains some 1500 mg of potassium per 100 grams, making it far richer in this mineral than any fruit or vegetable. A superb source of chromium it contains nearly 1400 mcg per 100 grams, which makes it incredibly dense in this mineral.

Its natural chromium content is perhaps the most impressive component. A mere two teaspoons contains nearly 100% of the minimum daily need for this mineral, which makes it richer than virtually any other natural food product known.

Natural calcium levels are high at 440 mg per 100 grams; compare this to whole milk at 120 mg per 100 grams. It is also an excellent source of naturally occurring vitamin C, containing some 150 mg per 100 grams (about 8 mg of crude natural vitamin C per teaspoon), making it far superior as a source of this nutrient to any fruit or vegetable, even orange juice. This high vitamin C content is to be expected from a truly mountain raised sun ripened substance. Thus, Resvital is a tremendously rich source of natural nutrients, and this is rare to find in herb/vitamin capsules. This is the original crude red grape food, completely sun-dried and totally natural. Resvital creates a new definition of what is a nutritional supplement.

The uniqueness of Resvital is related to the fact that the majority of nutrients in the grape are found not in the seed but in the skin, vine, and pulp. Thus, this formula provides not only the various flavonoids, such as the OPCs and resveratrol, but also an enormous density of nutrients.

There is yet another group of ingredients unique to red grape extract: organic acids such as tartaric and malic acids. According to Blumgarten these substances are effective stimulants for digestion and elimination as well as for the kidneys. This may be why grapes have long been utilized as a detoxification aid as well as kidney/digestive tonic.

Rosemary

Rosemary is a highly beneficial medicinal herb. Ignored by Americans as little more than a flavoring, it has an ancient history primarily as a medicine rather than a food.

The wisdom of the ancients regarding rosemary has recently been scientifically confirmed. Studies show that rosemary is among the most potent antioxidants known. This means that for survival purposes, it is infinitely more valuable than minor antioxidants such as vitamin E and beta carotene.

Rosemary is a potent antioxidant for all tissues. It possesses significant anti-cancer and anti-toxic powers. However, its antioxidant actions are geared more directly towards the brain and other tissues of the nervous system, which are dependent upon fat soluble antioxidants. Rosemary is one of the most readily absorbed of all fat soluble antioxidants. It efficiently finds its way into nerve tissues. It is rapidly absorbed via inhalation, through the skin, and via the digestive tract.

The easiest way to get the amount of rosemary needed to achieve these effects is via supplements, either herbal capsules or edible rosemary oil. Don't use rosemary extracts, that is standardized products. Duke notes that studies show whole plant supplements are more effective than single components or "standardized" chemicals as antioxidants.

Rosemary is listed among the most ancient of all medicinal herbs. For thousands of years it has been known particularly for its ability to improve the function of the mind. Ancient texts describe how concoctions of this herb were used to stimulate the mind, enhance mood, boost intellectual powers, and improve memory. In fact, it is most famous as a memory aid. Yet, it was also famous for combating disorders of the nerves as well as arthritis. Oil of rosemary is a concentrate of this herb's healing capacities. Condensed power is ultra-important in any crisis, including chronic disease. A condensed form of oil of wild rosemary is an active ingredient of the supplement, Neuroloft. This is a combination of wild rosemary, sage, gingko biloba, and St. John's wort. It is ideal for balancing brain and nerve function.

Modern research documents how rosemary works. Researchers describe it as having unusually high antioxidant activity, far greater than mere vitamins. Other researchers note that oil of rosemary is a strong inhibitor of viruses. Dr. Navarro found that the oil is highly protective for the liver, especially when it is damaged by toxic chemicals. French doctors determined that it actually doubled the output of bile, which helps purge the liver of toxins. Furthermore, this function of stimulating the flow of bile is helpful in human nutrition, because this substance is direly needed for the digestion of fat.

In the Middle East rosemary is used currently for digestive problems, but not just for the liver: it is applied for spastic colon, excess gas, heartburn, and indigestion. Europeans use rosemary as a circulatory stimulant. Chevalier describes its value in improving circulation, especially for the brain. Virtually all illnesses are associated with poor circulation. Topically, it is a great stimulant to the scalp, improving blood flow. Rosemary has an ancient history for fighting pain. In Europe it is still used for this purpose. Michael Tierra, master herbalist, notes that rosemary is of "great benefit in treating headaches," because it contains natural anti-pain compounds.

Rosemary is also an incredibly powerful anti-mutagenic substance. This means it combats virtually any toxic chemical which damages the genes. Thus, it is of lifesaving importance in the event of toxic chemical exposure. Researchers in England found that rosemary extract thoroughly protected the genetic material from chemical induced damage, partly by stimulating the synthesis of anti-toxic enzymes such as glutathione. The researchers concluded that rosemary can increase the body's ability to dispose of noxious chemicals.

Few natural substances offer this power. In fact, of over 140 fruits, herbs, and spices tested, rosemary was one of the rare few that proved to be a gene protector. The point is it is essential to take this substance in order to achieve guaranteed protection against toxic chemical exposures, radiation poisoning, as well as the stresses of everyday life in the modern world. The individual who wishes to be assured of protection against the poisonous future must have rosemary available, as edible oil of rosemary, as well as the bulk herb. The rat study by Dr. Milner at Penn State tells all: rats who were fed rosemary were twice as likely to escape being damaged by toxic chemicals than those who ate no rosemary.

Royal jelly

This is the food utilized by what is perhaps the most important creature on the Earth: the queen bee. Royal jelly is super-rich in vitamins, minerals, and enzymes. Plus, it contains the bonus of naturally occurring steroids, which are of enormous utility for the function of the human body.

Few people realize how critical royal jelly is. It is the only substance which leads to the distinction between the long-lived queen bee and regular bees. Incredibly, the queen lives 24 times as long as the regular bees, plus she is stronger and sexually potent. This explains why royal jelly is famous for halting impotence and improving hormone balance. It also explains its ancient use for rejuvenation, for healthier skin, and for halting aging. It is perhaps the most ancient of all beauty aids.

Modern research shows royal jelly has powerful effects upon adrenal function, and, thus, helps combat stress. This is largely because it is the richest source of a critical vitamin, pantothenic acid, which is essential for the proper function of these glands. Plus, it is high in naturally occurring steroids, that is cortisone-like substances. Adrenal weakness is due to cortisone deficiency. Symptoms of weak adrenals include exhaustion (which doesn't improve with sleep), nervousness, menstrual difficulties, depression or anxiety, digestive disturbances, chronic headaches, allergies, inability to handle stress, chronic upper back pain, sweaty palms, cold extremities, and cravings for salt and/or sugar.

In Europe royal jelly is famous for reversing adrenal failure as well as female sexual or menstrual disorders. For fighting fatigue, nervousness, or panic attacks royal jelly is essential.

Pantothenic acid is rare in most foods. The only common sources are liver and eggs; few Americans eat these. Thus, royal jelly offers hundreds of naturally occuring substances, just as God made them, plus the rare natural pantothenic acid, which is much more powerful and useful than the synthetic. Plus, royal jelly contains cofactors, such as lipoic acid and coenzyme A, which aid in the utilization of the vitamin. The consumption of royal jelly is an excellent means to achieve a daily intake of crude unprocessed pantothenic acid. Use nature's special remedies and gain ideal health, *just like the queen.*

Royal jelly is available in three forms: the lypholized powder, that is the dry capsule, the fresh liquid, which must be frozen or refrigerated, and the newly available stabilized liquid. The latter, which is a convenient means of consuming fresh royal jelly, is available as Royal Oil. This type can be conveniently consumed under the tongue for optimal effect. For capsules the fortified Royal Power, which is a combination of wild herbs and high potency royal jelly, is available. It contains a guaranteed potency of the active ingredient 10-hydroxydecanoic acid (10-HDA). Royal jelly is also available in AdrenoPower, which is the form sold to physicians. The Royal Power and the Royal Oil are the general royal jelly products, that is for those who wish to gain the many immense benefits of this substance. So, as a pure royal jelly supplement use the Royal Power and the Royal Oil. To determine the degree of adrenal weakness see the book, *Nutrition Tests for Better Health.*

Note: natural source steroids, such as those found in royal jelly, are harmless. These beneficial substances have been used for centuries.

Sage

An ancient proverb claims that if sage is consumed every day, the individual shall never grow old. During Medieval times the

English insisted that this herb was necessary for good health. These ancient findings are supported by modern research. Sage is one of the most powerful herbal antioxidants known. Researchers determined that when sage is added to food, the shelf life is extended tremendously—even longer than with synthetic preservatives. Could this same action occur within humans?

With the plethora of information disseminated about the protective effects of natural antioxidants, such as vitamin E, vitamin C, and wild berry extract, and grape skin/seed extracts it is revealing that an edible herb like sage is significantly more powerful in antioxidant powers than such foods. According to Taintu sage superceded virtually every substance tested in halting oxidation of fats. Edible sage oil from the wild spice is the type useful for human health. Sage oil is potent. Only small amounts are necessary, like 3 to 10 drops daily. Larger amounts may be needed to combat toxic chemical exposure. It can be freely used topically on wounds, cuts, abrasions, skin irritations, burns, warts, etc. It makes an excellent gargle for sore throats and can be applied to canker sores and cold sores as often as needed. Do not consume commercial or aromatherapy (i.e. clary) sage oils internally.

Sage is also a digestive tonic. It is particularly valuable for inflammation in the intestines, that is colitis and irritable bowel. Plus, it is soothing to the nerves of the digestive tract. Historically, herbalists have relied upon sage for diarrhea as well as intestinal parasites.

If the nervous system is out of balance, sage is perhaps the ideal tonic. It exerts tremendous calming action upon the nerves. Herbalists currently rely upon it for anxiety, nervousness, agitation. They even massage it into the skin to relieve muscle tension and pain. Furthermore, it is used for reversing depression and apathy, because of its ability to boost mood and stimulate the mind. Sage is an invaluable mind activator.

Sage is especially valuable as a hormone tonic. It gives great strength to the adrenal glands, which are responsible for controlling energy, the ability to fight stress, and the resistance to disease. In the modern era everyone needs an adrenal tonic. Sage also exerts powerful effects upon the sex hormone system. A partial list of conditions for which sage oil has been reported to be helpful includes:

- cold hands/feet or low body temperature
- immune decline
- sore throat/laryngitis
- fatigue and weakness
- adrenal weakness (and to combat high stress)
- respiratory conditions, particularly asthma and whooping cough
- insomnia
- hot flashes
- imbalances in menstruation/PMS
- infertility and impotence
- prostate disorders
- reducing of excessive sweating
- depression/anxiety
- agitation
- irregular menses
- hair loss
- dandruff
- aging skin
- graying of the hair
- muscular tension

What's more, sage is a beauty aid. Since ancient times it has been taken to reverse graying of the hair. Use it as a scalp/hair conditioner. Add it to facial tonics to greatly improve the tone/beauty of the skin. Sage is an astringent when applied to the skin, meaning it is a drying agent, counteracting excessive oiliness, scaling, and perspiration. However, since edible Oil of Sage is emulsified in extra virgin olive oil, it can be used on scaly and/or dry skin. For excessive graying use internally as well as externally. Along with rosemary sage is an active ingredient of Neuroloft.

Note: Sage oil should not be consumed by breast-feeding mothers, since it tends to slow milk production. Do not use commercial or aromatherapy sage oil. It may be high in adulterants and/or thujone, which is potentially toxic. Also, do not use sage oil if pregnant or nursing. Even so, remember, sage is an edible spice. Edible sage is the type consumed daily in the Mediterranean as a tea and tonic. Inherently, as a natural mountain spice it is safe for human consumption.

St. John's Wort

This is one of the most reliable anti-stress and nerve protective substances known. Since ancient times St. John's wort has been utilized to combat mood imbalances, mental stress, and depression. Yet, it was also regarded as sort of miracle cure for various wounds, including internal ulcers, skin wounds, burns, and cuts.

St. John's wort contains a wide array of unique compounds. It is an excellent source of flavonoids, which is made obvious by the fact that it consists largely of brightly colored yellow or yellow-orange flowers. According to the latest research the flavonoids, notably a compound known as *hyperforin*, appear to be the major active ingredients accounting for its brain-enhancing, wound-healing, and anti-stress actions. Chemically, these flavonoids act by helping the brain produce neurotransmitters such as serotonin, noradrenalin, and dopamine. The latter is required for blocking the ill effects of Parkinson's disease as well as Alzheimer's. In other words, St. John's wort contains chemicals which protect the brain from aging.

Crude St. John's wort contains a variety of natural compounds with potent biological activity. Wild-growing St. John's wort is much higher in active ingredients than farm-raised. The wild herb is rich in compounds known as *dianthrones*, which are relatively rare chemicals. Hypericin, St. John's wort's most highly touted active ingredient, is a dianthrone. The herb is also a good source of carotenoids, including certain types that combat toxic chemical exposure and cancer. What's more, recently it was discovered that St. John's wort is one of the few plants which contains a considerable amount of naturally occurring melatonin. This combined with the fact that it contains the calming neurotransmitter GABA (gamma amino butyric acid) largely explains its brain enhancing/anti-depressive properties. It is also high in essential oils. These oils are well respected for their potent wound-healing properties. This is why extracts of St. John's wort have been favorite remedies of herbalists for hundreds of years. The essential oil was famous in Medieval times for its wound healing properties. Wild St. John's wort oil is an active ingredient of Oreganol cream.

Unprocessed St. John's wort, rich in flavonoids, is a reliable natural remedy for defeating the mental stress associated with failure to cope or severe psychic pressure. It is also a dependable cure for apathy, grief, and depression. The key to achieving significant results is to select a St. John's wort product high in naturally occurring flavonoids. It was previously believed that a specific chemical, called hypericin, was the major component responsible for curative effects. However, Laakmann and Schellenberg, publishing in Germany, have thoroughly determined that it is the flavonoids that are mostly responsible for this herb's therapeutic powers. Essentially, if the product is low in flavonoids, it fails to work. This makes sense, since a plethora of research points to the critical role of flavonoids as the medicinal ingredients of plants.

Look for St. John's wort products which contain rather than merely standardized doses of hypericin the naturally occurring flavonoids. Also, be sure the St. John wort is wild, which is far more potent than the farm-raised. The label may not supply this information, because this data is so new. Unprocessed St. John's wort from wild plants is superior to farm-raised. Be sure that the supplier certifies that the product is made from the flowering tops rather than the lower stems. If possible, request an assay from the manufacturer describing flavonoid content.

Where this plant grows has a great impact upon its therapeutic powers. St. John's wort is a native of North Africa, Eastern Europe, and the Mediterranean. Thus, plants from these regions are top grade. In summary, the primary therapeutic powers of St. John's wort are as follows:

- combats depression
- balances mood
- aids in the healing of wounds (either the oil or pure herb)
- possesses anti-viral properties, particularly against herpes
- relieves stress and improves stress tolerance
- relieves head pain, particularly migraine/cluster headaches (the high flavonoid type only)

Note: for a guaranteed wild mountain-grown Mediterranean and high flavonoid St. John's wort, see Appendix A. Also, oil of wild St. John's wort is an active ingredient of the Oreganol cream, which is an ideal wound-healing remedy. The Oreganol cream is available at finer health food stores.

Salt

Salt is a lifesaving substance. This is particularly true during hardship. Natural salt, that is naturally occurring sodium and chloride, has never been a killer. The emphasis upon this is largely disinformation, primarily by the ultra-powerful refined sugar cartel. Even so, the medical profession caused it to appear as the enemy. Now medical scientists are withdrawing their salt warnings. The fact is they have admitted that aggressively removing salt from the diet is dangerous. Researchers publishing in 1998 in the prestigious British journal, *The Lancet,* found that the regular intake of salt had a slightly protective effect in preserving life and preventing sudden death. Dr. Alderman of New York's Albert Einstein Hospital provided definitive proof. He began studying the value of salt in heart patients. This was after discovering accidentally that heart patients who died suddenly had low salt levels. By giving salt to such patients premature deaths were essentially halted, and the survival rate increased by some 400%. In other words, individuals with the lowest levels of salt in their bodies were most likely to die.

In ancient times salt was traded as a valuable commodity, and in some regions it was equal in value to its weight in gold. There were specific health reasons it was so highly esteemed. Now it is known that the human body requires it, and if it becomes deficient, health can be seriously impaired.

Salt, as sodium chloride, is the most important electrolyte of the blood. In fact, 90% of the mineral content of the blood consists of it. This is why blood tastes salty. Salt is rapidly depleted from the body during periods of stress. It must be replaced or the health will suffer. Both extremely hot and cold weather cause salt depletion.

Certain individuals suffer from a condition which I've named the *Salt Wasting Syndrome.* I first discovered this dangerous condition in my clinic in Arlington Heights, Illinois. Some symptoms of this condition were identified and enumerated, but no one had previously recognized that it occurs within so many individuals. As many as 20 million Americans suffer from it. The condition is the result of the inability of the body to produce adequate amounts of adrenal steroids, specifically the salt-retaining hormone known as *aldosterone*. Thus, despite a normal or even above normal intake of salt, the individual loses it essentially faster than it is consumed. This may be represented by a low or low normal sodium and/or chloride level in the blood. This largely explains why certain individuals ravenously crave salt. It is a protective mechanism within their bodies that is in action. In the extreme salt deficiency can be serious, leading to vascular collapse and shock, perhaps death. Sodium is required for maintaining blood flow and pressure. Symptoms of salt deficiency include:

- exhaustion
- spastic muscles
- leg/foot cramps
- poor appetite
- headaches
- paranoia and/or psychotic behavior
- nausea
- confusion and/or irritability
- dizziness
- cold extremities
- sluggish circulation
- anxiety and depression
- impaired memory

Salt is a strength-providing nutrient. Plus, it is a preservative. What's more, it is an invaluable aid in combating stress due to its positive actions on the adrenal glands. It must be available as part of the everyday combat kit. Sea salt is the finest type to consume. Procure the highest quality sea salt available. Ideally, opt for salt which has undergone the least amount of processing, i. e. crude unbleached sea or land salt. Remember, all land salt was once sea salt.

Selenium

Selenium is perhaps the most important of all protective trace minerals. It is an exceptionally powerful activator of cellular defenses. It offers enormous utility for cellular function by keeping critical cells, such as white blood, spleen, and liver cells, in a heightened state of alert. It is particularly valuable for combating toxic chemical and heavy metal poisoning.

Selenium offers dependable anti-cancer actions. Some 100 studies point to its indisputable role in cancer prevention. A recent study by *JAMA* showed that simply taking this mineral in a dose of 200 mcg daily halves the risks for lung, colon, and prostate cancers. That is an incredibly powerful response for a single substance, making it perhaps the most protective mineral/nutrient against cancer known.

Besides prevention selenium may help destroy cancer after it develops. One study found that taking selenium dramatically improved survival in individuals with colon and/or rectal cancer. These results indicate that this mineral enhances the body's ability to ward off damage due to poisons of all types. This is largely because it is required for the production of an enzyme that protects every cell and organ in the human body from any insult: glutathione peroxidase. Researchers have shown that all living creatures have one element in common: they produce glutathione peroxidase. The enzyme is the initial defense for all animals from insects to humans against harmful stressors, including toxic chemicals, radiation, UV light, and free radicals.

Selenium is required for the cellular response against poisonous compounds. Without it, cells are readily destroyed. A lack of this mineral increases the potency of toxic chemicals. Researchers found that in the absence of this mineral the liver is readily damaged by synthetic chemicals, and when selenium is given the damage is minimized, even reversed. Their conclusion is that selenium protects the chromosomes from being damaged by toxic chemicals. Therefore, when glutathione levels are diminished, the tissues are easily traumatized. Selenium is responsible for regulating glutathione production, and, thus, a lack of it leaves the body highly vulnerable to toxic chemical-induced damage.

To boost glutathione synthesis take supplemental vitamin E, selenium, riboflavin, and vitamin C. These are the most important glutathione-increasing vitamins. Herbs and spices that boost glutathione levels include cumin, oregano, rosemary, and sage. Other herbs are helpful, but the aforementioned are the most aggressive and powerful. For instance, one study found that cumin oil alone increased tissue glutathione levels by nearly 700%, while rosemary boosted levels by some 400%. In this respect the multiple spice capsules, Oregacyn, are invaluable, since this is a combination of extracts of wild oregano, cumin, and sage. Taking the vitamins along with the herbs/spices dramatically improves the operations of the internal glutathione factories, giving the individual ideal health as well as the best chances for surviving a toxic crisis. Supplemental selenium and selenium-rich foods, such as Brazil nuts and garlic, may provide lifesaving protection in the event of a chemical exposure, radiation contamination, or sudden illness. If you are exposed to poisonous chemicals and/or radioactivity, take selenium immediately, at least 400 mcg twice daily. Be sure to consume only organically bound types, that is selenium chelates and/or selenium kelp.

Recently, an excellent type of organically bound selenium has become available. Researched at Rutgers University *selenium cruciferate* is a highly absorbable sulfur/amino acid-bound selenium. It is the type of selenium naturally found in high selenium vegetables like mustard greens, cabbage, broccoli, and kale. The selenium is in the form of selenomethionine and selenocysteine, which are the ideal types to consume. Selenium cruciferate is an exceptionally high grade nutritional supplement.

Selenium yeast is another high grade nutritional supplement. Here, the yeast binds the selenium, making it bioavailable. Selenium yeast and cruciferate are the preferred forms of this supplement. Sodium selenite, as well as selenious acid, is toxic:

do not consume these types. The fact is sodium selenite readily oxidizes human tissues, causing damage to the internal organs as well as the skin and nails. Today, in humans the primary source of selenium poisoning is the excessive intake of the selenite form. Look at all multiple vitamin/mineral and mineral tablet labels. If it says sodium selenite, do not buy it. A natural yeast-bound form of selenium, completely free of sodium selenite, is available at NutritionTest.com by calling 1-800-243-5242.

Large amounts of selenium are for short-term consumption only, like two or three weeks. The normal daily dosage is 200 to 600 mcg, depending upon the individual chemistry and/or level of exposure to toxins. Also, eat selenium-rich foods such as Brazil nuts, onions, and garlic. Yet, the point is in the event of a massive toxic chemical or radiation release, high amounts, like 1000 mg or more, of organically bound selenium taken daily on a short-term basis would be lifesaving.

NukeProtect may be even more ideal than mere selenium. This is because it is a combination of substances, which create antioxidant protection. The selenium in this formula is the highly absorbable selenium yeast, which is non-toxic. What's more, NukeProtect contains the entire gamut of nutrients and spice extracts for the protection against oxidative damage. For general health two capsules daily is sufficient.

Tomatoes

The tomato's greatest attribute isn't its vitamins. It is a compound known as lycopene, the component which gives tomatoes their brilliant red color. Researchers have determined that this pigment, which is chemically related to beta carotene, is as much as 10 times more powerful than beta carotene as an antioxidant. It is one of nature's most effective cancer fighters. Plus, it is a stimulant to the function of virtually every cell in the body. This is because lycopene aids in the transport of oxygen, which is the fuel that drives cellular metabolism.

Lycopene exerts strong protective effects against cancer, but it also protects against toxic chemical exposure. Researchers determined that when cells are placed under severe stress lycopene prevents their degeneration. Apparently, lycopene improves the ability of cells to communicate with each other, helping them block the formation of tumor cells. In other words, it helps cells remain in their normal configuration, preventing them from degenerating into malignant cells.

Lycopene is found in only a few foods, notably red sweet peppers, red grapefruit, watermelon, apricots, papayas, and tomatoes, the latter being the richest source. However, these foods eaten alone are not a reliable source of therapeutic amounts. This is because lycopene is fat soluble, meaning it must be dissolved in fat to be taken into the blood. To gain optimal lycopene power eat concentrated sources of tomatoes. Tomato juice is a good source, but it must be mixed with a bit of extra virgin olive oil. Plain sun-dried tomatoes or, preferably, sun-dried tomatoes in olive oil provide a huge supply of lycopene. Tomato paste is another option, but be sure to mix it in a bit of extra virgin olive oil before consuming. If you are exposed to toxic chemicals, eat a can of tomato paste blended with two tablespoons of olive oil per day. This tomato paste cocktail is perhaps the most convenient and powerful of all lycopene "supplements." It is preferable to get lycopene via food versus supplements, especially foods like cooked tomato sauce, which combine a source of natural oil with the lycopene. What's more, lycopene supplements may be largely genetically engineered. Before buying check with the company.

Vitamin A

Vitamin A is an important anti-stress agent. It strengthens immunity and boosts adrenal steroid synthesis. It is required for the formation of antibodies, which are essential for warding off infection. The antibodies protect the mucous membranes throughout the body from being attacked by pathogens. They are also needed to prevent allergic reactions.

Recently, researchers discovered that the regular intake of vitamin A impedes the growth of noxious viruses, particularly the herpes virus. In fact, a high vulnerability to herpes virus infection may warn of vitamin A deficiency. Researchers infected human cells with the virus. When the cells were "fed" vitamin A, the growth of the virus was dramatically reduced. The fact is vitamin A is the most powerful antiviral vitamin known. Early in this century researchers discovered that if the body was deprived of vitamin A, all cells and organs degenerated. Animals fed vitamin A-deficient diets became so frail that they looked as if they were starvation victims compared to the normally fed animals. Thus, during early research on this vitamin it became famous as the "growth factor." Indeed, now it is known that the growth of every cell in the human body is dependent upon it.

Vitamin C

In the early 1900s Dr. Szent-Gyorgyi, a Hungarian biochemist, discovered that a crude extract from the adrenal glands of animals cured a variety of disorders. He also produced a similar curative extract from paprika. Later, he discovered that vitamin C was the major active ingredient in these foods, or at least he thought so. When Dr. Szent-Gyorgyi purified the vitamin, it failed to produce the same curative effects. He concluded that crude extracts contain other components besides ascorbic acid accounting for the therapeutic properties. These substances were later named bioflavonoids.

Vitamin C and bioflavonoids are reliable, inexpensive remedies. Their uses are extensive, and they are among the easiest to take of all nutrients for combating toxic chemical exposure. They are universal toxin fighters, capable of reversing poisoning from virtually any compound. They reliably strengthen immunity.

Plus, they exert anti-stress powers, largely due to their ability to increase adrenal steroid synthesis.

Incredibly, vitamin C deficiency may be more common today than it was early in this century. According to a recent study in the *Journal of the American College of Nutrition* millions of Americans are deficient in this lifesaving vitamin. Random tests proved some 35% of individuals are lacking even the minimum requirement and up to 7% are severely deficient. The deficiencies were determined via blood testing. The point is in order for deficiencies to develop in the blood the individual must have been severely deficient. The fact is a large percentage of these individuals had signs/symptoms of borderline scurvy. What is perhaps most disturbing about these findings is the fact that this is occurring, even though nearly half of all Americans take synthetic vitamin C in multiple vitamins or other supplements. The conclusion is the synthetic vitamin is poorly utilized and/or metabolized. It may be that the synthetic C is rejected by the cells as compared to the natural type and/or that it is not retained within the cells properly. Obviously, only natural vitamin C from food or food extracts offers reliable, prolonged—and 100% safe—protection.

In a life-threatening crisis don't depend exclusively upon synthetic vitamin C. Rely instead on the immense powers of crude natural vitamin C plus the various flavonoids, the type only nature can produce. The vitamin C/flavonoid combination provides the individual with a type of condensed food, offering all of the unique benefits that only nature can provide. What's more, historically, only crude vitamin C sources have cured scurvy. Lemons and limes were used to reverse this disease in British sailors (17th century), pine needles cured it for Jacques Cartier and his men (16th century), and in Valley Forge wild strawberry leaves saved George Washington and his army. In scientific studies the natural ascorbic acid sources are the only time tested remedies proven effective.

Early symptoms of vitamin C deficiency are subtle and are rarely correctly surmised. Who would recognize as early warning signs fatigue, joint pain, joint stiffness, increased vulnerability to infections, slow recovery from illness, heat intolerance, and intolerance to exercise? A partial list of the symptoms of vitamin C deficiency includes:

• severe fatigue
• irritability
• depression
• weakness
• swollen and/or stiff joints
• aching of the joints
• easy bruising/fragile blood vessels
• petechiae
• swollen, bleeding gums
• frequent colds/flu
• increased vulnerability to respiratory infections
• poor wound healing

Vitamin C is absolutely crucial for lung function. The vitamin improves the breathing capacity of the lungs and aids in the destruction of any germs that may enter. What's more, it is of immense value for detoxification of the lungs in the event of noxious smoke or chemical inhalation.

Vitamin C is rapidly destroyed by smoke. If it is replaced quickly, damage from smoke can be minimized, perhaps eliminated. The fact is researchers at Cornell University found that vitamin C was among the antioxidants which dramatically improved lung function, reducing the risk of, perhaps preventing, lung diseases, including asthma, bronchitis, and emphysema.

Vitamin C's role in stress prevention is immense. It fights the toxic effects of stress upon both the immune and hormone systems. Dr. M. Levine, publishing in the New England Journal of Medicine, found that key immune cells do everything possible to concentrate vitamin C. The high level of the vitamin in these cells is apparently necessary, so they can combat germs and kill cancer cells. Levine then discovered that when stressed immune cells ingest even more vitamin C, which proves that stress destroys this vitamin. Major stress greatly depletes this vitamin to a degree that infections may develop. Plus, whenever the body is exposed to stress, cold weather, hot weather, or toxic chemicals, vitamin C is dumped through the urine.

Natural-source vitamin C exerts superior effects upon human tissues compared to the synthetic, plus it delivers a greater degree of biological activity. Note that virtually all the significant research performed on the preventive role of vitamin C in human disease has been done with food, which clearly demonstrates the omnipotent role of natural vitamin C in the healing process. Thus, for optimal results don't rely on high dosages of synthetic vitamin C, like 5 to 10 grams daily, but instead depend upon high quality crude sources of ascorbic acid and the associated bioflavonoids. Or, use a combination of the synthetic plus the natural.

A study done decades ago confirmed the unusual powers of natural vitamin C. The researchers found that vitamin C from natural sources was more powerful in its action than the synthetic type.

When the crude unprocessed ascorbic acid is combined with bioflavonoids vitamin C's powers are maximized. Bland writes in *Delicious Magazine (1992)* that vitamin C is always associated with bioflavonoids in nature and that at one time the latter were deemed so essential that they were named like a vitamin, i. e. *vitamin P*. He also notes that the flavonoids increase vitamin C's immune- enhancing powers. This makes sense, because bioflavonoids exert a wide range of crucial functions. They maintain strong blood vessels; without them, the blood vessels degenerate. They may well be the crucial factor for preventing hardening of the arteries. The critical vitamin-like nature of these compounds is emphasized by original books on nutrition, such as Cooper's *Nutrition in*

Health and Disease, which states that the bioflavonoids are necessary for the normal strength of the blood vessels.

Far more powerful than vitamin C alone bioflavonoids (or flavonoids) are potent antioxidants. Recent studies have shown that the effects of the combination of vitamin C plus bioflavonoids are far superior than the vitamin alone. What a mistake it is to isolate vitamin C. By doing so it is uncoupled from its functional associates to which in nature it is so intimately bound. For optimal benefits flavonoids should stay combined with the vitamin C. In a crisis depend upon crude ascorbate sources mixed with associated bioflavonoids. This type of agent will provide optimal results. Purely-C is the highest state of this technology available, combining top grades of flavonoids with their associated vitamin C molecules. This is a balanced formula and is far more therapeutic than the synthetically derived alternatives. Purely-C undergoes no adulterations and is free of synthetic vitamin C. It is guaranteed to be a true crude vitamin C/flavonoid source, like the type first discovered by Dr. Szent Gyorgyi. Its ingredients include rose hip and acerola powder, immature orange powder, immature tangerine powder, immature grapefruit powder, and red grape powder, all of which are the top natural sources of vitamin C and bioflavonoids. Purely-C is available in regular and non-citrus formulas in health stores, or to order direct call 1-800-243-5242. For more information see the company Website **www.oreganol.com**.

Vitamin D

Deficiency of this vitamin in Americans has reached epidemic proportions. As described by M. Thomas and colleagues in the *New England Journal of Medicine* as many as 40% of Americans are deficient, and this is despite the fact that many of these individuals are taking a daily multiple vitamin.

Vitamin D may not be a vitamin. It behaves within the cells like a hormone. The error in its definition makes sense. A vitamin is a substance that must be procured via the diet, in other words, it can't be produced in the body. Vitamin D fails to meet this definition, because if sunshine is available, the human body makes virtually all it needs.

Vitamin D is required for strong bones. It is needed to keep the teeth healthy and to prevent cavities. It is an impressive cancer blocker. It helps regulate cell growth. A regular supply is crucial for the maintenance of optimal health.

There are only two ways to get vitamin D: a well designed diet or, preferably, a combination of dietary sources plus exposure to sunshine. Only animal foods supply the vitamin. Top sources include eggs, butter, whole milk products, and fatty fish. Dark-skinned people require a more prolonged exposure to the sun than light-skinned individuals to achieve the same level of vitamin D synthesis. Individuals on strict diets and/or vegetarians are usually deficient. Vegans are usually grossly deficient in this vitamin. In this regard the deficiency can be so extreme that it leads to spontaneous fractures.

Sunlight is the ideal source for this vitamin. There is a warning: excessive sun exposure damages the skin, thus disrupting its ability to synthesize vitamin D. A few hours of indirect exposure, such as would occur from a long walk outdoors, is sufficient to procure daily vitamin D needs. Also, get your sun exposure before or after high noon. In fact, it's a good idea to stay out of the sun during the summer months from 11:00 a.m. to 3:00 p.m. However, if exposure to the sun during this period is unavoidable, be sure to wear a wide brimmed hat, which offers significant protection.

Vitamin E

Vitamin E is useful for dozens of situations. In emergencies it is a versatile aid for the healing of virtually any wound, especially burns, cuts, and abrasions. It is particularly valuable for the healing of sunburns. Taken internally, it boosts the body's solar radiation defenses. What's more, it strengthens the immune system and improves the lungs' ability to detoxify poisonous compounds. Vitamin E is also a potent circulatory tonic and should be taken regularly by anyone with a history of heart disease.

The best vitamin E to use as an antioxidant is the crude unprocessed type. There are two categories: the mixed tocopherols and the tocotrienols. The tocopherol type is the most well known; it is usually made from soybean oil. The tocotrienol type is made from palm oil. Both serve as excellent antioxidants. However, recent research indicates that the newer type, the tocotrienols, may be superior as antioxidants for protecting the body against poisonous chemicals than the tocopherols. Consume both types. However, soybean oil-derived vitamin E is now a poor option. This is because soybeans are genetically engineered, which creates contaminants. These contaminants are concentrated in the fats, and so the vitamin E, which is fat-soluble, is suspect. This may explain the recent association of the vitamin with an increased risk of sudden death. Natural sources of tocopherols and tocotrienols, that is natural vitamin E substances, which are non-gmo include red palm oil, crude pumpkinseed oil, cold-pressed sesame oil, rice bran, rice germ, rice bran oil, and nuts/seeds.

Cold-pressed sesame oil (Sesam-E), as well as the Pumpkinol, i. e. crude pumpkin seed oil, are top sources of natural vitamin E. These oils provide the full spectrum of vitamin E molecules in completely unprocessed forms. Both Sesam-E and Pumpkinol arel unique, since they are fortified with edible spice oils. Some 4 tablespoons provides 40 I.U. of crude vitamin E which in physiological status is equal to 400 I.U. of the typical supplement. As a natural source of the full daily needs of vitamin E take two tablespoons of each daily.

The antioxidant powers of vitamin E or, more correctly, the *vitamins* E are particularly valuable for protecting the skin and the lungs. Whenever these tissues are assaulted, it is necessary to increase the intake of this substance. Research points to the fact that the vitamin helps prevent scarring in the tissues when they are injured. Vitamin E has also recently been proven to offer valuable anti-aging properties for protecting the eyes. Individuals who regularly take the vitamin are much less likely to develop cataracts than those who fail to supplement. Even a small amount, like 400 I.U. every other day, was protective. Vitamin E's eye-protecting powers would be greatly accelerated through the consumption of herb and spice antioxidants, particularly oil of rosemary, oil of oregano, oil of cumin, and oil of sage. Many of these oils contain crude natural vitamin E.

CASE HISTORY
Mrs. P., a 75-year-old woman, went to her doctor because of failing vision. She was diagnosed with a cataract. A few months afterward she heard a radio program about the benefits of oil of oregano. She procured the product via mail (North American Herb & Spice Co.) and began regular consumption. Upon returning to her doctor, her eyes were examined by the head nurse. The nurse was shocked; Mrs. P.'s vision was normal and the cataract gone. The doctor rushed in and confirmed the exam and, like Mrs. P., gave the credit to her newfound remedy, oil of oregano, as well as OregaMax, which contains in micro-doses a variety of natural antioxidants, including gamma-tocopherol, the most biologically active form of vitamin E.

Vitamin E works synergistically with selenium. For optimal cataract protection take on a daily basis vitamin E, about 400 I.U. is usually sufficient, along with a daily dose of selenium, about 400 mcg. However, due to the potential for toxicity with commercial or 'chemical' vitamin E it is advisable to switch to natural sources. This is why Pumpkinol is ideal. To get the equivalent of 400 I.U. take 4 tablespoons daily. Again, the Pumpkinol, made from cold-pressed Austrian pumpkin seeds, is a full spectrum vitamin E supplement, which offers a nutritional profile completely different than the typical vegetable oil. Thus, truly, it is a whole food source of this nutrient.

Zinc

Zinc is newsworthy, largely because of the notorious zinc lozenges. The lozenges have been touted as a cure for colds. While they are not a cure, zinc is an important nutrient necessary for proper immune function. In this respect a regular intake helps strengthen immunity. This is because it is needed for fending off attacks by all types of germs. This explains why researchers, publishing in *Current Therapeutic Research*, discovered that zinc, as zinc acetate tablets, significantly reduced allergy and cold symptoms. The mineral is required for the synthesis of thymic hormones, which regulate immunity. What's more, zinc boosts the germ-killing capacity of white blood cells, plus it aids in the reproduction of these cells.

Perhaps zinc's greatest value relates to its role in wound healing. It is required for the synthesis and repair of all protein-based tissues, and that means skin, bone, muscles, and all other tissues in the human body. Zinc is also required for the daily healing of tissues from the damage that typically occurs as a result of aging and stress. This mineral is so critical that, without it, cellular repair and regeneration essentially halt. In fact, open wounds which fail to heal properly may signal a zinc deficiency.

If an injury occurs, take zinc. A reasonable amount is 75 to 100 mg of a chelated zinc product taken daily until the wound/injury heals. Thereafter, take 25 to 50 mg daily. However, in the event of exposure to heavy metals, radiation, or poisonous gases, take more, such as 150 mg daily for several days. Such a high content of zinc can only be consumed for a short period of time, about a week or two. The reason is that high amounts of zinc interfere with copper metabolism, causing a copper deficiency. This ill effect is easily neutralized by taking copper on a daily basis, about 4 mg. Maintenance doses of zinc of 25 to 50 mg daily are safe and do not deplete copper reservoirs.

This antagonistic action of zinc with other metals has its value: it is a heavy metal antidote. Zinc aggressively competes with a variety of metals for absorption. Perhaps this is because it is so crucial for cellular function. In other words, the cells aggressively bind it. It is highly specific for blocking the absorption of cadmium, a heavy metal which causes lung and prostate disorders as well as cancer. Zinc also blocks the absorption of lead and other heavy metals. Whether exposed to heavy metals, toxic chemicals, smoke, radiation, or toxic gases, the consumption of zinc is a necessity.

Zinc, as found in pumpkin seeds, is also a major nutrient for prostate health. Crude pumpkin seed oil is an excellent natural source of zinc. Yet, for reversing prostate disorders it is the oil which is most potent. Ideally, both the oil and the seed should be consumed together.

The history of this oil is fascinating. In 1773 the Austrian government deemed it so valuable that a directive was issued to protect it. The directive stated that it should be used only in salves, creams, and other medicinal products. Thus, it has been used as a natural medicine for hundreds of years.

This oil is concentrated, which makes it exceptionally nutrient dense. A mere quart of this extra virgin cold-pressed oil requires the seeds of 33 pumpkins to produce. The oil's deep dark green color illustrates its tremendous content of chlorophyll, beta carotene, and vitamin E.

Austrian pumpkin seed oil is a culinary delight. Drizzle it on salads, rice, whole grain pasta, and steamed vegetables. Add it to tomato juice, soups, and stir-fry dishes (just before serving). This is an easy way to reverse prostatic disorders, while consuming vital nutrients necessary for overall health. Yet, it is not just for the prostate. The fact is the Pumpkinol is also effective for balancing the health of the female glands, particularly the ovaries, uterus, and breasts. It is, essentially, a natural cure for cystic ovaries as well as fibrocystic breast disease.

Chapter 3
Nutrient Dense Foods

Food is critical to human survival. It must be carefully selected as a source of nutrients in order to maintain optimal health. The secret to procuring the greatest value from food is that it must be on the basis of nutrient density. Nutrient density is also critical for rebuilding the body when it is afflicted with disease. This is because disease creates the requirement for an excess of nutrients. The fact is nutritional density is the key for securing the most beneficial life-protecting—and lifesaving—value for food.

Density makes sense. In the modern world there is no room for error. In this fast paced world it is critical to gain as much power per pound from foodstuffs as possible. This is particularly true in a crisis, where stress and chaos reign. The human body needs fuel to thrive. It demands the most efficient fuel possible. Plus, efficient food/fuel sources help the individual maintain strength, energy, and mental balance at a time when the world may be enveloped in turmoil (it already is). The individual can keep calm and strong with power-packed nutrient dense foods. That is the individual's greatest advantage for superiority in difficult times.

In a crisis or high stress period it is crucial to consume food that provides the greatest nutritional value per calorie. Food must nourish the body. It must aid in satiety. In other words, it must satisfy the body's needs. This is true physically, emotionally, and mentally. It must fuel the tissues, organs, and cells. It must nourish the body and in no way detract from its nourishment. In a crisis there is zero margin for error. A trendy or unscientific approach to food could prove disastrous. The foods selected in this section are guaranteed to provide the greatest density of nutrients per pound for fueling improvement of general health as well as for crisis survival.

A brief review of human physiology, as well as food chemistry, is necessary in order to comprehend nutrient density. The human body survives by converting food into energy. This process occurs continuously in every cell in the body. Human cells are capable of combusting, that is burning, three sources of fuel: carbohydrates, proteins, and fats. Only one of these is an efficient source of fuel: fat.

Think about it. What was used in ancient times as fuel? It was oils such as whale blubber and olive oil, both of which were used in lamps. Today, it is crude oil that provides fuel oil and gasoline. This is the fuel humanity relies upon for survival. The same is true for the cells of the body. In contrast, wood, which is less efficient than oily fuels, is mostly carbohydrate. Wood burns quickly, while oils burn more gradually. The fact is human cells crave fat as a source of fuel, and this issue must be thoroughly understood in the event of a crisis. There is no time for inefficiency, and in order to increase the odds for the preservation of health the individual must select food scientifically. To achieve a virtual guarantee for survival, utilize high density fuel sources, that is fatty foods, as one of the primary foodstuffs.

Protein is the second most important food, but it is not because of fuel efficiency: it is an excellent source of nutrients, particularly the all-important amino acids. A good thorough protein source contains dozens of different amino acids. Protein offers dual benefits, because its amino acids can be used as fuel, but they are also needed to rebuild and repair cells, which is why this food is so essential.

Carbohydrates also serve an important role. However, with few exceptions they offer a relatively lower density of nutrients and fuel than fats/protein. Certain carbohydrate- rich foods play a crucial role as a source of food, particularly for children. Plus, carbohydrates, such as wild rice, brown rice, lima beans (the best of all beans), rolled oats, dried fruit, carob molasses, and honey, are easy to feed children, plus they are well tolerated, with a low risk for allergic reactions. A few unusual carbohydrates, such as teff, amaranth, and quinoa, are highly nutritious and well digested, but they are less commonly available. Perhaps the greatest value of carbohydrates is that many of these foods are easy to store for prolonged periods: hence, the survival value of brown/wild rice, lima beans, raw honey, and dried fruit. What's more, they are easy to administer, especially for children and the elderly. The top quality carbohydrates for the maintenance of optimal health are listed throughout this section.

Brazil nuts

These nuts are a nutritional treasure chest. The problem is they tend to spoil. If storing, preserve in the freezer or in air tight containers. Add a natural preservative to the container, like a sprinkling of antioxidant spices: oregano, cumin, rosemary, cayenne pepper, coriander, or thyme. Or, add a few drops of P73 oil of oregano or oil of rosemary/sage to the container. Oil of oregano is important, because Brazil nuts tend to mold, and the oregano combats food molds.

Brazil nuts are the top source of selenium. A few Brazil nuts easily provide the minimum requirement. Thus, since selenium is crucial for combating chemical or radiation poisoning, Brazil nuts may act like a lifesaving food/medicine to eat aggressively in the event of toxic chemical contamination. They are also one of the few dependable sources of chromium and are an excellent source of potassium as well as phosphorus, plus they are a top source of vitamin B_6. Furthermore, they are so rich in fatty acids for fuel and fiber that just a few Brazil nuts completely satisfy hunger.

Carob molasses

The carob tree, growing wild in the Mediterranean, may well be the manna of the Bible. While the word carob as such doesn't appear in the Bible, according to the biblical scholar B. Montague-Drake there is no doubt that it is referred to in Luke 15:16. Carob is derived from the Arabic, *kharoub*, indicating the medicinal and food value it maintained during the scientific revolution of the Islamic Empire of the Middle Ages. Then, scholars listed dozens of medicinal uses for this God-blessed plant. The fact is St. John's diet, that is the "locust and wild honey," probably did not consist of sugar-coated insects; it was instead the locust bean plant, that is the wild carob pod, whose beans are to this day known as "locust beans." Have you ever seen the listing on the ingredients of processed foods, "locust bean gum?" That is an extract from the hard seeds (beans) of carob pods.

While carob powder is popular in the United States, in the Mediterranean carob is eaten as syrup or molasses. The molasses is produced by boiling the pods into a thick syrup or concentrate. What remains is a sweet easy-to-digest carbohydrate that is far preferable as a sweetener and/or source of food to chocolate syrup or sugar. For instance, sugar and corn syrup are pure carbohydrate, containing no nutrients, whereas carob contains a significant amount of nutrients, notably iron, calcium, and potassium.

In the Mediterranean carob molasses is used as a food rather than merely a sweetener. It makes an ideal replacement sweetener for any sugar. Its chocolate-like taste is warming and nourishing, yet, it is devoid of the typical nervous system toxicity of the cocoa bean. Use it instead of sugar on cereals. Add it as a malt-like fortifier to hot whole milk. It may be taken as a quick source of energy, ideally added to whole organic milk. Carob molasses has a dependable medicinal use: it is a non-toxic, non-habit forming laxative. However, it appears to help normalize the bowels rather than induce only a temporary laxative action. Carob is a top source of naturally occurring antioxidants, which help protect the body from aging. This is another reason to consume the molasses.

To make your own locust and honey, that is protein and carbohydrate, survival food add a few nuts, milk, or cheese to carob molasses. Enjoy a treat meant for the prophets. To order wild Carob Molasses call 1-800-243-5242.

Fruit, dried

Dried fruit can be a valuable fruit, mainly because it is a source of concentrated energy. However, in drying certain nutrients are concentrated, particularly vitamin C and potassium. Plus, it provides natural sugar in a highly digestible form.

Perhaps the greatest value is in the concentration of naturally occurring vitamin C and bioflavonoids. The fact is rather than the sugar content this is why it is valuable for survival. Select low sugar fruit for drying, since they contain a greater density of important nutrients than high sugar fruit such as oranges and apples. The high amount of simple sugars is detrimental, providing only hyper-energy but offering little longevity nutrition. Remember, it is the nutrients in the fruit, that is the enzymes, vitamin C, folic acid, and flavonoids, that offer the greatest survival power.

While sugar may be somewhat valuable as a source of energy/fuel, it is the nutrients, such as vitamin C, bioflavonoids, and carotenes, which will offer the greatest protection against disease and injury. Thus, because of its nutrient content primarily, fruit is a necessary ration and those which pack the greatest nutrient density are preferable. This is why only the most nutrient dense of all fruit are listed.

This chart lists the fruit items with the greatest nutritional density. Fruit with a high fiber content, such as papaya, pears, strawberries, and kiwi, are more filling and less caustic for individuals with blood sugar problems and/or diabetes than low fiber fruit. The most nutrient dense fruits include:

Fruit	Primary Nutrients
kiwi	folic acid, vitamin C, enzymes
papaya	folic acid, vitamin C, beta carotene, enzymes
mango	folic acid, vitamin C, beta carotene, enzymes
pears	pectin and potassium
strawberries	pectin, vitamin C, potassium, ellagic acid
blueberries	manganese, anthocyanidins
grapefruit	vitamin C, potassium, lycopene (if red)
peaches	beta carotene and potassium
apricots	beta carotene, iron, potassium
fresh pineapple	enzymes and potassium
cantaloupe	potassium, folic acid, vitamin C
watermelon	lycopene, potassium, beta carotene

Certain high sugar dried fruits are relatively high in nutrients. Apricots are exceptionally nutrient dense. They are high in sugar, but the type they contain is readily metabolized. They are a superb source of beta carotene (and, therefore, vitamin A). What's more, they are super-rich in potassium and contain a fair amount of protein, which is unusual for a fruit. Thus, they should be a part of crisis food intake.

Always purchase dark or sulfite-free apricots. Sulfites are a type of chemical bleach used to keep apricots from turning dark. This chemical is a major cause of allergic reactions, and asthmatics are particularly reactive to it. Figs, another high sugar fruit, are also a tremendous source of nutrients. They provide a greater amount of calcium than any other fruit, plus they are rich in iron and potassium. Both figs and apricots are useful and convenient survival and health-giving fruit.

Herring

This is a super-rich food for survival as well as daily nutrition. This is because herring contains superb amounts of fat soluble vitamins, B vitamins, protein, and fatty acids. Two cans of herring provide a complete array of nutrients in the form of fatty vitamins, B vitamins, protein, minerals, and fuel fats, enough for an entire day—perhaps longer. The only thing it lacks is vitamin C. The fatty acids in herring are readily digested, offering fish oils, fat soluble vitamins as well as fuel calories. Herring plus dried fruit or tomatoes is a nutrient dense meal.

Honey

Honey provides fuel, that is calories, and nutrients, plus it is a lifesaving medicine. It is a relatively inexpensive natural remedy with a versatility unmatched by modern drugs. Knowing the therapeutic powers of honey is a must for those who wish to have the survival advantage for the future.

The bees use honey for food, but they also know it is a means of keeping the hive sterile. Germs cannot flourish in it. This is because of a phenomenon known as *hydroscopicity*. Honey is low in moisture. Thus, it attracts moisture. Germs are over 90% water. If a germ is deposited in honey, it becomes dehydrated and, therefore, dies. This is because the honey siphons the moisture out of it. The same occurs when pure honey is applied on the tissues all germs die. Incredibly, it kills virtually any germ found on the tissue, usually in a matter of seconds. This is true even of drug-resistant types. However, as confirmed by British and European research this attribute only applies to the truly crude and raw types of honey.

Honey also contains relatively large amounts of organic acids, which are natural antiseptics. Some honeys are high in hydrogen peroxide, a potent germicide. This may explain why it has been discovered that honey virtually sterilizes any wound, even those which fail to respond to antibiotics. A recent study published in the *British Journal of Surgery* found that wounds treated with honey became sterile, even those that failed to heal with antibiotic therapy. In certain instances the honey packs sterilized the wounds within a few hours. Some of these festering wounds were several years old. The honey applications cured over 80% of the wounds. However, only crude unprocessed honey exhibited this effect.

In England honey is currently used in burn wards. It is applied because it dependably sterilizes the wound, plus it speeds healing, minimizing or eliminated scarring. I use it on burns and find it highly effective. In contrast to other common forms of sugar, such as white sugar, brown sugar, and Karo syrup, honey is a fair source of vitamins and minerals. Dark honeys are the richest types, containing considerable amounts of potassium, magnesium, and calcium. Dr. Paavo Airola indicated that honey not only provides calcium but also aids in its absorption and retention in the body.

Wild honeys are by far the best ones medicinally. These honeys are produced by bees that visit exclusively wild medicinal plants. Such honeys are utterly rare today. Currently, only a few types are available, and all of them are harvested in a limited supply. Some examples include Wild Oregano honey, Mediterranean Wildflower honey, Wild Fir Tree honey, and Wild Thistle honey. These are extracted from beehives found in the Mediterranean mountains. To order these completely raw and unfiltered honeys call 1-800-243-5242 or in Canada, 1-866-drspice. On the Web these honeys are available at tunies.com and P73.net. The fact is the wild Mediterranean honeys, produced by bees that are never fed sugar, are the finest honeys known. They are truly medicinal honeys, meeting the Qur'anic definition of being "medicine for humankind."

In the Middle East wild raw honey is relied upon to settle upset stomach and resolve diarrhea. It is also used for intestinal disorders and chronic infections. The honey bees that produce these rare honeys are never fed sugar. All of the honey is produced from plant nectar and sap. There is another unique type of honey made from tree blossoms, although these are only partially wild: Mediterranean Orange Blossom honey. This honey is collected by bees which visit the medicinal neroli or sour orange tree. The tree produces a highly aromatic nectar. Thus, the honey is also highly aromatic. These unique health-enhancing honeys have never before been available in the United States. Wild Oregano and Thistle honeys, as well as Mediterranean Orange Blossom honey, are available by calling 1-800-243-5242. In Canada call 1-866-drspice.

Pesticide use in the United States has essentially decimated the wild bee population. Plus, there is only minimal wild territory left. Thus, the highest quality wild honeys for internal consumption must be imported. For topical application there are a number of excellent wild or naturally created raw honeys. Any crude raw honey serves as an effective topical wound antiseptic. However, for internal use opt for the wild imported honeys, which are truly medicinal.

Jerky or canned meat

Have you ever wondered why the Native Americans made every effort possible to make dried meat? They knew it was among the most sustaining and nourishing of all foods and that it would help them survive difficult times, exposure to the elements, and unpredictable winters.

Jerky is one of the most nourishing of all foods, plus, if properly prepared, it lasts virtually forever. Dried meat is rich in nutrients, providing protein, vitamins, minerals, electrolytes, and fatty acids. In other words, short of vitamin C, meat contains everything necessary for survival. Meat is nourishing for another reason: it sustains the individual, more so than any other food. This is because it is rich in all eight amino acids, which are required as nourishment by every cell in the body.

One of the main reasons meat is so essential is that it provides a unique category of nutrients in a complete form: the electrolytes. These critical nutrients are required for the most essential functions of the human body. The most basic body processes, including heart nerve activity, brain/spinal nerve firing, nerve conduction, hormone production, temperature regulation, blood flow, and blood pressure, are dependent upon them. These electrolytes are sodium, chloride, bicarbonate, potassium, magnesium, and iodine. Few foods contain them as a unit. Vegetables are lacking in them, as are fruit. Nuts contain a few of them, but these foods are severely lacking in sodium, iodine, and chloride. Beans are virtually devoid of these nutrients. However, meat boasts the entire category and salted meat is even more complete. Milk is the other major source.

Meat is particularly important for teenagers and growing females. A recent study published in *The Physician and Sports Medicine* (November 1998) showed that by avoiding red meat, young girls are developing severe protein and mineral deficiencies. In particular, the teenagers studied were extremely deficient in iron and zinc, and meat is the prime source of these nutrients.

Types of jerky include those made from beef, turkey, and fish. Regarding beef and poultry only truly organic and/or vegetarian-fed animals can be used. Be sure to purchase only types made without nitrates. What's more, only truly organic grass-fed animals can be used. A nitrate-free turkey jerky of excellent quality is made by Shelton's turkey farms. Here, only free-range turkeys are used. If making your own, be sure to add plenty of tangy spices, as these act as natural preservatives. Canned meat products in their own juices is another option, that is, again, if it is organic.

Mackerel

A can of mackerel is so nutritious that it can help you survive for an entire day or perhaps longer. This fish is so rich in nutrients that it rapidly satisfies the appetite, providing prolonged strength and energy as well as the sensation of fullness.
Canned mackerel (with the bones) is a top source of calcium and phosphorus, both of which are needed for energy production. It is an excellent source of fuel fatty acids, plus its fatty acids aid circulation and, thus, is highly nourishing for individuals living in cold climates. Mackerel is an excellent source of B vitamins, notably pyridoxine, niacin, and biotin. It is also an excellent source of vitamin D, which is very difficult to procure in the diet. Be sure to drink the juice of the mackerel; it is rich in fat soluble vitamins as well as fish oils.

Whole milk, dried/powdered

It would be difficult to find a more useful, nutritious, and vitamin-packed food than powdered milk. The individual can essentially live on powdered milk, with a bit of vitamin C, for prolonged periods, perhaps years. It is a complete food, offering virtually every vitamin/mineral and, certainly, every amino acid needed.
    It is the amino acids that are essential for survival. Without them, the organs readily degenerate. Milk is one of the few foods which offers a complete array of necessary fat, carbohydrate, and protein as well as a full array of vitamins and minerals. This is why the individual can live adequately for prolonged periods on milk supplemented with a bit of fruit and/or a crude vitamin C/flavonoid supplement such as Purely-C. Here is an interesting nutrient dense food. Mix a tablespoon of Purely-C (several opened and emptied capsules) with a pound of milk powder. To fortify it even more add a tablespoon or two of Resvital (red sour grape powder). This creates a vitamin C-fortified whole food capable of indefinitely sustaining life.
    Be aware that cow's milk allergy is relatively common, affecting as many as one in three individuals. If you are allergic

to milk, rely on meat, poultry, and fish as the primary source of protein. Only organic milk should be used.

Nuts, seeds, and nut butters

This category offers among the most nutrient dense and satisfying of all foods for survival. All nuts are useful for body sustenance. Excellent choices for nutrient density include almonds, pecans, filberts, pistachios, sunflower seeds, and Brazil nuts. However, peanuts are perhaps the most versatile, because this nut (actually legume), is the more readily digested than virtually any other type. Plus, it offers an exceptional density of certain nutrients found in lesser amounts in other nuts/legumes.

Other nuts (mixed nuts)

All nuts offer a huge density of nutrients. Almonds, filberts, pecans, Brazil nuts, and pistachios are all top food sources. While high in fat, the type of fat they contain is incredibly healthy. A study conducted by Massachusetts researchers determined that the natural fat of nuts actually helped prevent heart attacks and had no ill effects upon the body. Nut eaters had significantly less heart attacks than those who avoid nuts.

Nuts store well, however, there is a risk they will grow mold. To help prevent this, store them in the freezer or refrigerator. Sprinkle your favorite spices or spice mixture over the nuts. You may choose to add a few drops of an antiseptic edible herbal oil to the nut container, i.e. oil of wild oregano, oil of rosemary, oil of cinnamon, oil of sage, oil of bay leaf, oil of cilantro and coriander, etc. One study found that when antioxidant spices were added to vegetable oils (nuts are a type of vegetable) the shelf life was increased by as much as 900%.

Peanuts and peanut butter

The peanut is one of the most nutrient dense foods known. It is not a true nut, instead being a legume. Certain individuals fail to tolerate legumes, and in this case other non-leguminous nuts, such as pecans, filberts, and almonds, may be preferred. However, for those who tolerate it, peanut butter or peanuts are exceptionally nutritious and easily digested. It is like a type of vegetable steak. In the form of peanut butter it keeps indefinitely. It may be preserved for even longer periods by adding antioxidant oils such as rosemary, sage, and oregano oils.

Peanuts are rich in a variety of nutrients, making them an ideal food for quick energy. They are also ideal for daily nourishment, since they pack a greater array of nutrients than virtually any other snack/food short of milk products and fresh meats. Peanuts also contain surprise components such as the flavonoids resveratrol and myoinositol. The myoinositol helps combat nerve damage and is anti-diabetic. Resveratrol is perhaps the most powerful naturally occurring anti-cancer substance known. The value of these unique naturally occurring substances in peanuts is notable. Researchers at the University of Alabama found that diabetics with nerve damage improved significantly simply by incorporating peanuts and other myoinositol-rich foods into the diet. Peanuts are also an excellent source of vitamins and minerals, many of which are difficult to procure in the diet in large quantities. Both peanuts and peanut butter contain a high density of thiamine, niacin, pantothenic acid, and biotin as well as vitamin E, copper, and potassium. Few if any other nuts/legumes can match such nutrient density. However, the crude red sour grape compound, that is the Resvital, is the most potent and biologically active source of naturally occurring resveratrol known.

Aflatoxin contamination is a significant problem with peanuts/peanut butter. This danger can be ameliorated by the addition of antifungal spices, which are a particularly agreeable addition to peanut butter. Certain spice oils neutralize aflatoxin. Simply add a few drops of Oreganol P73 oil or oil of cumin to the peanut butter and mix thoroughly. This will halt and/or reverse mold/aflatoxin contamination. Oregacyn/Oreganol P73 will also relieve any toxic symptoms due to this substance.

Unfortunately, today, peanut butter and jelly sandwiches are often not allowed in schools. If the jelly could be replaced, perhaps, with honey this is far more nourishing than many of the things children eat today. With the addition of spice oils the reaction to the aflatoxin and/or mold spores does not occur.

Rice bran and rice polish

This is far more nourishing than any other grain-like food. Grain allergy is common. However, allergic intolerance to rice, which is a seed instead of a grain, is rather rare.

Compared to other types of bran the type from rice is high in protein. In fact, it is one of the few vegetable proteins that is nearly comparable to milk in protein value. The digestibility of rice bran protein is reportedly as high as 75%. The oils in rice bran are highly digestible. In fact, the composition is similar to that of olive oil. Rice bran oil is also high in plant sterols, which are vegetable types of cholesterol. These substances possess natural hormone-like powers, and this explains the hormone balancing effects of rice bran.

Rice bran/polish is among the finest sources of natural vitamins and minerals. The types of vitamins and minerals it contains are easily absorbed. It is one of the best natural sources of natural niacin. It is also exceptionally rich in pantothenic acid and biotin. Rice bran or polish is the top source of magnesium and phosphorus in addition to supplying a good amount of manganese, potassium, and chromium.

Rice bran and polish are so rich in food nutrients that it may limit the shelf life. It is a whole food, and, thus, it is vulnerable to spoilage. However, if unopened, the shelf life is at least two years.

Nutri-Sense is a supplemental source of natural rice bran and rice polish. Pure granular lecithin and fortified ground flaxseed are added to balance the formula. Nutri-Sense is a complete formula, providing immense natural source nourishment for the body. The human body requires nourishment, and Nutri-Sense provides natural source vitamins, minerals, amino acids, and fatty acids in a form which is readily absorbed.

The vitamins and minerals in Nutri-Sense help activate the cells and increase energy. Because it is a food rather than a synthetic supplement, Nutri-Sense has a limited shelf life and should be refrigerated after opening and consumed on a daily basis. Use it, don't try to store it forever.

Salmon

Canned salmon is highly nourishing for all age groups and is one of the most convenient nutrient-rich foods available. It is an excellent source of amino acids, fatty acids, B vitamins, and minerals. In other words, it is a complete food.

Salmon may be regarded as sort of the nutritional cadillac of all fish. It is inordinately rich in fish oils. This oils offer dozens of benefits to human cellular function. Salmon is also exceptionally high in vitamins. It is one of the few fish which contains a rather complete array of B vitamins, and it is exceptionally rich in niacin, pyridoxine, and pantothenic acid. What's more, it is one of the few excellent meat sources of vitamins D and E, both of which are difficult to procure in the diet. For instance, muscle meat is essentially devoid of such vitamins. Because it contains bones, canned salmon is one of the best food sources of calcium, containing a greater amount per ounce than milk.

Alaskan wild salmon is the superior choice versus Atlantic or fresh water salmon. Wild salmon is richer in the critical essential fatty acids than the farm-raised types. Wild Norwegian and Icelandic salmon are other superb choices. Salmon is one of the most nutrient dense of all foods. It may be relied upon to help balance nutritional needs. However, there is a warning: the excessive consumption of salmon increases tissue levels of mercury. Unfortunately, due to pollution fish are now contaminated with this toxin. Thus, salmon intake should be limited to a maximum of one serving per week. The exception may be high quality Alaskan wild salmon. For pregnant women the intake should be restricted to a maximum of one or two servings per month. However, wild salmon is always preferable to farm-raised. Rather than eating excessive amounts of salmon or other large fish during pregnancy, organic beef, turkey, or chicken may be consumed as a protein source. For fish, sardines may be selected.

It is possible to neutralize or purge the mercury that accumulates through fish consumption. This is through the intake of the potent liver- and heavy metal-purging formulas, that is LivaClenz and GreensFlush. The GreensFlush is a wild greens formula, while the basis of the LivaClenz is wild spices. To purge the heavy metals and to cleanse mercury residues take one dropperful of each twice daily. For significant mercury or heavy metal overload increase the dosage to three droppersful twice daily. Whenever consuming salmon or other large fish, take two droppersful with any such meal.

Sardines

This is a totally condensed food, ideal for quick nutrition. It is a meal in a can, a day's food in a tin, a survival package. Sardines possess everything required for the basic needs: amino acids, fatty acids, B vitamins, and minerals. They are also the top source of nuclear nutrients, that is RNA and DNA. Thus, with the exception of vitamin C, two or three cans of sardines provide the daily necessary ration.

Buy sardines packed in mustard, tomato sauce, or pure olive oil. Another option is sardines packed in their own fish oils, known as sild sardine oil. The latter is the most nutrient dense of all sardines, and offers a unique aromatic flavor. It is the natural sardine oils which gives this fish their intense flavor. The best sardines are made by the King Oscar company.

Unfortunately, lately I have noticed while shopping that sardines in their own oil are hard to procure. Sardines in sild oil were routinely available a few years ago. Perhaps the makers have been influenced, rather, corrupted, by the low-fat craze and have halted shipment or production. With consumer persistence, the demand can be created for this preferred and nutritionally rich type of sardine so that it will be returned to the shelves. Since they are a smaller fish sardines are less likely to be contaminated with mercury than, for instance, salmon or tuna. Thus, they can be eaten more often, like two or more times weekly.

Tuna

This is one of the most easily digested, nutritious, and filling of all foods. It is virtually pure protein, with a small percentage of fat. The highest grade is white or albacore tuna, this type being richer in omega-3 fish oils than the regular variety. The main vitamins in tuna are niacin and pyridoxine, of which it is a top source. Always select tuna packed in pure water, not the oil-packed varieties. Again, there is great concern regarding mercury contamination. Since tuna is one of the most extensively mercury-contaminated fish, the consumption of tuna should be limited to two servings per month and for pregnant women perhaps only one serving per month. When eating large fish, such as tuna and salmon, always take simultaneously the GreensFlush. This wild greens formula purges mercury from the body. With every serving of tuna or similar ocean fish take four droppersful of the wild greens formula daily.

One of the great things about tuna is that when it is eaten, it fills you up. It is essentially pure protein. However, to make it even more filling pour a tablespoon or two of pure extra virgin olive oil into the container. This gives the tuna an irresistible aromatic flavor. Add to this a few chopped green onions, which provides vitamin C, and pour on vinegar for a tasty and nutritious treat.

Vegetables, dried

As a disaster medicine vegetables offer little sustenance value. They are high in moisture and low in solid nutrients such as protein, fatty acids, and vitamins. However, they are relatively high in minerals and are, of course, a top vitamin C source. Vacuum packed and/or dried vegetables have an indefinite shelf life. These types of vegetables are far more nutrient dense than the canned varieties. Even so, certain dried vegetables offer a significant amount of mineral salts, which are much needed for reversing cellular stress.

Nutrient dense vegetables ideal for drying include:

- turnips
- radishes
- red and green sweet peppers
- zucchini and yellow squash
- parsley root
- parsnips
- tomatoes (actually a fruit)
- sweet or regular potatoes

Wild and brown rice

Botanically, wild rice is neither rice nor grain. It is the seed of a water grass known as *Zizania aquatic*. It is one of the few items in the supermarket which may be regarded as a sort of wild organic food. Of all starches rice is perhaps the easiest to store, least likely to mold, and most nourishing. Plus, in contrast to commercial grain, it rarely causes allergic reactions.

Wild rice is an excellent source of fiber. The type it contains is soluble fiber, which means it is gentle on the gut. Researchers have found that this type of fiber helps the natural bacteria thrive, providing them with fuel. This explains why the regular consumption of wild rice greatly aids bowel function.

Wild rice is higher in certain nutrients than brown rice, notably fiber, niacin, riboflavin, silicon, phosphorus, and iron. The fact is it is several times richer in niacin and riboflavin than brown rice.

Wild and brown rice store readily. Cooked rice is highly nourishing for all age groups. Blend a 50/50 mixture of wild and brown rice and cook in mineral water. The broth remaining is extremely nourishing, being high in both B vitamins and minerals; be sure to drink it or use it as a soup base, never waste it.

Wild rice is one of the most sustaining of all types of carbohydrate sources. The protein and starch it contains are easily digested. This makes it an excellent food for children. It is also very nourishing for the elderly. Use it as the preferred grain type starch for a high level of nourishment without risk for allergy or intolerance.

Food preservatives

In disasters the individual must be armed with methods to protect food, that is to prevent it from spoiling. Normally, refrigeration serves this purpose. It protects the food by stalling oxidation and germ growth. Yet, the possibility exists that the electricity could be disrupted and refrigeration cut off. Most individuals would regard this as a total loss, with all the food being discarded. Though this may astonish many individuals, there are measures to take which may preserve the food without refrigeration. In other words, the food doesn't have to spoil. Think about it. How did the people of ancient times, the Native Americans or the settlers of North America, keep food from spoiling? How did they manage without constantly contracting food poisoning? Now there are available substances capable of preserving food, extending the shelf life far beyond what was previously believed possible. These substances are natural antioxidants and antiseptics. If the oxidation can be blocked and germ growth halted, food may be kept virtually indefinitely, as these are the only chemical processes capable of spoiling it.

Only natural preservatives are safe for use in humans. While they are no replacement for refrigeration, if there is a disruption in common conveniences, they could prove invaluable.

Natural preservatives may be divided into two categories based upon the degree of efficacy: major and minor. Major preservatives are preferred, because of their dual action: they kill germs and halt oxidation. Minor antioxidants primarily slow oxidation and may offer a mild antiseptic action. Do not add chlorine or hydrogen peroxide to food. These are caustic chemicals capable of causing organ damage. Use only natural preservatives or antiseptics such as the following:

Major preservatives

- bee propolis
- wild oregano herb
- oil of oregano
- oil of rosemary
- oil of sage
- wild sage herb
- oil of cumin and cumin herb
- oil of bay leaf
- cloves
- salt

Add any of the above liberally to food and beverages.

Minor preservatives

- ascorbic acid—helps prevent spoilage of meat, fruit, and vegetables
- oregano herb—greatly retards food spoilage with modest but effective antifungal and antibacterial action. Halts spoilage of dry and wet foods. Great for sprinkling on fresh vegetables.
- cinnamon powder—mild antiseptic especially useful for meat

and starches. Its antioxidant action impedes food spoilage (cinnamon oil is also highly useful)
- vitamin E—strictly an antioxidant for fats, meats, fatty foods, etc.
- red grape powder—an incredibly useful antioxidant; also blocks mold contamination.
- lemon juice—mild antiseptic; prevents fruit and vegetables from oxidizing
- vinegar—a tremendous preservative; impedes oxidation of any food; prevents microbial growth
- cayenne, black pepper, and peppercorns—mild antiseptic

The fact that oil of oregano, particularly the wild spice extract Oreganol P73, kills germs is fully documented. It was Georgetown University, 2005, which demonstrated the effect. As published in *Molecular and Cellular Biochemistry* the P73 material utterly destroyed five major bacteria, including strains of klebsiella and tuberculosis. Previously at the University the oil was proven to destroy Candida albicans as well as drug-resistant staph, the latter being demonstrated in the animal model. There is no drug with comparable activity. Even the FDA, generally hostile towards herbs, proved its efficacy, demonstrating that oil of wild oregano killed eight food-borne pathogens, including salmonella, molds, pseudomonas, and E. coli. Even germs which may contaminate foods from rodents, for instance, Yersinia, the same species which causes plague, were destroyed.

Chapter 4
Wilderness Foods

The purpose of this section is to share my personal knowledge of wilderness foods. Only a finite percentage of Americans are capable of foraging for food. First, it is virtually impossible to procure enough food from foraging. The energy it takes to collect it is greater than what it will provide. However, it is reasonable to presume that certain industrious individuals are capable of finding food outside of supermarkets and health food stores. The key is to realize what could realistically be foraged. In other words, in this section you will learn what are the wild or rural foods you can find without herculean efforts.

I frequently forage. It is a relaxing hobby. I do most of my foraging while on trips in remote regions, where the plant materials I pick are relatively free of pollution. Yet, I also frequent berry bushes or trees within a few miles of my home. Remember, sun-ripened wild fruit is always superior nutritionally to the commercial varieties. Foraging is a healthy hobby, if you know what to look for. When foraging, beware of one major enemy: ticks. Be sure to check the body for ticks after any wilderness jaunt.

The greatest problem is that there is little wild food available. The exceptions are rather remote regions, such as the woods of northern California, Oregon, Washington State, Minnesota,

Michigan, Wisconsin, and Maine as well as certain Appalachian states, where individuals are accustomed to foraging. In Canada foraging is realistic, especially in the regions of lakes and forests in the far north. Thus, perhaps 5% of North Americans live in regions ideal for foraging. However, for the other 95% a few industrious individuals could procure food, perhaps through hunting and fishing.

In rural regions there may be a plethora of wild foods such as wild asparagus, berries, and various edible animals. Yet, even in the wide open space of America's rural regions feeding a family from the wild would be extremely arduous, perhaps impossible. Note that the American Indians were readily exterminated simply by disrupting their access to their normal food production/hunting procedures.

If the natives failed to survive at the turn of the century in the wilderness, how realistic is it that massive amounts of Americans could do so? The fact is only the most astute, knowledgeable, and savvy individual could successfully feed off the wild without the support of the commercialized convenience world.

Because of this only the most rudimentary wild edible substances, which are highly accessible to relatively large numbers of individuals, are described. In other words, the foods in this section are selected because they are familiar to nearly everyone and, thus, the majority of individuals can apply this information rapidly, without becoming an herb expert. Plus, there can be no chance for confusion with non-edible or even poisonous plants. Thus, everyone, from small children to the elderly, can safely follow the advice in this section.

Perhaps of greatest significance is the fact that these wild plants can be procured to add nutrition to the daily menu. Wild foods are far richer in vitamins and minerals than commercial foods. For instance, wild dandelion greens may contain as much as five times more vitamin A (as beta carotene) than greenhouse-grown varieties, and, in addition, up to ten times the potassium levels.

Dandelion greens

These are not difficult to find. They are right in a person's neighborhood. They are most edible during the spring and early summer. The best greens are the young leaves, which may grow under the older leaves. Older leaves are fibrous and inedible, that is they are mostly cellulose. Be sure the dandelion greens that are picked are from an area not sprayed with pesticides.

Dandelions are extremely rich in nutrients, far richer than any common vegetable. They are extremely high in beta carotene as well as vitamin C. For B vitamins they pack a greater density of riboflavin and niacin than any common vegetable. They contain a legion of critical minerals, particularly iron, calcium, phosphorus, magnesium, and potassium. What's more, they provide both protein and essential fatty acids.

Dandelion greens are highly protective for the body's most critical organs: the liver and kidneys. In Germany they are relied upon for liver cleansing, while in France they are highly touted as a natural diuretic. Simply pick the greens, wash thoroughly, and cook or eat raw. Sprinkle with lemon juice or red grape powder if desired. Dandelion greens are a complete food.

Fishing

This is one of the easiest types of all foraging. Virtually everyone knows how to fish. Provided it is from a relatively unpolluted region the nice thing about fishing is that anything which is caught is edible. Prepare basic fishing gear with reliable artificial lures just in case food sources run scarce. Remember, bait, such as worms, amphibians, and insects, can always be found.

To catch fish, everyone knows that the proper gear is required. Yet, the most important component is neither hook, line, nor sinker. Rather, it is belief. You must believe you will catch fish; you must be confident. They are there, and they are hungry. You must know this. Believe you will catch them, and you shall. This is more important than any gadget or technique.

Fishing is a relaxing, enjoyable hobby, plus it may provide valuable nutrition for the table. Nothing supercedes the taste of freshly caught fish. Be sure to cook your catch in spices, which offer both the benefit of great flavor plus stimulation of digestion.

Apples, pears, plums, and peaches

There are millions of wild trees (and innumerable abandoned orchards) bearing tasty fruit, although the produce may not appear as lovely as that in the grocery store. Be sure to remove fruit from only public or wilderness land. Don't enter private orchards without permission. If you desire food, simply ask. Most growers are generous with excess produce. Note: pears are one of the most readily digested of all fruit; an entire family can virtually live off of a well-endowed pear tree for several days, perhaps weeks. Plant fruit trees if you can, because every tree is a blessing for the future of this planet.

Mulberries

Virtually every block in the northern United States has within it a mulberry tree or, perhaps, a child who can find one. The mulberry may be the top survival berry. This is because it is high in a special chemical which helps reverse virtually any type of poisoning: resveratrol. Plus, mulberries are a good source of vitamin C and potassium, which are also needed for detoxification.

Don't wait for a disaster to strike to collect mulberries. This is one of the most nutrient-rich of all berries, available to virtually everyone. These sun-enriched berries are far more nourishing than the rather bland nutrient poor varieties found in the supermarkets. Plus, mulberries offer significant anti-toxic and anti-cancer powers. If you pick an excess, they may be dried in the sun or in an oven under low heat. This way you can eat them continuously.

Wild strawberry leaves and berries

This exotic plant, rare today, once filled the meadows, forests, and clearings of virtually every Eastern, Southern, and Midwestern state in the country. It grew like a weed. Native Americans filled baskets full of this fragrant fruit, devouring it as an exotic treat. The leaves of the wild strawberry plant were respected by the primitives for anti-diarrheal powers. The medicinal power of wild strawberry leaves is largely due to its high content of tannic acids. The berries are rare currently, unless the individual lives in the remote reaches of Canada, Montana, Michigan, Minnesota, Maine, and Alaska. They may also be found in the wild meadows of Nebraska and Wisconsin. The fresh leaves are super-rich in vitamin C.

Strawberry leaf tea is one of the most nourishing of all beverages. Fortunately, this is commercially available as Wild Power Tea. Brew this tea and add hot milk and honey for a pleasant flavonoid-rich drink. This was the brew that saved George Washington and his men at Valley Forge from dying of scurvy. Native Americans taught them to dig beneath the snow to discover the leaves, still green and vitamin/flavonoid rich.

Drink Wild Power Tea for a taste of an original, nourishing Native American formula. It is highly refreshing and makes a perfect evening hot drink or daytime cool beverage.

Wild blueberries and huckleberries

Once found in dozens of states these beautiful berries are extremely nourishing, exotic in taste, and even filling. They are more rare now and only found in remote areas such as in the wilderness regions of northern California, Washington State, Oregon, Michigan, northern Minnesota, northern Wisconsin, Alaska, and Maine.

These berries' richest component is a group of chemicals called anthocyanidins, the substances responsible for their brilliant color. The anthocyanidins are potent cancer fighters, plus they aid vision, a fact which explains the visually endowed bears' preference for them. Wild blueberries are an excellent source of potassium and a good source of vitamin C. The leaves are also nutritious, being high in vitamin C, flavonoids, and potassium. Add the leaves to hot water and let steep; the tea is a reliable cure for diarrhea as well as diabetes.

Wild raspberries and blackberries

These are the most abundant of all wild berries and are particularly abundant in Midwestern states as well as the East Coast. They are found nearly everywhere in Canada. Thus, they are one of the easiest of all wild foods to procure. Wild raspberries/blackberries are a good source of vitamin C and are super-rich in flavonoids. The leaves and berries of these plants are excellent digestive aids and are curative for mild diarrhea. Raspberry leaf tea is a dependable aid for female complaints, particularly menstrual discomfort or excessive menstrual bleeding.

Wild grapes, grape shoots, and grape leaves

Wild grapes are rarely used by Americans, yet they are perhaps the most prolific of all wild berries, although, in fact, they are a type of fruit. All parts of the plant are edible. The young shoots or curls are a top source of vitamin C and are pleasantly tart in taste. However, the grapes themselves are particularly high in the vitamin. The leaves, that is the young ones, are entirely edible, either raw or soaked in vinegar water. They too are an excellent source of vitamin C as well as resveratrol. While extremely tart, wild grapes are an excellent source of vitamins, minerals, and flavonoids. A handful provides the minimum daily need for vitamin C and potassium. They ripen in late August and September. Grapes, organic or wild, are so nourishing that for cleansing fasts they are frequently used as the sole food.

Rose hips

These can be found everywhere, even in flower gardens and parks. However, the best ones come from wild rose bushes, which are also prolific. Rose hips are the best source of vitamin C of any North American plant. They are edible primarily after the first few frosts. They may be dried and immersed in boiling water; this helps extract the vitamin C. They are also rich in protein, essential fatty acids, and vitamin E, the latter being found in the hard seeds lodged within the pulp. Rose hips are also a mineral concentrate, providing large amounts of iron, phosphorus, and potassium.

If you have access to the wilderness, gather rose hips after the first frosts. Dry them and store in the freezer. Add the dried hips to any herbal tea or grind them and add to soups or sauces. Fortify your food through the addition of vitamin C- and flavonoid-rich wild rose hips. Your health will improve as a result.

Nuts

Virtually everyone has made at least one attempt to collect nuts from the wild. The most common wild nut trees are black walnuts, hickory nuts, hazelnuts, butternuts, and pecans. Extracting the nuts from their shells is arduous. However, the meats are delicious and highly nourishing. If there is no food to be found, locate nut trees and fill bags full. This will provide dense nourishment for survival, especially in the event of the onset of difficult winters.

Nut oils provide the perfect fuel for the cells of the body in combating cold temperature. Plus, nuts are an excellent source of essential fatty acids, so direly needed for the health of the hair, skin, and nails. Thus, a handful of wild or plantation nuts provides immense nutritional support, especially for combating the ill effects of cold weather. Recently, scientists have proven that regular consumption of nuts significantly reduces the risks for cardiovascular diseases.

Other wilderness foods

There are hundreds of other foods which may be harvested from the wild or from public lands. This chapter is merely an attempt to guide individuals to the most prolific and easily accessible of these. Perhaps the individual could add to this list significantly with certain items of favorite wild nourishment. Wild asparagus, onions, garlic, chicory, lamb's quarters, yellow dock, sumac berries, rice—the list is endless. Just remember to leave some behind for reseeding and for forage since the wildlife must also have food.

Chapter 5
The Illnesses

There are tens of thousands of illnesses which afflict humankind; no book can cover them all. However, the purpose here is to describe those illnesses which will commonly occur during human difficulties or crises and which are most likely to cause discomfort, disability, disease, and even death in the event of human catastrophe. It is to select the most common illnesses that will pose problems. It is to provide the tools to prepare in the event medical care either falters or is unavailable.

The conditions are listed alphabetically to allow for the quickest possible reference. Plus, the objective is to use the most simple terms possible, ones that the average individual would readily recognize. For instance, instead of using the medical term gastritis, "Stomachache/pain" is listed. Instead of hypertension, "high blood pressure" is listed. Plus, treatments are constructed with a priority towards crisis management. Yet, the treatments are also invaluable for reversing chronic disease. Again, instead of listing "arthritis," which is a chronic disease and is usually not a crisis, "joint pain" is listed. However, the information regarding joint pain is useful to the arthritic. What's more, within many of the listings the most common and easy-to-recognize signs and symptoms have also been noted. This is so the condition may be readily diagnosed.

Here is the objective: to provide the individual with the most powerful, versatile, and easy-to-use remedies available. In an emergency there is no time to think, only to react. This book provides the tools to react effectively to difficult or dangerous situations.

Whether for everyday disasters, chronic health problems, toxic chemical exposure, or acts of Nature the individual needs a quick reference to determine what to do. This chapter serves precisely this function.

Unless otherwise mentioned all amounts listed represent adult dosages. For children or tiny individuals the amount can be reduced by at least half or perhaps two thirds.

Abdominal pain

The problem with abdominal pain is that it might be a mild incident amenable to simple measures, and it could also be a medical or surgical emergency. There are circumstances where sudden abdominal pain is non-surgical. For instance, pancreatitis, that is inflammation of the pancreas, causes severe abdominal pain, but surgery is rarely required. While sudden abdominal pain is usually a medical emergency requiring immediate physician supervision, in a disaster it may be impossible to procure medical or surgical care. In other words, the hospitals and doctors' offices may themselves be disabled or destroyed.

Methods of combat against abdominal pain

- Seek medical care immediately. Give no food or drink: only pure water at most.
- Keep the individual warm; cover with blankets if possible. Lay the individual on his/her right side.
- Rub essential oils on the body, but avoid harsh touching or pushing on the abdomen; gentle rubbing to apply the oils is allowed. Rub the oils on the back, face, and neck as well as the soles of the feet. Concentrate on rubbing the spine, buttocks,

and feet. Repeat the essential oil rub often. The best oils for this purpose are pure wild oil of oregano, oil of lavender, oil of bay berry, oil of rosemary, and oil of sage.
- Oil of ginger (emulsified in extra virgin olive oil) should be the first substance to consume. If tolerated, it will greatly ease inflammaton of the internal organs and combat stomach and intestinal distress. Note: for children use the Kid-e-Kare Tumi-eez. Take 2 or more drops under the tongue or in a small amount of water as often as needed.
- Take P73 wild oil of oregano, as researched by Georgetown University, the type emulsified in extra virgin olive oil. The safest method is to avoid taking anything into the stomach. Thus, take the oil under the tongue, one or two drops as often as necessary to halt the pain. In severe abdominal pain this may induce vomiting. However, the vomiting itself may be therapeutic. Often, this safe edible herbal oil will halt the pain rapidly, perhaps within minutes. This remedy may prove lifesaving in case medical care is arrested. The oil may be rubbed on the abdomen and/or spine.
- If food/beverage can be taken by mouth, begin with simple remedies that relax the digestive tract. Make tea from fresh ginger root. This is soothing and pain relieving. Oil of fennel and rosemary are also highly relaxing to the gut. Add a few drops in hot water or juice and sip until pain is relieved. Remember, significant abdominal pain unrelieved by simple remedies requires immediate medical attention.
- If supplements can be taken by mouth, try Infla-eez and/or Oregacyn Digestive. Both are well tolerated and are highly effective in reversing digestive disorders and/or pain.

Special Note: in this and all subsequent illnesses described in this book several natural cures are listed. For more information see Appendix A.

Things to avoid

- don't eat anything for at least 24 hours, in other words, rest the gut until the symptoms improves. At most, sip on pure water (perhaps with a few drops of oil of edible ginger and a small amount of raw honey.
- don't take aspirin or other anti-pain/anti-inflammatory drugs.

Aching feet

No one can afford the agony of aching or tired feet. The feet may be revitalized with essential oils. Rubbed topically, the oils quickly ease foot pain. They are also well absorbed from the porous skin of the feet, invigorating the entire body. Burning of the feet may warn of vitamin deficiency, notably a lack of vitamin B_5 (pantothenic acid). Royal jelly is a top natural source of this vitamin.

Aching feet combat kit

- Infla-eez rubbing oil—rub on feet vigorously.
- Oreganol P73 (Super Strength is best)—rub on soles of feet. Also, take 2 drops twice daily in juice or water.
- oil of lavender—rub on soles of feet as desired.
- Royal Oil (high potency liquid royal jelly—take 1 or 2 teaspoons twice daily.
- Royal Power premium-grade royal jelly (as a rich source of naturally occurring pantothenic acid)—3 capsules twice daily.

AIDS

The problem with AIDS is that virtually anyone, no matter what is his/her status, can become infected with this frequently fatal infestation. Thus, an infected individual may, if injured, liberate the germ in secretions or blood, and whoever comes in contact may become infected. This is how most health workers contract the disease. However, this mode of transmission is comparatively rare. The vast majority of individuals develop AIDS from sex. Obviously, IV drug abuse is the other major cause, as is blood transfusions, perhaps vaccines. Yet, homosexual acts are the most common perpetrators of this disease. With this disease in many instances the individual is essentially a cesspool of infection.

In a crisis setting individuals may come in contact with blood from injury victims. It is crucial to protect the body from such a potential disaster, since AIDS is largely transmitted by blood. The Oreganol P73 oil of wild oregano is a potent germicide capable of neutralizing the AIDS virus. What's more, Oreganol kills candida, a major complication of this disease.

AIDS combat kit

- Oreganol P73—rub on any open wound or region which may be infected by the virus or which is contaminated by human blood or secretions. Also, take 10 or more drops under the tongue three times daily. For full blown AIDS use the SuperStrength, 5 or more drops under the tongue three times daily. plus 20 or more drops twice daily in juice or water.
- oil of rosemary—take 20 drops twice daily.
- Oregacyn multiple spice capsules—take 2 or more capsules twice daily.
- NukeProtect—take 3 or more capsules twice daily.
- OregaMax—take 8 or more capsules daily.
- Infla-eez—take 3 or more capsules on an empty stomach twice daily.
- Oreganol P73 Juice—take 1/2 ounce three times daily.
- Rosemary Essence (research shows that rosemary inhibits the HIV virus)—take 1/2 ounce three times daily.

Foods that help
- protein-rich foods, such as fresh meat, nuts, whole milk products, yogurt, fermented soy, and fish, are invaluable, since this is a protein/tissue-wasting disease.
- garlic, onion, leeks, cinnamon (contain antiviral compounds)
- raw almonds (as a source of protease inhibitors)

Allergic reactions

Allergic reactions plague modern humanity. For instance, as many as one in three Americans have food allergies to such a degree that they suffer with daily symptoms. It is significant enough to be allergic to certain foods, but the problem today is that people are exposed to tens of thousands of synthetic chemicals, all of which can provoke allergic reactions. Some of the most pervasive of these allergy-causing chemicals include MSG, sulfites, aspartame, saccharin, and food dyes.

Allergic intolerances lead to hundreds of symptoms. Some of the primary symptoms include:

- hives or other sudden rashes
- shortness of breath and/or swelling in the throat
- sinus attacks
- itchy skin
- urinary discomfort
- headaches
- irritable bowel
- heartburn/indigestion
- diarrhea
- bloating after eating
- fatigue
- mood swings and/or irritability
- depression
- agitated behavior (especially in children)

- constipation
- colitis attacks

Hives are one of the major signs of allergic reactions. If you develop them, it is a signal that your body is reacting to something you have ingested, either a food or a drug.

Allergic reaction combat kit
- Oreganol P73—take 2 or more drops under the tongue as often as needed daily; also, take 5 drops as frequently as necessary in juice or water. What's more, rub the oil on any skin reaction.
- OregaMax capsules—take 2 or more capsules twice daily.
- Royal Power premium-grade royal jelly (unless allergic to bee stings)—take 3 capsules three or more times daily.
- organic selenium—take 200 mcg every 8 hours until symptoms abate. Then, take 200 to 400 mcg daily.
- pantothenic acid (capsules, not hard tablets)—take 500 mg three or more times daily.
- Infla-eez—take 2 or 3 capsules several times daily until the reaction is eliminated.

Things to avoid
- synthetic food dyes and artificial flavorings
- processed food
- nitrated meats
- drugs, including antibiotics
- NutraSweet and saccharin

Angina (see also Heart attack)

This is heart pain, which is believed to be caused by a lack of oxygen to the heart muscle. Yet, it is closely correlated to mental stress, especially anger and hostility. Relaxation and peace of mind is the antithesis of this condition. Put simply, if your heart muscle hurts, your inner heart, that is your soul, also hurts.

The role of hostility in the cause of heart disease has been confirmed by medical science. Researchers publishing in the *American Journal of Cardiology* determined that hostility and anger specifically damage the arteries of the heart, the very ones responsible for preventing angina.

Technically, angina is a type of pain that occurs over the left side of the upper chest, i.e. over the heart, which may spread to areas of what are known as referred pain. The nerves to the heart interconnect to other regions like the jaw, left side of the arm, upper back, and neck. This is why anginal pain may strike any of these regions. Much of the pain may be related to a deficiency of oxygen. In other words, the arteries supplying the heart are diseased and fail to deliver sufficient oxygen. This results in chest pain.

Physical disorders play a primary role in this condition. The arteries of the heart may be narrowed. The blood is often too thick, impeding oxygen/nutrient delivery. Also, the hormonal system may be disrupted, especially if the individual is under stress. Infection is also a factor, with the arterial walls and heart both being commonly infected. The responsible germs include all categories: viruses, bacteria, fungi, and parasites. What's more, dietary factors play an enormous role. Smoking and alcohol consumption greatly aggravate this condition. To correct the angina procure a thorough evaluation by a physician (hopefully one with a nutritional orientation), and take the following remedies:

Angina combat kit

- oil of rosemary—5 drops under the tongue several times daily during an attack; as a regular amount, take 5 to 10 drops daily.
- oil of oregano (the edible type, i. e. Oreganol P73)—take 2

drops under the tongue as often as necessary.
- Rosemary Essence—as a circulatory tonic, take 2 or more ounces daily.
- Resvital powder (to regenerate the arteries)—take 4 capsules three times daily.
- Infla-eez (uncoated) a powerful enzyme formula for cleansing the arteries and reducing systemic inflammation—take 3 capsules three times daily on an empty stomach.

Foods that help
- squash, pumpkin, zucchini, and yellow squash
- garlic, onions, leek, shallots
- nuts and seeds
- colorful berries
- rich-colored hot spices, especially cayenne and turmeric.

Things to avoid
- caffeine, chocolate, iced tea
- alcoholic beverages and beer
- nitrated/processed meats
- cigarette, cigar, and pipe smoke
- stress, hostility, anger, and apathy

Anthrax

This is a severe acute disease caused by a bacteria called *Bacillus anthracis*. It usually occurs on farms, but urban outbreaks are possible. There have been no major epidemics of this disastrous illness in recent history, but there have been outbreaks. In Ontario, Canada (1998), dozens of individuals contracted this condition in its less fatal form, that is the type that attacks the skin. In the United States during 1998 there were numerous incidents of purported anthrax spore releases, mostly in public buildings. All were false alarms. Then, in 2001 the drill turned real. Someone in the government released anthrax spores, causing the deaths of several individuals, including postal workers. Through a racially-charged letter, Muslims were falsely stigmatized. Quickly, it was determined that there was no Islaamic 'terror' and that, rather, it was an inside job. Government-issue anthrax poisoning became a reality.

Exposure to anthrax spores is nearly always fatal. The problem is that when the spores are inhaled in large numbers, the germs multiply rapidly in the lungs, suffocating the individual. It is the weapon of germ warfare. Thus, there is no medical defense.

An outbreak of anthrax remains a significant possibility, especially since the development of active infection in Canada. While antibiotics are useful for the skin manifestations, they offer no certain protection in the event of spore release. Thus, the individual must rely upon natural remedies as an adjunct. The fact is natural cures, particularly the edible essential oils, would prove lifesaving in the event of an anthrax outbreak. A study by Georgetown University proved that a blend of wild oregano oils, known as P73 Oreganol, stopped the growth of anthrax bacilli. A combination of wild oregano, cumin, and cinnamon (i. e. Oregacyn capsules) was even more effective than oil of oregano. To date spice oils are the only known substances which effectively halt the growth of this germ. Those which are most effective are oregano, cumin, garlic, and cinnamon oils.

Anthrax combat kit

- oil of oregano (Oreganol SuperStrength)—apply topically to skin lesions. If spore contamination/lung infection occurs, massive amounts will be needed, like 40 to 80 drops daily in juice or water. Also, take a few drops under the tongue as often as every five minutes.

- oil of cumin (cumin also halts the growth of this germ)—take 10 to 20 drops daily in juice or water.
- oil of bay leaf—take 10 to 20 drops daily in juice or water.
- Oregacyn Respiratory—take 2 capsules several times daily.
- raw garlic/onion—consume as much as possible.
- Black Seed-plus—take 3 capsules four times daily.
- protective mask and clothing (plasticized jackets/suits, gloves, etc.)

Foods that help
- raw onion juice—a cup twice daily
- raw wild oregano honey—6 or more tablespoons daily

Arsenic poisoning

Heavy metal poisoning is one of the modern world's most monumental disasters. This occurs largely in industrial workers, yet, it can also develop in unwitting victims who live near pollution-generating industrial complexes.

Poisoning by arsenic is far from remote. This heavy metal is a component of a variety of industrial chemicals, notably insecticides, fumigants, weed killers, fruit sprays, and rodent poisons. The highly toxic arsenic gas is transported every day on the railways and roads of North America. As a result of its rather ubiquitous nature thousands of cases of chronic arsenic poisoning occur every year. Symptoms of arsenic poisoning include:

- metallic taste in the mouth
- numbness and tingling in the nerves
- odd skin lesions, which are dry and excoriated
- muscular weakness and/or paralysis
- confusion
- headaches, usually chronic

- burning sensation in the limbs
- nausea and vomiting
- loss of appetite
- weight loss
- vague abdominal pain
- petechiae (tiny skin hemorrhages)
- watery diarrhea (may be severe and prolonged)

Arsenic detoxification kit

- organic selenium—take 200 mcg three times daily.
- calcium and magnesium—take 1200 mg of calcium and 600 mg of magnesium daily. Do not use magnesium oxide. It is poorly absorbed and usually causes diarrhea if taken in large amounts.
- GreensFlush—take 20 or more drops twice daily. If exposure is severe, double or triple this amount.
- Oreganol P73 Juice—take 1 ounce twice daily. If exposure is severe, double this amount.
- LivaClenz—take 10 to 20 drops twice daily. If exposure is severe, double or triple this amount.
- NukeProtect—take 3 or more capsules twice daily.
- Resvital powder—take 2 capsules three times daily.

Aspergillus infection (Aspergillosis)

This is a potentially devastating infection from a bizarre fungus (mold), which lives primarily in soil. This fungus was once thought only to attack weakened or immune-compromised individuals. Yet, even today relatively healthy individuals are developing the infection.

Aspergillus is a filamentous fungus, meaning it grows in tiny filaments or threads. These threads can invade virtually any tissue in the body, but they have a preference for attacking the sinuses, lungs, and heart valves. However, they also readily invade the skin, nails, external ear, nasal mucosa, vagina, and even the bone marrow. Cancer patients are its greatest victims. Globally, some 300,000 cancer patients die yearly from aspergillosis, candidiasis, and other fungal infections. There is a virtual disaster occurring in America regarding this germ. According to bone marrow transplant expert Dr. Elias Anaissie aspergillus is invading individuals from a ubiquitous source: drinking water. He describes how tap water is loaded with the fungus, explaining that "chlorine doesn't touch aspergillus." He is so concerned about this that he recommends hospitalized patients receive sponge baths instead of showers, which aerosolize the germ. Scientific studies confirm Dr. Anaissie's concerns: simply turning on a sink can liberate enough aspergillus in the air that it can be detected six feet away. The fact is in numerous hospitals in Western countries aspergillus outbreaks are routine. Nurses and doctors suffer from extreme infestations, which cause potentially life-threatening infections of the lungs, blood, and other internal organs.

While there are no drugs which destroy this germ, Nature provides the answer. P73 Oreganol decimates it. As described by European researchers as little as a tenth of a percent concentration (a drop or two in a few ounces of water) halts and prevents its growth. A mere one percent concentration obliterates it.

Aspergillus infection combat kit

- P73 oil of oreganol (SuperStrength is best)—take 2 to 5 drops three times daily under the tongue. Take 5 to 10 drops twice daily in juice or water. Note: also rub the oil of Oreganol around sinus region and the nose, or place a small amount on a Q-Tip and apply in nose (for sinus/lung fungus). Before drinking add a drop or more of oil of oreganol to any suspect water.
- OregaMax capsules—take at least 3 capsules twice daily. For stubborn cases take 3 capsules three times daily.

- Resvital—take 3 capsules twice daily.
- black seed capsules (Black Seed-plus)—take 3 capsules twice daily. Note: aspergillus infection may cause symptoms which mimic the common cold.
- GreensFlush wild greens formula—2 or more droppersful twice daily

Things to avoid
- refined sugar, wheat products, rye products, wheat grass
- chlorinated tap water
- brewer's and baker's yeast

Asthma

This is one of the gravest epidemics facing the Western societies. This is because in the past one hundred years, despite medical care the death rate from this disease has nearly tripled. As many as 1 in 15 individuals in North America suffer from asthma, an incredibly high number. Yet, for asthmatic victims the greatest desperation results because of the fact that the medical profession offers no cure for this potentially disastrous illness. It is ironic that an orthodox medical journal, *Hippocrates Magazine,* states "there is no cure for asthma." This is despite the fact that Hippocrates himself, working in the 5th century B.C., apparently cured it with herbs.

Mold allergy and/or infection is the most likely cause for today's asthma epidemic. It is rarely suspected or diagnosed by physicians. Molds are also an indirect cause. They poison the immune system, leaving it vulnerable to attack by other germs. What's more, mold, as well as yeast, directly infects the bronchial linings, often causing this disease. Other major factors include chemical sensitivity, air pollution, food allergy, and immunization reactions. Common symptoms of asthma include:

- chest tightness
- wheezing
- coughing
- inability to take a clear deep breath
- inability to exhale completely
- sensitivity to chemicals, fumes, and odors

Asthma is largely due to fungal infection. This is why this disease can be cured with large doses of wild oregano extracts, notably the Oreganol and the triple spice compound, Oregacyn respiratory.

Asthma Combat Kit

- Oreganol P73—take 3 or more drops under the tongue twice or more daily.
- Oregacyn respiratory—take 2 or 3 capsules twice or more daily.
- black seed capsules (Black Seed-plus)—take 2 or more capsules three times daily.
- Purely-C—take 3 capsules twice daily.
- Oreganol P73 Juice—take one ounce twice daily in juice or water or straight.
- Royal Power herb-fortified royal jelly—take 3 capsules twice daily to boost adrenal function.

Things to Avoid

- tartrazine (yellow dye #5) and other synthetic food dyes
- MSG and sulfites
- white sugar

Athlete's foot and/or jock itch

These aggravating, unrelenting conditions afflict tens of millions of North Americans. Every manner of cream, powder, and formula is applied to the feet/groin in an attempt to cure it. Yet, it is easy to eradicate. Athlete's foot is caused by a fungus, which invades and feeds off the superficial layers of skin on the feet. This fungus eats keratin, the protein which makes up skin. It also feeds off of sugar, which is delivered to the skin from the blood. It is usually contracted from moist contaminated public places such as school showers, gymnasiums, bathtubs, and bathroom floors. Jock itch is caused by the same fungus.

Athlete's foot/jock itch combat kit
- oil of oregano (Oreganol P73, SuperStrength is best)—rub on feet, morning and night. For jock itch dilute (three to five drops in a teaspoon of myrtle or olive oil). Apply once or twice daily. Also, take 3 or more drops under the tongue twice daily.
- Garlex natural garlic antiseptic—take 20 drops twice daily; also rub topically, as needed.
- OregaBiotic natural antibiotic—take 20 drops twice daily; also rub topically, as needed.

Things to avoid
- don't go barefoot in public places
- synthetic socks, which retain moisture and germs (use cotton or wool instead
- white sugar and sweets feed the fungus, making eradication difficult

Back pain

Back pain and injury are perhaps the most common causes of disability in the United States today. In a crisis back pain is an utter disaster. Who can afford to be crippled at a time of difficulty?

Many of the drugs which fight pain are caustic to the stomach and intestines. Thus, their unsupervised use may cause more harm than good. This is why it is more appropriate to rely on natural remedies to combat disaster-related pain than to use drugs. Use home remedies combined with appropriate exercise to rebuild the back and eliminate the pain.

Back pain combat kit
- bromelain/papain (uncoated capsules, i.e. Infla-eez)—take 2 to 4 capsules three times daily on an empty stomach.
- oil of oregano (SuperStrength is the best)—rub topically on painful region. Take 5 to 10 drops twice daily in juice or water.
- Resvital powder—take a teaspoon twice daily in juice or water.
- Purely-C (natural vitamin C supplement)—take 3 capsules twice daily.
- OregaMax capsules (for naturally occurring trace minerals for building bone)—take 2 to 3 capsules 3 times daily.

Foods that help
- raw almonds
- fresh papaya including seeds
- cayenne pepper, oregano, and sage

Other ideas
- don't sleep on the stomach; preferably, sleep on the right side
- squat low before lifting heavy objects; lift with hips and thighs
- don't eat foods to which you are allergic

Bed sores and other skin ulcers

Bed sores are open wounds that afflict primarily the elderly and infirm. They are caused largely by constant pressure against the tissues, the result of immobility. These sores notoriously fail to heal despite aggressive medical treatment, which includes massive antibiotic therapy and surgical debridement.

Varicose ulcers, also known as stasis ulcers, are similar to bed sores in appearance. They are due to poor blood flow as a result of sluggish venous return. In other words, the blood stagnates in the lower extremities, leading to infection and/or ulceration. A history of varicose veins increases the risk, as does diabetes and atherosclerosis.

Because their circulation is so poor, diabetics frequently develop ulcerations in the extremities, particularly in the legs and feet. The ulcers easily become infected, which may lead to gangrene.

Medical treatment for bed sores usually fails. What's more, repeated dosages of antibiotics damage the immune system, causing deep-seated fungal infections, both in the wound(s) and internal organs. This is why yeasts are frequently cultured from these wounds, although they are usually regarded as a source of "secondary infection."

Fungi thrive on diseased and/or dead tissue. In a forest molds and mushrooms do not grow on healthy trees. They grow prolifically on diseased, dying, or dead trees. In other words, fungi attack the sick and debilitated. The same applies to human tissues. This is why they attack chronic wounds.

Oil of oregano, as well as other essential oils such as rosemary, myrtle, and lavender, is the agent of choice for the topical treatment of bed sores, varicose ulcers, and diabetic ulcers. In particular, oil of wild oregano exhibits both antibacterial and antifungal activity. It is ideal for use on open wounds, since it penetrates deep into injured tissue and coats both healthy and diseased portions. It helps sterilize the wound and its secretions. It disperses pus. Plus, it helps speed the healing of these difficult-to-cure wounds.

Oil of oregano is the first choice for bed sores or other poorly healing open wounds. It should be utilized topically as well as internally. Usually, only small amounts are needed topically. Other oils may be of even greater value for speeding healing, notably the oils of rosemary, myrtle, lavender, and bay leaf. The oils can be administered simultaneously with medical therapy. They should routinely be applied on open wounds which are being treated with systemic antibiotics. If the wound is too sensitive, rub the oils on the surrounding skin. This speeds healing, eradicates infection, and prevents further infection from developing.

The aforementioned oils are the active ingredients of Oreganol cream. This cream is more gentle on wounds, as well as inflamed regions, than the oil. The fact is this is the ideal form to use for inflamed skin disorders such as eczema, dermatitis, rosacea, and psoriasis. This cream also contains honey, as well as propolis, which speeds wound healing.

Oregano oil's superiority over antibiotics lies largely in its potent action against fungi. Fungi are parasites; in other words, they are opportunists. They invade weakened and diseased tissues. Healthy tissue is immune to them.

If the infection is destroyed, open sores heal rapidly. In other words, it is the infection which is delaying the healing. Nutritional deficiency may also play a role, as a lack of vitamins A, C, B_5, B_6, and essential fatty acids greatly impedes wound healing, as do deficiencies of zinc, iron, and selenium. Merely replacing the deficient nutrients greatly accelerates wound healing.

Skin ulcerations must be regarded seriously, especially in the chronically ill. In diabetics open wounds may proceed to more serious conditions: gangrene and amputation. If the infection can be rapidly eliminated, the wound will heal quickly, and the crisis will be resolved.

Bed sore/open wound combat kit

- Oreganol (P73)—apply topically as often as needed and take internally, 5 to 10 drops twice daily. Rub on skin surrounding the wound. To accelerate wound healing apply honey over the oregano oil.

- crude raw honey (wild oregano or Mediterranean wild flower are best)—apply topically on wound site and cover.
- Oreganol cream—for wound healing; apply as needed; rub on skin surrounding the wound.
- Infla-eez capsules—for wound healing, take two or more capsules on an empty stomach.
- Purely-C—for stimulating cartilage and skin regeneration; take 3 capsules twice daily.
- Royal Power—for stimulating wound healing, take four capsules twice daily.
- Resvital powder—take two teaspoons twice daily.
- selenium—take 300 to 600 mcg daily until wound heals.

Bee stings (see also Killer bees)

About 1 in 200 people is severely allergic to bee stings. Yet, every individual is vulnerable to suffering from the painful stings of these creatures. What's more, there is a new threat, the killer bees, which can cause fatality in virtually anyone, allergic or not.

Bee stings are the most common type of insect bite in the northern United States and Canada. In the southeast fire ants are the primary stinging insect. Repeated stings by fire ants make the individual more vulnerable to bee sting hypersensitivity. Conversely, individuals sensitive to bee stings are usually highly sensitive to fire ant stings.

For the vast majority of individuals bee stings are easy to resolve. Simply apply an antivenom herb extract to the sting site. The best antivenom herbs are oil of oregano, juice of raw garlic, and juice of raw onion. Oil of oregano (i. e. Oreganol P73) is perhaps the most aggressive and potent of these. However, if this is unavailable, simply crush raw garlic or onion. Apply the maceration to the sting site. Eradication of pain and swelling should be immediate. For those with severe reactions the therapy should be more aggressive; call for medical help immediately. Symptoms of life-threatening bee sting shock include:

- hives
- throat tightness
- inability to talk (swollen vocal cords)
- inability to swallow
- coughing spasms and/or wheezing
- weakness and/or dizziness
- loss of consciousness
- severe swelling at the sting site

If any of these symptoms develop, seek medical care immediately. However, edible oil of oregano, (i. e. Oreganol P73) is an absolute lifesaver in this scenario, as is demonstrated by the following:

CASE HISTORY
Mr. J. was vacationing in Vale, Colorado, when his worst nightmare occurred: he was stung in the neck by a bee. The problem is Mr. J. is highly allergic to bee stings, and just a few months prior he nearly died from a sting. Rapidly, he developed a severe toxic reaction; his neck swelled up enormously, and he collapsed almost immediately. Fortunately, an herbalist was in his presence. This brave soul grabbed his bottle of oil of oregano (North American Herb & Spice Co.), placed several drops in Mr. J.'s mouth and rubbed it on his neck. Within minutes Mr. J. was revived; his neck swelling was halted, in fact, it was reversed. By the time the ambulance arrived, he was completely well and did not require further care. This immensely valuable herbal substance, the wild oil of oregano, saved his life.

What to do in a bee sting emergency:

Get medical help immediately, and:
- remove the stinger if possible
- saturate the sting site with oil of oregano or garlic/onion maceration
- for severe toxic/systemic reactions give oil of oregano by

mouth (only use the edible kind by North American Herb & Spice: do not use aromatherapy oregano oil or cheap imitations internally)
- apply ice to the wound, that is if the swelling fails to recede
- seek medical care if necessary (or available)

Bee sting combat kit
- oil of oregano—apply this lifesaving oil directly to the sting site. Repeat as needed. The oil also helps dislodge the stinger. Also, take 5 or more drops under the tongue as needed.
- garlic cloves—crush and apply maceration to the wound (not necessary if oil of oregano is available).
- Garlex antitoxin oil—apply several drops on the wound/sting as needed.
- tweezers (for removing the stinger)

Killer bee combat kit (see also Killer Bees)
Same as the aforementioned, however:
- if the bees are still attached, pour oregano oil on them; this will kill them or drive them off. If a spray bottle is handy, add the oregano oil to it; pump-spray the bees. Or, use the ready-to-use Germ-a-CLENZ and spray directly at any attacking bees. These oils burn their eyes and scent glands, destroying them. Pump-spray the air all about you to drive them off.
- take oil of oregano under the tongue and/or squirt into the mouth, as much as possible.

Bell's palsy

This condition, which afflicts tens of thousands of Americans yearly, is caused by paralysis of a nerve that controls the muscles of the face. The muscles simply refuse to work, because the nerves supplying them have become disabled. It is caused by a virus, which attacks the nerve, causing inflammation and swelling, disrupting the function of the nerve. Ultimately, it is the swelling that causes the problem, because this places great pressure on the nerve, blocking the flow of nerve impulses.

The involved nerve controls the strength of the muscles of the face, but when it is infected, this function fails. This explains the typical symptoms of Bell's palsy. Each side of the face has one of these nerves, and, since only one side of the facial nerve is infected, only one side is damaged. Bell's palsy symptoms include inability to wrinkle the brow, inability to close the eyelids (the eye stays open), inability to make a voluntary facial expression (like a smile), numbness of the face and lips, pain behind the ear, and excessive tearing. Aggressive treatment of this condition is necessary, because unless the swelling is reduced and the virus killed, permanent damage is likely.

Bell's palsy combat kit

- oil of oregano (Oreganol P73–use of the SuperStrength may be necessary)—rub over the check, facial bones, and behind the ear on the affected side. Take 5 or more drops under the tongue several times daily until the problem is solved.
- oil of rosemary—2 drops under the tongue 5 times daily. Take also 10 drops in juice or water twice daily.
- Royal Power premium grade royal jelly—take 3 to 4 capsules twice daily.
- vitamin A eye drops—for dry or exposed eyes
- Infla–eez—take 2 or 3 capsules three times daily on an empty stomach.

Bite wounds

At some point fully half of all North Americans will be bitten by some type of animal or another person. Such wounds may induce great physical and emotional trauma but also readily become infected. Certain infections are life threatening, notably tetanus and rabies. However, the latter can be prevented if the bite is treated immediately with antiseptic compounds and/or immunizations.

According to Presutti, writing in *Post Graduate Medicine,* dog bites are the most common type, accounting for as many as 2,000,000 bites per year. With their powerful jaws dogs can greatly traumatize the tissues, because they are capable of exerting hundreds of pounds of pressure. Thus, their bites may puncture the skin but may also bruise or traumatize deeply, even to the bone. Cat and human bites also readily become infected.

Bite combat kit
- oil of oregano (i. e. Oreganol P73)—apply liberally to wound as often as necessary and take 2 drops under the tongue twice daily.
- oil of lavender—apply to wound liberally as often as necessary.
- Oreganol cream—apply to wound; dramatic for inducing healing and for softening skin (i.e. preventing scarring).
- vitamin E (internally and externally to prevent scarring).
- Infla–eez (uncoated potent fruit enzymes)—take 3 or more capsules twice daily on an empty stomach.

Bladder infection

Bladder infections are a preventable, in fact, curable catastrophe. Known medically as cystitis, these infections cause an enormous degree of disability. Untreated, they can lead to serious kidney infections. Yet, natural remedies are proven to cure this condition.

The majority of infections are caused by bacteria, E. coli being the most notorious. Yeasts are also a common cause, especially in individuals who have taken repeated doses of antibiotics. One of the greatest risk factors for recurrent bladder infections is mechanical invasion of the bladder. Thus, individuals who have had prolonged surgeries resulting in catheter placement and/or anyone who has had scopes inserted in the bladder or penis has a high risk for infection, particularly by yeasts. If the individual has been previously catheterized and is suffering from recurrent kidney or bladder infections, it is virtually assured that yeast infection is the cause.

Bladder infection combat kit
- oil of fennel (a great urinary flushing agent)—take 5 to 10 drops twice daily.
- oil of wild oregano—take a few drops under the tongue three times daily and 5 to 10 drops in juice or water twice daily.
- wild oregano capsules (OregaMax caps)—take 3 capsules three times daily.
- CranFlush—take 20 drops several times daily or as directed.
- red grape powder (Resvital)—take 4 to 6 capsules three times daily (or 1 teaspoon three or four times daily).

Foods that help
- Welch's Grape Juice
- cranberry juice concentrate or pure unsweetened cranberry juice
- wild (raw) oregano honey
- watermelon (natural urine- and bacteria-flushing agent)

Things to avoid
- citrus juice
- caffeine, coffee, tea, and iced tea
- sugar and chocolate

Bleeding gums

Bleeding gums are a warning sign of nutritional deficiency, indicating a lack of vitamin C and/or bioflavonoids. In the extreme, bleeding gums represent an early sign of scurvy.

When the gums break down, they are readily invaded by germs. The germs must be destroyed for the gums to heal and the bleeding to be stopped. Antiseptic herbs, such as cloves, bay, oregano, and tea tree, especially their oils, are effective and safe for reversing this condition.

Bleeding gums combat kit
- oil of oregano (Oreganol P73)—rub on gums, a.m. and p.m; also, use on toothbrush.
- Purely-C—an all-natural vitamin C capsule, take two or three capsules twice daily.
- folic acid—take 5 mg daily.
- OregaMax capsules (also a source of gum/teeth-nourishing trace minerals such as calcium, zinc, and magnesium)—take 2 or 3 capsules twice daily.
- Resvital—take 1 teaspoon or 4 to 6 capsules daily.

Things to avoid
- white sugar (causes the degeneration of the bone that sets the teeth, the enamel, and the gums)
- soda pop (phosphoric acid and sugar destroy enamel and damage bone)

Bleeding wounds

What can be done if an individual is bleeding to death? Certainly, the person must be rushed to the hospital. Yet, the more common disaster is minor to moderate bleeding, which is treatable.

Only a few natural substances act as clotting agents, that is they halt bleeding. When applied topically, these agents stop bleeding, while speeding the healing of wounds. These substances include garlic, onion, and essential oils. Phenol-rich oils, particularly the edible oil of wild oregano (Oreganol P73), are the best naturally occurring clotting agents. Simply drizzle

The Illnesses 141

the oils on the wound. You may need to apply slight pressure (with a clean cotton ball or bandage). When applied to the skin, oil of oregano is an aggressive clotting agent. The fact is oil of wild oregano helps normalize blood clotting. Yet, when taken internally it balances the blood clotting mechanism, preventing internal bleeding. Repeat as needed until bleeding halts. The effects are virtually miraculous. For shaving cuts it is a lifesaver.

Bleeding wounds combat kit

- P73 oil of oregano (SuperStrength is best)—add directly to the wound/cut; if bleeding fails to stop immediately, apply firm (but not excessive) pressure until it stops.
- Purely-C—to heal any wound and help minimize bleeding take 2 to 3 capsules twice daily. For severe bleeding take 2 or more capsules every half hour or every hour.
- red grape powder (Resvital)—a tremendously valuable circulatory aid and clotting normalizing agent. Take 2 to 4 capsules every few hours. For more severe problems take 6 capsules several times daily or a teaspoonful several times daily. The powder is an astringent and, thus, may also be dusted on the wound.
- Oreganol cream—apply to wound and on surrounding skin.
- PropaHeal—apply to wound and on surrounding skin, a tremendous wound healing aid.

Note: the best method (outside of surgical intervention) for stopping bleeding from a gushing wound is heavy pressure by applying, preferably, sterile gauze or a clean cloth. Pressure plus essential oils is highly effective.

Blood clots

Blood clots are of two types; the type that is within the surface tissues, that is in the veins just under the skin, or the deep type, which cannot be felt or seen and which is in the deep veins or organs of the body. Both of these are medical emergencies, although medical treatment for the superficial type is often minimal.

Blood clot combat kit

- wild oil of oregano (Oreganol P73, Super Strength is best)—rub over involved area. Take 5 to 10 drops under the tongue several times daily.
- high dose bromelain/papain (i. e. Infla-eez)—take 2 or more capsules 3 to 6 times daily, preferably on an empty stomach.
- onion juice—if the clot is in the leg or arm, soak a cloth in onion juice and wrap around involved area. Drink a cup of the juice daily.
- Resvital powder—a heaping teaspoon 2 or 3 times daily in juice or water.
- Purely-C—to help normalize blood clotting take two capsules of this all-natural vitamin C twice daily.
- Sesame-E—as a source of natural vitamin E to regulate blood clotting, two teaspoons daily.

Foods that help

- sardines, salmon, albacore tuna, mackerel, and herring (consume as much as possible—fatty fish oils help dissolve clots).
- onions and garlic (raw)
- papaya and its seeds
- raw fresh pineapple

Boils

There are two types of boils: carbuncles and furuncles. The distinction is that carbuncles are infections within the sebaceous glands of the skin, while furuncles are infections within the hair follicles. The latter condition commonly occurs in men with heavy beards, who shave frequently. Shaving traumatizes the delicate facial skin. This allows germs to gain entry to the hair follicles, in which they multiply.

Black males are particularly susceptible to the development of extensive boils, largely due to ingrown hairs on the face and other regions. These boils often occur in large numbers on the cheeks and/or neck and are quite disfiguring.

Most furuncles and carbuncles are caused by staph and/or strep infections. Infection by yeasts may be a contributing factor.

While boils are often painful and/or disfiguring, they are not regarded as a serious condition. However, if left untreated, they may persist for weeks or months. Systemic antibiotic therapy usually fails to eradicate them. The drugs can't penetrate the site of the infection. Plus, the infections are often caused by antibiotic-resistant microbes, staph and strep being the most notorious of these. People who live in close quarters, such as athletic teams or hospitalized patients, may suffer from outbreaks of staphylococcal boils.

Boil combat kit

- oil of oregano (Oreganol P73)—apply to the involved sites; take also 5 to 10 drops internally daily.
- Oreganol cream—highly effective, apply to involved areas.
- oil of myrtle—apply to involved areas.
- Sesam-E (as a source of mixed tocopherols)—take 1 or 2 teaspoons daily.
- Infla–eez—take 2 or more capsules twice daily on an empty stomach.
- primrose or borage oil—take 4 capsules twice daily.
- Germ-a-CLENZ natural spice mist—spray on infected area 2 or more times daily.

Foods that help
- papaya plus the seeds and/or dried papaya spears
- sunflower seeds, raw
- fatty fish of all types

Things to avoid
- caffeine, coffee, chocolate, tea, iced tea
- deep fried foods

Bone infection (osteomyelitis)

This infection usually occurs as a consequence of trauma or surgery. Typically it is caused by bacteria, which lodge in the bone, destroying it. Most commonly, it develops in leg bones. Smokers and diabetics have the highest risk.

The hallmark for this disastrous illness is an open wound or a hole in the skin, which drains pus or other secretions. This is called a draining sinus; the opening may be large or small. This is apparently the body's way of exuding the toxins, which have accumulated within the bone. The usual culprit is staph, although Pseudomonas, a very obnoxious and difficult-to-kill microbe, may also cause it. It may also be caused by tuberculosis. Bone infection may develop without trauma or surgery. No one is sure how this happens, but this certainly signifies that the immune system is dysfunctional: the bones are normally sterile.

Bone infections nearly always result when compound fractures develop in disaster circumstances. This is because there is no means to keep the tissues sterile.

Bone infection combat kit
- The site should be cultured and the appropriate antibiotics taken (if available).
- Oreganol SuperStrength—take internally and put on or into the wound.

- oil of wild lavender—rub over and/or in wound
- oil of bay leaf—take 10 to 20 drops twice daily.
- wild oregano herb (OregaMax capsules)—take 3 or more capsules twice daily.
- Infla–eez high potency enzyme formula—take 3 or more capsules three times daily on an empty stomach.
- OregaBiotic multiple spice capsule—take 3 capsules three or more times daily.

Bronchitis

As described in *Patient Care*, January 1996, medical doctors claim that they don't know the cause of bronchitis. What's more, they state that antibiotics are virtually useless for curing it. Taber's Medical Dictionary defines bronchitis as "inflammation in the bronchial tubes." There must be a cause of the inflammation; in fact infection is the primary factor. Fungal infection is the main culprit. Food allergies are a secondary but important cause. Eliminating the inflammation certainly helps resolve this condition. However, if the bronchial tubes are infected, the offending germ must be destroyed in order for resolution to occur. This is where the wild oregano extract, that is the oreganol P73, is invaluable. It reverses this condition largely by destroying the offending fungi.

Patients are commonly bombarded with multiple doses of antibiotics in an attempt to cure the disease. However, according to current research fungi and viruses are the primary cause of bronchitis, not bacteria. Plus, the condition may be caused or aggravated by food allergies. Even if bacteria are involved, they are usually immune to antibiotics. Thus, antibiotics usually aggravate this condition, since these drugs worsen allergic tendencies and fungal infections.

The approach to treatment must be totally different than the current method. This illustrates the value of using natural antiseptics and anti-inflammatory agents, both of which combat the causes of this condition.

Bronchitis combat kit

- oil of oregano—take 2 drops under the tongue, as often as necessary. Take also 5 drops three times daily in juice or water.
- OregaBiotic wild multiple spice capsules—take 3 capsules three times daily.
- oil of rosemary (for opening up lung passages)—rub on chest and take 5 to 10 drops twice daily.
- Orange Blossom Essence (i.e. white coffee) or Rose Petal Essence—add 2 tablespoons of either one to hot water as a tea; drink as often as needed.
- Purely-C—take 3 capsules three times daily.
- oil of lavender—rub on chest and under nose; take 2 drops under the tongue twice daily (for this purpose use only the edible oil of lavender emulsified in extra virgin olive oil). May also be inhaled directly into the nose. Or, for children use the highly effective Kid-e-Kare rubbing oil, and rub all over the body, especially on the chest, forehead, and feet.

Foods that help

- horseradish, freshly grated if possible
- raw onion and garlic
- onion/garlic/meat broths
- raw honey

Things to avoid

- milk products, especially butter and cheese
- chocolate
- wheat and rye

Bruises

This condition results from trauma which is sufficient enough to break blood vessels. The broken blood vessels allow the leakage of blood into the tissues, leading to the reddish-brown or purplish color of the bruise. In some individuals bruises develop without obvious trauma. This is an early sign of scurvy and represents a significant deficiency of vitamin C and bioflavonoids. It may also tell of fungal infection in the gut. The fungi crowd out the good bacteria, such as Lactobacillus, which are responsible for synthesizing a special clotting factor: vitamin K. Killing the yeasts allows the return of the good bacteria, thus helping to normalize vitamin K synthesis. Thus, easy bruising may be a warning sign of vitamin K deficiency as well as fungal infection.

Bruise Combat Kit

- oil of oregano (P73 Oreganol)—apply topically to dissipate the bruises (it works for this rather dramatically).
- Purely-C—as a source of naturally occurring vitamin C take 3 capsules three times daily.
- oil of rosemary (rich in flavonoids)—take 5 to 10 drops twice daily.
- Wild Power Tea—drink one or two cups of this brew daily.
- oil of myrtle (rich in flavonoids)—take 2 to 5 drops twice daily and rub on the involved region.

Foods that help

- tangerines and grapefruit (and their juices, eat the inner rind)
- watercress, arugula, and spinach
- frozen unpasteurized orange juice (this is usually made from ripe oranges, which are higher in vitamin C than the so-called fresh ones)
- rose hip tea or, preferably, essence of rose petal tea

Burns

Burns are among the most traumatic of all injuries, both physically and mentally. If a burn covers a small surface area, like a bit of the finger, the trauma is tolerable. However, if it covers large areas, like a part of the arm or torso, this creates great stress. In the extreme shock may develop. If the burn is caused by a noxious chemical, such as lye or bleach, the shock is due to severe trauma to the tissues and also the absorption of the chemical through the skin and/or inhalation. The point is burns are not merely a surface injury, they impact the entire body. Any burn covering more than an inch is highly traumatic to the body. The pain alone is enough to create shock in certain individuals.

Burn combat kit

- oil of oregano (Oreganol P73)—apply to the region liberally, and take a few drops under the tongue as often as necessary.
- Oreganol cream—apply to region as needed.
- oil of wild lavender—apply to region as needed.
- aloe vera—apply to region (usually after applying essential oils)
- high potency enzyme therapy (i.e. Infla–eez)—for large scale burns to reduce swelling and trauma, take 3 capsules several times daily on an empty stomach.
- Wild Oregano or Mediterranean Wild Flower honey—apply to any burn either by itself or after applying essential oils. This is a highly effective salve, even for the most severe burns.
- Infla-eez antiinflammatory enzyme—2 or 3 capsules twice daily on an empty stomach.

Things to avoid

- bandages that stick to the skin. It is preferable to leave the wound open.

Canker sores

These are usually induced by food intolerance, that is food allergy. Sensitivity to chemicals in the foods, as well as prescription and/or nonprescription drugs, is another cause. Certain researchers believe that infection plays a role in canker sores and that strep or perhaps viruses are partly to blame. However, food allergy is the number one provoking factor. British researchers found that wheat was the major canker sore-inducing food. Other allergenic foods include rye, corn, yeast, milk products, eggs, beans, citrus fruit, shrimp, peanuts, and chocolate.

Canker sore combat kit

- wild oil of oregano (Oreganol P3)—apply to involved region and take 2 drops under the tongue twice daily.
- oil of rosemary—apply to involved region and take a few drops twice daily in juice or water.
- Royal Power—take 3 capsules twice daily.
- oil of sage (soothing; anti-pain)—apply a few drops on involved region.
- folic acid—take 3 or more mg twice daily.
- Infla–eez antiinflammatory enzymes—3 capsules twice daily.
- NukeProtect antioxidant formula—2 capsules twice daily (contains natural selenium, which helps combat these sores).

Things to avoid

- all grains, especially wheat (flour products are the #1 offender)
- milk products, especially butter
- citrus fruit and juices
- nuts, beans, and legumes

Carbon monoxide poisoning

This is primarily a problem of smoke inhalation. With a hidden carbon monoxide leak, such as might occur from a leaky furnace, by the time it is noticed it is usually too late to apply a natural remedy.

In the early 1990s I experienced a near fatal carbon monoxide event. While on a fishing trip in the remote wilderness, our group stayed in a rudimentary cabin. One of the members, an adolescent, almost created a catastrophe. Tired of the endless barrage of mosquitoes, he thought that by plugging up the outside vent to the heater he would block them from entering. With the vents blocked the cabin filled with carbon monoxide. Asphyxiated during the night we awoke well after fishing time in a stupor, tired and incoherent. Fortunately, one of the windows was cracked, otherwise it is likely that everyone in our party would have died.

Tens of thousands of Americans develop chronic carbon monoxide poisoning. This type of poison can cause severe or disconcerting symptoms. For instance, boaters are at high risk. This is particularly true of boats with enclosed cabins. Fishermen who troll using gas motors are at risk. Smoke inhalation from fires is a major cause of carbon monoxide toxicity. Perhaps the greatest cause is a type of chronic contamination which results from low-level leaks. This is usually from oil furnaces and gas stoves, which seep carbon monoxide into homes, causing chronic illness. This is not a rare disease, and as many as 100,000 Americans suffer some degree of carbon monoxide poisoning every year.

The medical treatment of carbon monoxide exposure is oxygen, the ideal form being an oxygen chamber. Such facilities are unavailable in most hospitals and will be inaccessible in the event of major crises. Symptoms of carbon monoxide poisoning include:

- headache (one of the earliest signs and may be severe)
- fatigue
- weakness
- incoherence
- dizziness
- nausea or upset stomach
- apathy
- muscular exhaustion
- cherry red complexion

Note: the above symptoms are often mistaken for the flu.

Carbon monoxide detoxification kit

- oil of rosemary—take 5 drops under the tongue several times daily plus 10 drops in juice or water twice daily.
- Rosemary Essence—drink an ounce several times daily.
- Oreganol P73 Juice—drink an ounce several times daily.
- Oregacyn respiratory formula—2 to 3 capsules every hour with juice or until symptoms are eliminated twice daily.
- beta carotene—take 50,000 I.U. of natural source beta carotene twice daily.
- vitamin E as Pumpkinol and/or Sesame-E—take 4 tablespoons daily until condition resolves.
- NukeProtect—take three capsules three times daily.

Foods that help

- tomato paste mixed with olive oil
- pumpkin and butternut squash
- red radishes (and their tops if possible; make radish juice from the tops and drink a cup daily)

Things to avoid

- exposure to smoke or fumes; even a tiny amount can be disabling, also, avoid nitrated/processed meats.

Chapped lips

This annoying condition is rarely ameliorated with lip balms alone. Actually, this condition may be caused by nutritional deficiencies. Deficiencies of essential fatty acids, folic acid, riboflavin, and vitamin A may all play a role. To treat this condition take a multiple vitamin containing vitamins A, folic acid, riboflavin, and vitamin C. Take also essential fatty acids, for instance, primrose or flax oil. Use a natural herbal-based lip balm. Take additional folic acid, 5 mg daily.

Other invaluable substances include healing essential oils such as oils of bay berry, myrtle, and lavender. Also, use the Oreganol cream, which is rich in tissue healing emollients, applying as needed. This is very effective for healing severely chapped lips.

Chicken pox

This is one of the most contagious of all diseases. It is caused by a virus: the Herpes virus. The chicken pox (herpes) virus usually attacks children, who have no immunity to it. If an outbreak occurs, fully 80% of all non-immune sensitized individuals exposed to it will become infected, including adults. However, it usually strikes children ages 4 to 8 years. Infants are occasionally infected, and it can be quite serious in this age group. Ironically, chicken pox in adults is usually more severe than in children; life-threatening pneumonia is often a consequence. Adults exposed to the virus while taking steroid therapy are at the highest risk for severe infections, since cortisone of all types may provoke the infection and drive it deep into the tissues. If the infection is severe enough, brain damage can occur (usually in children/infants).

Chicken pox combat kit for children
- oil of oregano (Oreganol P73)—take 1 drop under the tongue or in juice or water every three hours. Rub on chest, thighs,

buttocks, and/or soles of feet. **Note:** only the Oreganol P73 has been proven safe for children and infants.
- Kid-e-Kare rubbing oil—rub on chest liberally as well as on the soles of the feet; also, rub vigorously on the buttocks. Do this at least twice daily. This is a highly effective way to eliminate disconcerting symptoms such as fever, sweats, and chills, as demonstrated by the following:

> Young Jason had a severe fever of 104.0 degrees. He also had the chills. Doctors failed to prescribe any medicine, advising bed rest and a wait-and-see attitude. At night the mother rubbed the Kid-e-Kare rubbing oil on the child's forehead and chest. The next morning the child awoke, the fever fully broken, and said, "I feel like dancing."

- Purely-C—take 2 capsules three times daily.
- OregaMax capsules—take 2 capsules three times daily.
- wild oregano honey—take a tablespoon three times daily.

Chicken pox combat kit for adults

- oil of oregano—take 2 drops under the tongue every hour until condition improves; then 2 drops every few hours.
- OregaMax capsules—take 3 capsules three times daily.
- Purely-C—take 3 or more capsules three times daily.
- Royal Power—take 3 or more capsules twice daily.

Things to avoid

- soda pop and sugar
- chocolate: absolutely none of any kind

Chlorine gas/liquid poisoning

Chlorine is a highly noxious substance, which is extremely corrosive to human tissues. Millions of tons of chlorine gas and liquid chlorine are transported by rail car and truck yearly. Other millions of tons are stored in factories and depots. Chlorine gas/liquid spills are relatively common events in the United States, afflicting thousands of individuals every year. The unfortunate people who live near factories, as well as industrial workers, are the usual victims.

Note: a chlorine spill and resultant gas cloud is extremely dangerous. Be aggressive in taking antioxidants such as wild oil of oregano, edible oil of rosemary, oil of cumin (i. e. oil of cumin, a special formula for reversing liver toxicity), Oregacyn respiratory capsules, and NukeProtect, which contains the highly protective selenium and numerous other antidotes; this may save your lungs and perhaps your life.

Chlorine exposure combat kit
- gas mask and protective clothing
- Oregacyn respiratory—fully lifesaving, take 1 or more capsules as often as needed.
- oil of rosemary—take 20 drops under the tongue every hour. Also, rub on any suspect lesion.
- oil of oregano—take 2 drops under the tongue every few minutes to prevent respiratory collapse.
- organic selenium—take 200 mcg every six/eight hours. Use this dosage only for emergencies; take vitamin E, 1200 I.U. daily.
- Purely-C—take 2 capsules every hour.
- oil of sage (a powerful antioxidant and lung protector)—take 2 drops under the tongue every half hour.
- Essence of Sage—drink two or more ounces daily until the exposure ends.
- NukeProtect—take 2 capsules every hour until symptoms ease.
- Resvital—take 2 or 3 capsules every hour.
- GreensFlush—take ten drops under the tongue as needed.

Cholera

This is a highly contagious intestinal infection caused by the obnoxious pathogen, *Vibrio cholerae*. Currently, cholera is responsible for hundreds of thousands of deaths yearly, mostly in poor countries. Yet, outbreaks could occur anywhere. This is because cholera is a waterborne disease, and the responsible germ could contaminate any water system.

A bout of cholera could probably kill virtually anyone. The germ viciously attacks the intestines, particularly the small bowel. It causes bile-stained, profuse, watery diarrhea, plus vomiting, which is usually violent, and severe intestinal cramps. Nothing seemingly can stop the diarrhea. The stools have what is known as a "rice in water" appearance. Yet, if the organism is killed, the diarrhea will stop. Unstopped, the individual usually dies from dehydration.

The infection notoriously fails to respond to even the most heroic medical efforts, thus illustrating the importance of natural therapies. A variety of natural substances have been shown to halt diarrhea and destroy noxious germs. These remedies include oil of oregano, oil of cumin, oil of cinnamon, raw honey, garlic, and natural (normal) flora. Such spice extracts are the components of the respiratory formula, Oregacyn, as well as the OregaBiotic.

It was Eli Metnickoff, the man who popularized yogurt, who did the cholera challenge. After taking large amounts of yogurt over a period of time, he drank a dose of cholera. He failed to contract the disease. Thus, his system was apparently protected by the natural Lactobacillus which he had consumed via the yogurt.

There are no effective drugs or vaccines for this condition. Thus, the individual must depend upon natural cures. If you contract cholera, don't eat anything, in other words, rest the gut. Seek medical attention. Sip on clear fluids, and use the natural remedies described herein. Be aggressive with these remedies: your life may depend upon it.

Cholera combat kit
- wild oregano honey—take large amounts, like a quarter cup three times daily. Continue the honey therapy for at least 3 days. This is the most effective honey for diarrhea.
- oil of oregano (SuperStrength is best)—take a few drops (3 to 10) under the tongue repeatedly until the diarrhea slows down or halts.
- LivaClenz—take 5 to 10 drops internally several times daily.
- High grade Lactobacillus acidophilus and bifidus (i. e. Health-Bac high implantation bacterial supplement)—if 1/2 teaspoon taken in warm water throughout the day.
- papaya seeds—if this can be held down, pulverize and add to water. Or, take papain-based antiinflammatory enzymes, i.e. Infla–eez, 3 capsules twice daily.
- raw garlic—this is irritating to the gut but may be the only remedy available. Thoroughly chew cloves and eat repeatedly.

Foods that help
- garlic/onion broth
- vinegar
- raw honey (Wild Oregano Honey)
- orange blossom tea
- rose petal essence

Other ideals
- rest the gut as much as possible; use raw honey/vinegar, broths, and teas for fluid replenishment.

Cold exposure (coldness of the body, hands, feet, etc.)

Exposure to cold weather and the resulting cold body temperature are a great concern in human crisis. Could significant crises afflict this country so that common conveniences, such as heating and shelter, are unavailable? This happened in 1998 during the great ice storms in the upper northeastern United States and Canada. What would individuals do—how would they behave—if they were unable to keep warm, that is if the common conveniences of everyday life are disrupted? Perhaps some individuals might even harm others to gain their security.

Cold body temperature protection/combat kit

- oil of oregano (Oreganol P73)—take 2 to 4 drops under the tongue three times daily. Rub on face and hands a few moments before going outside.
- cayenne pepper—add to food; sprinkle on socks to prevent frostbite.
- oil of cold-pressed garlic (i. e. Garlex) — ten drops under the tongue as often as needed.
- onions, raw—eat one bulb daily.
- OregaMax capsules (contain wild oregano, garlic, and onion) —take 2 or more capsules twice daily.
- Thyroset—take 4 capsules (about 1000 mg) of arsenic-free kelp daily.
- oil of sage (highly warming)—if possible, make oil of sage tea by adding several drops to hot water. Also, take oil of sage, 5 to 10 drops daily.
- oil of cilantro plus coriander (highly warming)—take 5 to 10 drops twice daily.

Foods that protect

- sardines, salmon, albacore tuna, mackerel
- crude extra virgin olive oil
- salted roasted nuts
- fresh beef (as steaks, chops, roasts, stews, broth—marrow soup is particularly nourishing, the fattier it is the better it is for cold protection)

Cold sores

Cold sores are caused by a virus, specifically the Herpes virus type I. This virus apparently resides in the majority of Americans, parasitizing the cells of the nervous system. Usually, it remains dormant, hiding deep within the nerve tissues. However, when the individual is subjected to extreme stress or is taking certain medications, such as cortisone or chemotherapy, the virus migrates through the nerves and into the skin. This results in extensive inflammation and, thus, severe pain. The key treatment is the use of wild oil of oregano, that is the Oreganol P73, which destroys this virus.

Cold sore combat kit

- oil of Oreganol—apply immediately and repeatedly, directly to the lesion when you feel the tingle. Take 2 or more drops under the tongue several times daily or until the lesion clears.
- lysine—(more of a preventive than a cure) 500 mg as needed.
- Royal Power premium royal jelly (to combat stress and reverse adrenal weakness)—take 2 capsules every few hours.
- OregaMax—take 2 capsules every few hours.
- PropaHeal (oil of propolis)—apply directly to the lesion repeatedly. This is highly antiviral.

Foods that help

- anything rich in all eight essential amino acids, that is beef, chicken, fish, eggs, and milk products
- fatty fish such as sardines, salmon, albacore tuna, and mackerel
- fresh whole milk mixed with honey

Things to avoid

- chocolate (a major cause of cold sores)
- peanuts and peanut butter
- refined vegetable oils and deep-fried foods, especially the so-

called brominated vegetable oils
- MSG
- nitrated meats
- food dyes

Colds

This condition may be caused by viruses. It may surprise many people but colds can also be caused by fungi. The medical profession has taught that colds are always caused by viruses. Yet, recently, it has been determined that mold infections cause the same symptoms as seen in colds. The fact is allergic intolerance to mold or infection by yeasts/molds may be the primary cause of this disorder.

Cold viruses attack primarily the nasal passages, sinuses, and throat, that is the upper respiratory tract. They parasitize the cells in these regions. They also attack the lymph glands, notably the tonsils, adenoids, and lymph nodules. In the event of cold symptoms these regions should be treated with essential oils and other remedies aimed directly at the site of infection. This is done by taking the hot-tasting essential spice oil under the tongue, through inhalation, and/or intranasally. What's more, a recent study proves that the special respiratory spice extract Oregacyn killed 100% of all cold viruses in a mere twenty minutes.

Cold combat kit

- oil of oregano—a powerful, effective remedy; take two drops under the tongue several times per day. For severe colds take two drops under the tongue every hour, and rub around the sinus region and/or apply it directly to the inner lining of the nose. Because of its immense antifungal action, this is an outright cure for the common cold.
- raw honey plus vinegar—use this often as a food and tonic until the cold dissipates.

- OregaMax capsules—take 3 capsules three or more times daily.
- Purely-C—take 2 or more capsules every hour.
- Oregacyn respiratory capsules—take 2 or more capsules several times daily.

Foods that help

- fresh juices, especially vitamin C-rich ones like tangerine, papaya, grapefruit, and strawberry juice
- organic meat or poultry broth with onion and garlic
- canned tomato juice; drink two quarts daily

Things to avoid

- white sugar and/or chocolate; these are disastrous foods to consume during a cold
- milk products
- nitrated meats
- white bread and/or pasta

Colic

This term is a bit of a misnomer, because it appears to define a colon problem. Yet, the term is used for any type of spasm in the abdomen. Today, it applies almost exclusively to children.

Childhood colic is usually a minor problem. The objective is to settle the stomach or intestines so the child (and parents) can rest. Essential oils are the optimal agent for this purpose. They possess considerable powers to relax the stomach and intestines, quickly reversing spasticity and/or pain. There is no medical treatment for baby colic, which is further reason to utilize natural cures.

Colic combat kit

- Kid-e-Kare rubbing oil—rub on the soles of the feet, over abdomen, and on buttocks.
- oil of oreganol—rub on soles of feet and over abdomen.

- Oreganol P73 Juice—give a small amount, like a tablespoonful, to halt colic.
- Essence of Neroli Orange—gentle, but effective; give a teaspoon or more in goat milk, formula, or juice.
- edible oil of fennel—used since antiquity, a famous English remedy; two or three drops daily should be sufficient.
- Kid-e-Kare Tumi-eez—rub all over the body as needed, especially the abdomen and forehead.

Things to avoid

- caffeine, chocolate, sugar, coffee, and cow's milk

Colitis attacks

This category covers a wide range of bowel disorders, which may collectively be grouped under this heading. These disorders include irritable bowel syndrome, spastic colon, Crohn's disease, and ulcerative colitis.

These conditions are plagues of modern civilization. They are directly due to erroneous diet. Food allergies and infection also play an important role. Emotional distress is another major cause of colonic disorders. Stress, despair, and worry, as well as guilt, all are largely to blame. Why these emotions specifically attack the bowel is unknown. However, there is a direct connection between large nerves, which are influenced by the emotions, and the gut.

Colonic illnesses are manifested by severe toxicity affecting the entire digestive tract, although the colon suffers the brunt of the damage. Symptoms include diarrhea as well as constipation, cramps, spasticity, mucous in the stools, bleeding in the stools, hemorrhoids, nausea, and bloating. Untreated, it may lead to infections throughout the body and, ultimately, colon cancer.

Colitis combat kit

- oil of oregano—take 2 drops under the tongue several times daily. Plus, take Oreganol gelcaps, two caps twice daily.
- OregaMax capsules—take 2 or more capsules three times daily.
- oil of sage (a relaxant to the gut and aids the coping mechanism —the adrenals)—take 5 drops twice daily in hot water.
- Oregacyn Digestive–highly effective, take 2 to 3 capsules with each meal.
- oil of rosemary (blocks spasticity and nourishes the gut wall) —take 5 to 10 drops twice daily in juice or water.
- oil of fennel or oil of ginger (highly important for normalizing the gut)—3 to 5 drops twice daily.
- wild oregano honey—3 or more tablespoons daily.
- GreensFlush–ideal for cleansing toxins and stimulating natural bowel activity, 2 to 3 droppersful under the tongue as needed.

Things to avoid

- all sources of caffeine
- refined sugar and corn syrup
- wheat and flour products of all types
- beans and legumes
- milk products of all types, especially milk, ice cream, and butter

Concussion

One of the most common human injuries, concussion is especially prevalent in children. It is caused by direct trauma to the skull. In mild cases no damage is done. However, with extreme injury temporary or permanent brain damage may occur. This may be manifested by insomnia, headaches, amnesia, and even permanent neurological deficit.

Concussion combat kit

- oil of lavender—rub all over face and head, especially under the nose. Rub on soles of feet. Do this repeatedly until an improvement in consciousness is noted. For children use instead the highly aromatic Kid-e-Kare rubbing oil and rub on forehead and chest, as well as the soles of the feet and spine, as needed.
- oil of oregano (P73 only, that is the safe spice oil)—rub on chest and face; take 2 drops under the tongue several times daily until condition improves.
- Purely-C—take 2 capsules every hour (especially valuable to prevent internal bleeding).
- Infla–eez antiinflammatory enzymes—3 capsules three times daily on an empty stomach.
- Essence of Neroli Orange—gently activates and stimulates brain function and eases stress; add 2 tablespoons to hot water and sip. Repeat as needed.
- Neuroloft—take 2 capsules twice daily, a major neurological aid (if unavailable use the Oreganol P73 Juice).

Things to avoid

- loud noises and bright light; Note: keep the individual in a dark quiet room until help arrives.

Conjunctivitis

In September 1998 hurricane George struck the American South like a hydrogen bomb. It blasted through the U.S. Virgin Islands destroying thousands of homes and displacing tens of thousands. One of the consequences was the spread of infection, and conjunctivitis was top on the list. As a result of the hurricane pink eye incidence was 30 times higher than normal.

Conjunctivitis is defined as inflammation or irritation of the eye membranes that cover the whites of the eyes and also the membranes of the inner eyelid. A red inflamed eye is the same as conjunctivitis. It is commonly caused by infection, particularly bacteria and viruses. Thus, most cases of red eye signal infection. Red eye can also be caused when foreign objects become trapped in the membranes of the eyes such as particles of dust, sand, metal, or wood. Even so, when such particles are trapped for prolonged periods, infection often develops. If there is a discharge that tends to form a crust, especially if foul smelling, infection of the eye or inner eyelid is assured. Red irritated eyes which itch usually signal allergic reactions. Exposure to toxic chemicals, especially if they are airborne, may be a major cause of red or inflamed eyes. Signs and symptoms of acute bacterial conjunctivitis include:

- burning
- automatic tearing
- irritation
- yellowish, yellow-green, or pus-filled discharge
- swelling of the eyelids

Viral infections of the eyes are potentially catastrophic. This is because viruses spread easily, and viral conjunctivitis may become epidemic, especially in medical facilities or in institūtions housing large numbers of people. Careful hand washing reduces the risk of transmission. Typical symptoms include red eyes, watery discharge, swelling of the eyelids, and sensation of something in the eye. Such infections are usually contagious for at least one week.

Viral eye infections may be caused by herpes, and this can become dangerous. Never use cortisone creams in the event of viral/herpetic eye infections, as this may cause the virus to spread, permanently damaging and scarring the eye.

Conjunctivitis combat kit
- oil of oregano (Oreganol P73)—take 2 drops under the tongue twice daily. Rub a small amount on cheeks under the eye (be sure to avoid any direct contact with eyeball. Use only edible oil of wild oregano emulsified in extra virgin olive oil). Remember, it travels.
- oil of wild lavender—rub on forehead and cheeks around eyes (but not in eyes). Note: in children use Kid-e-Kare rubbing oil.
- vitamin A eye drops—add one drop in involved eye twice daily.
- Purely-C (as a source of crude natural vitamin C and bioflavonoids)—take 3 capsules twice daily.
- Essence of Rose Petals—as an eye wash use as needed.

Constipation

Constipation is a disease only of modern civilization. In this condition the colon fails to efficiently eliminate wastes. Symptoms of constipation include abdominal pain, bloating, gas, headaches, bad breath, and fatigue. When movements finally occur, the stool is usually hard and dark. A good definition is having less than a bowel movement per day. Extreme constipation is having less than a bowel movement per week.

It has been proposed that a lack of dietary fiber is the primary cause of constipation. Yet, this is only one factor. Food allergy and chronic infections are the other major causes. Dehydration is another important factor. Perhaps the most neglected issue is the fact that constipation may be a key sign of intestinal infection. Parasitic infection is a major cause of constipation. The bulk of the parasites itself may plug up the bowel, making it difficult to have a movement. Yeast infections can also cause chronic constipation. Here, in order to ease the constipation the yeasts/parasites must be killed.

There has been a gross overemphasis upon using harsh laxatives, whether chemical or herbal, in an attempt to cure constipation. The problem is that the bowel becomes damaged from the aggressive powers of many laxatives, and, as soon as these agents are halted, the constipation returns. If you use herbal laxatives, they should only be taken for a short period for purposes of detoxification, not every day.

Constipation combat kit
- oil of oregano—take 2 to 5 drops twice daily in juice or water.
- OregaMax—take 3 capsules two or three times daily.
- red grape powder (Resvital)—take 4 capsules three times daily (or take a heaping teaspoonful twice daily).
- Nutri-Sense—take 3 heaping tablespoons twice daily in juice or water.
- Oregacyn Digestive—take 2-3 capsules with meals.
- Thyroset (helps stimulate/enhance colonic muscle function)—take 4 capsules daily.
- GreensFlush wild greens drops—2 to 4 droppersful twice daily.
- wild oregano honey—take 3 tablespoons twice daily.

Foods that help
- Nutri-Sense drink/food mix or ground flaxseed
- papaya plus the seeds
- wild rice (and/or rice bran)
- wild rosemary (or Hercules Strength capsules)
- carob molasses—a highly effective gentle, non-habit forming bowel aid. Add this to the Nutri-Sense for a natural means of balancing colon function.
- rye and oats

Note: be sure to increase fluid intake, and drink at least 6 large glasses of water daily.

Things to avoid

- refined sugar
- anything made with white flour and/or hydrogenated oils

Cough

A cough may be a rather mild problem. However, it may also become a disability. A persistent cough is one of the most disabling of all symptoms. It is tiring, as well as damaging, both to the lungs and nerves. Persistent deep coughs may also damage internal organs, particularly the esophagus and/or stomach.

A cough is a sign that lung function is compromised. This is usually due to an infection, although chemical poisoning as well as allergic sensitivity may provoke it. Persistent cough with no obvious cause may also warn of cancer. However, usually, it signals chronic infection by bacteria, fungi, viruses, or parasites. Currently, mold/yeast infection of the lungs represents perhaps the number one cause of chronic cough. This is especially true of a dry or ticklish cough with or without clear mucous.

Cough combat kit

- oil of oregano—take 2 or more drops under the tongue three or more times daily. Also, rub on chest, around sinuses, and under nose.
- Oregacyn respiratory formula—2 capsules twice daily.
- black seed extract (Black Seed-plus)—3 capsules three times daily.
- oil of bay leaf—rub on chest and face; take 2 to 5 drops twice daily.
- OregaMax capsules—take 3 capsules twice daily.
- Oreganol P73 Juice (highly warming)—1/2 ounce as often as needed.
- Thyroset (arsenic-free)—to boost metabolism take 4 or more capsules daily.

- oil of sage—take 5 to 10 drops twice daily in hot water.

Foods that help
- wild sage herb (for making tea)
- iodine-rich foods such as sardines, salmon, halibut, etc.

Things to avoid
- milk products and chocolate
- wheat and other commercial grains (may provoke a type of mold sensitivity)

Cracks at the corners of the mouth

This painful condition is strictly caused by a vitamin deficiency. However, once the cracks develop they may become invaded by germs, notably yeasts. The primary deficiency is riboflavin, although niacin and folic acid deficiencies may play secondary roles.

Vitamin/herbal cures
- royal jelly (i. e. Royal Power), naturally rich in riboflavin (500 mg capsules)—take 4-6 capsules daily.
- GreensFlush (as a source of natural riboflavin)—two droppersful twice daily.
- oil of propolis, i.e. PropaHeal (soothing; stimulates healing)—apply topically.
- folic acid—take 5 mg daily.
- Nutri-Sense fortified natural B vitamin mix—two tablespoons in juice, water, or in a home-made shake twice daily.

Foods that help
- organic liver (the top source of riboflavin)
- organic whole eggs or egg powder (fair source of riboflavin)

- almonds or almond milk (good vegetable source of riboflavin)
- organic whole milk yogurt, whole milk, or milk powder (rich in riboflavin)
- watercress, spinach, and avocado
- wild rice and its broth

Croup

Croup is a respiratory crisis demanding immediate medical attention. It is a childhood condition manifested by odd breathing sounds or a cough resembling a bark. The child may also appear to be suffocating or wheezing. There is also loss of voice, difficult breathing, weakness, and rapid pulse. Croup may eventually be determined to be a type of diphtheria secondary to immunization reactions. The fact is this illness, which may be provoked by immunizations, is often manifested by membrane formation in the throat, similar to that seen in diphtheria.

In children this is one of the most serious respiratory infections. Obviously, it requires medical support. Even so, natural remedies are of immense value. This is emphasized by *Taber's Medical Dictionary*, which states that "antibiotics (and other drugs) are of no...benefit." The following amounts apply to young children.

Croup combat kit

- oil of oregano, (Oreganol P73)—a drop under the tongue as often as tolerated, but no more than 10 drops daily. Rub additional oil on buttocks, chest, or soles of feet.
- Kid-e-kare rubbing oil—rub on face, chest, buttocks, and soles of feet.
- Kid-e-kare throat spray—spray on back of throat as often as needed.

- Kid-e-kare antiseptic gelcaps—take 1 or 2 gelcaps as needed.
- raw honey—give as many tablespoons as possible.
- Thyroset (arsenic-free)—give as many capsules as possible (add to juice, etc.)
- Wild oregano honey—take twice daily.

Foods that help
- clear vegetable or meat broths
- Kiwi fruit and papaya
- Raw wild honey

Things to avoid
- chocolate and refined sugar
- junk food of any type

Cuts/lacerations

The average American's arsenal for combating injuries is pitiful. Usually, it consists of noxious smelling drug store items, which offer little versatility. After many years of usage few Americans have any confidence in these items, the results being just as disappointing as the odor. The familiar names include hydrogen peroxide, hexachlorophene, antibiotic ointments, rubbing alcohol, and iodine. These agents are poor choices in a crisis. What's more, they are incapable of aiding wound healing. In fact, they may impede it.

Natural substances greatly accelerate wound healing. What's more, many of these agents, notably oregano, bay leaf, bay berry, propolis, honey, lavender and rosemary oils, bee propolis, and raw honey, offer germ-killing powers. Some of them, like oils of oregano, lavender, and myrtle, contribute significant painkilling properties. Such oils are components of Oreganol cream. This cream kills a wide range of germs, while soothing inflamed tissues. It also helps prevent scar formation.

Natural cures for cuts, lacerations, and other open wounds
- oil of oregano (P73 only)—apply as needed; take a drop or two under the tongue.
- raw honey (manuka or wild oregano)—apply to wound, perhaps over the essential oils. Cover with bandage or leave uncovered.
- Oreganol cream—apply to wound as needed.
- red grape powder, i. e. Resvital (a tremendous astringent)—take 6 or more capsules daily to aid in wound healing.
- Kid-e-Kare Ow-eez, ideal for children—apply to any wound as often as needed; helps eliminate pain as well as inflammation.

Cyanide poisoning

Cyanide is perhaps the most poisonous of all chemicals. In minute quantities it is fatal. As little as a tenth of a gram can kill a grown man. Much has been disseminated regarding the toxic effects of consuming cyanide, for instance, cyanide-laced drugs. However, a far greater crisis is the disastrous consequences of inhaling it in the form of cyanide gas. This is what happened with the catastrophe of the Union Carbide plant in Bhopal, India; tens of thousands were killed and maimed as a result of the "accidental" release of cyanide gas. Decades later, still, the victims are suffering. These gases are known chemically as hydrogen cyanide or hydrocyanic gas.

Thousands of tons of cyanide gas are transported by rail or truck in the United States every year. Plus, this lethal chemical is stored in chemical bins throughout the country. A release in a metropolitan area, as occurred in India, could kill thousands within minutes, while leaving other uncountable thousands permanently diseased. The disease resulting from cyanide gas exposure is gruesome; corrosion of the lungs, leading to permanent disability—a slow writhing brutal death due to suffocation.

With the exception of a gas mask and special protective clothing there is no means of fully guarding the body from exposure to cyanide gas. This is because cyanide compounds are rapidly absorbed throughout the tissues. After entering the lungs cyanide is quickly absorbed into the bloodstream. It also penetrates the skin, ultimately entering the blood and internal organs. There, it poisons the cells and organs thoroughly. It does so by halting the ability of the body to transport and use its most critical substance: oxygen. Without this life-giving substance, death rapidly ensues. However, while cyanide gas releases are rare, there is a more insidious factor: smoke inhalation. Modern building materials are cyanide-laced. Thus, many fire-related deaths may in fact be due to the inhalation of cyanide gas, which is rapidly liberated during fires.

In the event of a massive release of cyanide gas the logistics of self-protection are overwhelming. Here is the protocol: immediately don a mask, wear protective eye covering, and wear a plastic/resilient suit. If the latter is unavailable, wear a blast jacket, rain coat, or similar plasticized outerwear. Quickly mobilize away from the site of exposure or stay indoors, closing all doors and windows. Secure the building as air tight as possible. Take megadoses of the anti-toxic antioxidants, particularly spice oil concentrates as well as the highly potent NukeProtect. It is critical to rely also upon the wild oregano essence, that is the Oreganol P73 Juice, to neutralize acute toxicity. Signs and symptoms of cyanide poisoning include:

- burning of the eyes and respiratory passages
- shortness of breath and breathing distress
- petechiae (small hemorrhages on the skin)
- nausea and vomiting
- almond-like odor from the breath and skin
- severe convulsions and/or seizures
- cherry-red color of the skin

- faintness, dizziness, fainting, and/or collapse
- sweating

Note: acute cyanide poisoning usually results in death within 20 minutes and, thus, many of these symptoms are rarely seen. Cyanide poisons the body by irreversibly binding to red blood cells, preventing them from delivering oxygen to the tissues. Without oxygen, survival is impossible, and death results precipitously. However, if protective gear is rapidly donned, sudden death may be averted. In this case the aforementioned symptoms may appear, because, no matter how well the individual is protected, a certain degree of exposure will occur. If any of these symptoms develop after toxic chemical exposure, seek medical attention immediately (if possible).

If exposure of any sort occurs, take huge amounts of antioxidants. Take the doses repeatedly, in other words, be aggressive. This is the only chance of survival.

Cyanide exposure combat kit

- Oregacyn respiratory—two capsules as often as necessary, perhaps every hour or even every half hour.
- oil of rosemary—take several drops under the tongue every few minutes.
- oil of sage—take a few drops under the tongue every few minutes. Also, take 20 additional drops internally twice daily.
- Essence of Sage—drink an entire bottle or more.
- Oreganol P73 Juice— a critical component, drink an entire bottle or more.
- LivaClenz (for detoxification of the cyanide through the stool)—take 10 or more drops every hour until danger abates.
- red grape powder (Resvital)—take 4 to 6 capsules every hour (or one teaspoon each hour) or more.

- NukeProtect—take 2 or more capsules every hour (such a dosage is for emergencies only).
- Purely-C—take 3 or more capsules every half hour or every hour.

Dehydration

This is a disorder not just of fluid loss, but it also represents the loss of critical elemental substances. Known as electrolytes, these substances include sodium, chloride, magnesium, and potassium. Usually, sodium and chloride are the main electrolytes lost in dehydration.

One of the main issues with dehydration is to know what are the signs and symptoms. This is because dehydration is one of the most underdiagnosed of all illnesses. The problem is no one suspects it, and, thus, it is frequently missed. This is particularly true of the elderly, who often fail to take care of themselves properly. In heat waves dehydration is a major cause of sickness and death in this population.

Hot weather is a major factor in causing dehydration, as is prolonged fever. The latter causes rapid fluid loss through both the skin and lungs. With fever, dehydration may develop in as little as a few hours. Diarrhea may rapidly lead to it, as can vomiting. If vomiting, diarrhea, and fever all occur concurrently, dehydration will develop quickly, as will electrolyte loss, that is the loss of critical blood-buffering components such as potassium, sodium, chloride, and bicarbonate. This combination of fluid and electrolyte loss can be deadly.

Diabetics and/or individuals taking diuretics are at the highest risk of developing life-threatening dehydration. Laxative abuse, that is the chronic use of laxatives, may also precipitate it. Major symptoms of this condition include:

- dry mouth or eyes
- lack of tearing

- dry skin
- constipation
- confusion
- agitation and/or hallucinations
- lack of urination or little urination

Dehydration mainly occurs in the elderly and in small children. If these individuals become sick, it is a good rule to evaluate them often for signs of dehydration.

Dehydration combat kit
- water (mineral water is best)
- juices (non-citrus juices such as grape, peach, pear, apricot, papaya, and fresh vegetable are well tolerated and highly nourishing)
- clear soup or soup broths provide both fluid and electrolytes
- high water foods are exceptional for replenishment; eat watermelon, cantaloupe, honeydew melon, radishes, turnips, red sweet peppers, tomatoes, and cucumbers.
- sea salt—once the fluids are replenished this helps prevent water loss. Note: some dehydration is due to salt deficiency, and water balance cannot be maintained unless salt is administered.
- Royal Power—strengthens the adrenal glands, which are responsible for fluid balance.
- oil of rosemary and sage (also for strengthening the adrenal glands)—take 5 drops of each twice daily.

Things to avoid
- all sources of caffeine (it is a dehydrating agent)
- alcoholic beverages (they are diuretics)
- antihistamines and anti-pain drugs, including aspirin, ibuprofen, and acetaminophen

Dengue fever

This disease is caused by a virus. It is transmitted by a mosquito that lives almost exclusively in the tropics. However, the mosquito is an inhabitant of the southern United States and has been found in significant numbers in Louisiana and Texas. In fact, in the 1920s, an outbreak of this disease, affecting some 750,000 individuals, occurred in Texas.

As described in *JAMA* in Central America dengue fever is currently an epidemic. However, it could also strike in epidemic proportions in North America, particularly in the Deep South. It should always be suspected as a possible cause of illness for those becoming sick after traveling in the tropics, particularly Central and South America. In fact, any traveler to Central/South America, as well as southeast Asia, could contract it.

Dengue fever is one of several hemorrhagic fevers which occurs frequently in the tropics. It is essentially a mild form of Ebola. One helpful fact in establishing the diagnosis is that the mosquito which transmits it usually bites during the day. Usually, dengue is represented by a disconcerting illness that dissipates within two weeks. However, the hemorrhagic type is a killer, and in those who contract it up to one in five die.

Modern medicine claims that nothing can be done to prevent these deaths and that "supportive" care is the only option. Do not make this assumption. The condition should be treated aggressively with nutrients and herbs that block the damage, plenty of fluids, as well as with natural anti-infective agents.

Dengue combat kit

- oil of oregano SuperStrength—take large amounts; 5 to 20 drops under the tongue every few minutes; 20 drops (which fills a gelatin capsule nicely) internally every hour if necessary. Rub the oil on the face and buttocks (a means of rapid absorption into the blood through the skin). Or, take Oreganol gelcaps, about 2 twice daily.

- Purely-C all-natural vitamin C—for maintaining blood vessel and immune strength, two or more capsules twice daily.
- Oreganol P73 Juice—2 ounces twice daily.
- oil of propolis (i. e. PropaHeal)—take 10 to 20 drops every hour or two.
- oil of rosemary—10 drops twice daily.
- juice of raw onion (yellow onion is preferable)—drink a cup or more per day. It may be enhanced with radish juice.
- OregaMax capsules—as many as can be swallowed.

Foods that help

- vitamin C rich juices may help curb hemorrhaging; otherwise, rest the system of food.
- raw honey—useful for curbing diarrhea.
- Resvital powder—also helps halt hemorrhages.

Things to avoid

- blood thinners, including aspirin.
- non-steroidal anti-inflammatory drugs (i.e. arthritis/pain medication).
- stagnant water: if possible, be sure to eliminate all sources of it near the home, since this is where mosquitoes breed.

Dermatitis

This is defined as inflammation and/or irritation of the skin. It is represented by a rash, which often occurs on the skin in circumscribed patches. In extreme cases the entire body may be enveloped in it.

There are dozens of types of dermatitis, and there are just as many causes. The most common cause is allergic reaction. Reactions may be to foods, but the most likely culprits are chemicals. Dermatitis is an exceptionally frequent side effect of drugs. Foods which commonly provoke allergic dermatitis include milk products, refined sugar, chocolate, wheat, rye, and corn.

Dermatitis combat kit

- oil of oregano—dilute in extra virgin olive oil or cocoa butter and apply. If the region is too sensitive, take the oil internally, 10 or more drops daily. Internal consumption is the main method for eradicating chronic dermatitis.
- Oreganol cream (top agent for wound healing and for aiding irritated skin)—rub on irritated skin twice or more daily.
- premium-grade royal jelly, i. e. Royal Oil (to acidify the skin and regenerate the adrenal glands)—take 1/2 teaspoon twice daily.
- OregaMax capsules—take 3 capsules twice daily.
- primrose or borage oil—take 6 or more capsules daily.
- oil of bay berry—a natural emollient, rub a few drops on any irritated region, as needed.

Things to avoid

- lye-based soaps and detergents of any kind. Wash clothes in hot water; add 10 or more drops of oil of oregano and/or oil of lavender; use baking soda or other non-caustic washing agents.
- milk products, apple juice, and citrus fruit
- refined sugar, chocolate, and caffeinated beverages

Diabetes and diabetic attacks

Rarely found in primitive societies, diabetes is the scourge of the Western world. It afflicts tens of millions of Americans. It is one of the top five causes of death nationally.

This is a disease of poor diet. With diabetes, the human body is unable to properly metabolize food, especially sugar.

However, infection may be a contributing factor. Yeast and fungal infections rampage within diabetics.

If diabetics suffer blood sugar attacks, they must be fed. However, candy bars are not the answer. They should be given food; certainly, fruit or fruit juice will suffice to prevent fatality. Yet, blood sugar-balancing herbs, such as extracts of cumin, cilantro, coriander, and artichoke, work equally as well as the sugar. Grape, carob, or pomegranate molasses are superb alternatives to sugar as emergency aids. However, again, it is best to improve the body's ability to control the blood sugar levels in order to avoid catastrophes. For instance, red sour grape (Resvital) provides natural chromium, direly needed for blood sugar regulation. Nutri-Sense contains natural thiamine and niacin, which are crucial for proper sugar metabolism.

Recently, certain spices, notably cinnamon and fenugreek, have been shown to dramatically lower blood sugar, greatly improving the diabetic condition. Tested in a specialized trial Oregulin is one such spice extract. It proved equal to insulin in its anti-diabetic powers. It efficiently reduced blood sugar as well as blood pressure. This spice oil combination essentially eliminated Syndrome X, that is insulin resistance. It proved capable of reducing blood sugar, while normalizing blood pressure.

Oregulin also speeds weight loss. What's more, it helps lower blood pressure. These actions are dramatic proof that this natural medicine reverses insulin resistance. In contrast, insulin therapy frequently leads to an in increase in arterial damage and, therefore, blood pressure.

Diabetes combat kit

- oil of myrtle—take 5 drops twice daily.
- Oregulin blood-sugar regulating spice oil (with cinnamon)—take 1 or 2 capsules with each meal. This is of utmost importance, proven to normalize insulin function.
- oil of oregano—5 or more drops daily under the tongue or in

juice or water.
- OregaMax capsules—take 2 or 3 twice daily.
- Nutri-Sense protein/B drink mix (made from nutrient-rich rice bran, polish, flax, etc.)—take 3 heaping tablespoons in juice, milk, or water as an anti-diabetic B vitamin-rich nourishing agent.
- Resvital crude red sour grape powder—take 1 to 2 teaspoons twice daily.
- Oreganol P73 Juice—highly active in reversing this pathology, 1/2 ounce or more daily.
- Royal Power high grade royal jelly—4 capsules every morning.

Foods that help
- artichokes
- cumin seed
- cilantro leaves
- sea salt (add to food liberally; salt doesn't cause diabetes, but sugar does)
- blueberries
- cinnamon

Things to avoid
- chocolate as well as all foods containing refined sugar
- refined flour, rice, barley, oats, and corn meal
- orange, pear, apricot, and apple juice
- pancakes, waffles, bread, and pastries

Diaper rash

This is not simply a rash; it is an infection of the skin, usually caused by yeasts. The baby may be a carrier for yeasts and may have vaginal and/or intestinal overgrowth. It is best to avoid drugs in children and, rather to utilize natural agents such as lactobacillus and antifungal spices. Acidophilus bacteria and other normal flora inhibit the growth of yeasts. One ideal type is the European-source Health-Bac, which readily implants into the human intestines.

Edible herbs with antiseptic actions are highly antifungal. Research by Cornell University, published in 1998, documents how certain edible herbs, particularly onion, garlic, and wild oregano, destroy fungi. These herbs/foods are safe for pregnant and/or nursing mothers. Plus, in the proper form they are safe for infants. OregaMax is a wild oregano, garlic, onion formula available for all ages. It also contains an edible unique wild Mediterranean berry called *Rhus coriaria* (mountain sumac, unrelated to poison sumac). Wild oregano is the main active ingredient. A study published in the *International Journal of Food Microbiology* found that wild oregano in an amount less than 1% completely killed all fungi tested against it. In the Mediterranean the OregaMax formula is consumed by children of all ages. This is the maximum strength wild herb, the whole herb, versus the distilled oil. For children old enough to eat solids merely mix the contents of two or more capsules per day in food to ward off yeast/fungus infections. For younger infants mix the OregaMax into raw honey or cereal; one or two capsules daily should suffice. Breast-feeding mothers may take the OregaMax, 6 or more capsules daily, to benefit the infant. The point is wild oregano, as well as garlic, onion, and mountain sumac, are foods. What's more, these herbs are safer for human use than many of the substances freely given to children such as aspirin, acetaminophen, and even soda pop. However, do not give raw garlic to infants; it is too caustic. What's more, commercial oregano is irradiated and contains residues of thermonuclear ions. Thus, it would not be appropriate to give it to infants (or anyone else). The oregano in OregaMax is entirely wild and is never irradiated. It may be taken for any of the wide range of fungal infections afflicting infants and children. OregaMax may be purchased at health food stores, or to order direct call 1-800-243-5242.

If the mother is breast-feeding, she too may require treatment with antifungal agents and/or acidophilus cultures. Breast-feeding mothers should avoid consuming drugs whenever possible, since these chemicals will be transferred into the breast milk and passed on to the baby. Yet, the same is true of natural substances, even natural bacteria.

Once the friendly bacteria are ingested, they populate the mucous membranes of the gut. Additionally, they may be absorbed into the bloodstream. From here they are concentrated in breast milk. Noxious microbes may also be transported from the bowel into the blood and end up in the milk. These facts emphasize the importance of treating both the mother and the infant in preventing Candida overgrowth. In this regard both OregaMax and the oil of oregano (Oreganol P73) are completely safe for lactating mothers.

Breast milk is a derivative of the mother's diet, and whatever she eats/drinks and whatever medicine she takes will be in it. Thus, breast-feeding mothers, as well as infants, should strictly avoid the intake of drugs if possible.

Care should be taken on how to cleanse the involved skin of diaper rash. A thorough rinsing with lukewarm water usually suffices; add a small amount of a gentle type of essential oil to a warm wash cloth (oil of bay berry, oil of rosemary, oil of myrtle, etc.). Avoid using harsh soaps, as they usually cause further irritation. The skin is acidic and most soaps are basic, and they tend to alter it towards a basic pH. This encourages the growth of fungi as well as pathogenic bacteria.

Diaper rash combat kit

- oil of oregano (an excellent antifungal)—dilute this by adding 5 drops in a tablespoon of olive oil; apply as needed. However, before using it on sensitive baby skin be sure to read the label carefully. Do not use aromatherapy oregano oil or *Thymus capitus*, that is the so-called full strength or undiluted types. The latter is a dangerous oil and, unfortunately, is common in

inferior or imitation brands. These may burn the baby's sensitive skin. It may not be a permanent burn, but, nonetheless, such a reaction should be avoided. It is possible that inferior types of oregano oils might contain synthetic ingredients. Be certain the product used contains only natural oil of oregano extracted from the wild plant (i. e. the P73 Oreganol). Use only the type(s) emulsified in extra virgin olive oil (must say on the label *guaranteed wild* oregano oil, wild crafted, or 100% wild; North American Herb & Spice, Vivitas, Vitamin Shoppe, and Physician's Strength are the best sources). Do not use commercial oil of oregano on babies skin.
- OregaMax capsules (for the mother or child)—take one or more capsules daily.
- Oreganol 6% cream—the ideal form of wild oregano for sensitive skin, apply sparingly to the irritated skin as needed. Must be applied carefully; may cause temporary burning on genitals.
- oil of wild lavender—apply to the irritated skin as needed.

Things to avoid

- refined sugar and candies of all types
- harsh soaps
- perfumed diapers

Diarrhea

This is perhaps the most disconcerting of all illnesses. The fact is uncontrolled diarrhea may rapidly lead to severe dehydration, perhaps death. In fact, diarrhea causes untold millions of deaths worldwide, especially in primitive or poor countries.

Uncontrolled diarrhea is particularly disastrous in children. In fact, diarrhea is perhaps the primary cause of childhood illness, and it kills millions of children every year, primarily in poor countries. While in a catastrophic circumstance diarrheal illnesses pose potentially serious problems, nationally, fewer than 1,000 children die every year as a result of this condition. The fact is virtually all childhood deaths from diarrhea are preventable.

If diarrhea afflicts large numbers of people, there must be an obvious source for the infection. Either the food or water must be contaminated. Attempt to determine what this source is to avoid re-infection. Germs which commonly cause food and waterborne epidemics include hepatitis viruses, E. coli, Salmonella, Shigella, Camphylobacter, trichinella (pork worms), Vibrio (the cause of cholera), Giardia, and Cryptosporidium. All can cause fulminant life-threatening diarrhea.

Diarrhea combat kit

- wild oregano or thistle honey—consume as much as necessary, up to a pound per day (diabetics must omit this one).
- oil of oregano—a few drops under the tongue repetitively. Also, take a few Oreganol gelcaps internally daily.
- Oreganol P73 Juice—drink 2 ounces three times daily or more often if necessary.
- HerbSorb (Eastern aromatic spice and intestinal tonic formula) —take 3 capsules several times daily.
- OregaBiotic natural and safe antibiotic—take two or more capsules twice daily or as needed.
- Infla-eez (as a roto-rooter type agent for destroying parasites, a major cause of diarrhea)—take one or more capsules as needed. Helps halt diarrhea.

Foods that help

- raw honey is (easy on the gut)—wild oregano honey, rich in much-needed potassium, is ideal.
- clear meat or chicken broths
- onion/garlic broth
- ginger root tea

Things to avoid
- chocolate and refined sugar
- solid foods
- apple and orange juice

Diphtheria

According to Miriam Tucker, senior writer for *Family Practice News*, diphtheria is "alive and well"...in the United States. Thus, unfortunately, this scary disease has yet to be eradicated despite immunizations. In fact, modern medicine bragged that the organism was essentially eliminated from the populous. Yet, as described by Dr. W. A. Orenstein in *Family Practice News*, June 15, 1998, an epidemic of this dreaded disease remains a significant possibility. Diphtheria is primarily a throat disorder, that is an infection of the throat by a bacteria. This bacteria not only invades the throat but also produces a potent toxin, diphtheria toxin, which can cause damage throughout the body. Because it is so rare in the United States, it may be easily missed. This increases the risks for a serious outbreak.

The typical symptom is a sore throat with a membranous tissue attached on the mucous membranes that develops beyond the tonsils. This membrane may extend all the way into the lungs. Other symptoms include swollen neck lymph nodes, low grade fever, chills, and hoarseness. Suspicion should be high for diphtheria if the typical symptoms develop in individuals traveling to Russia or the Orient. While a diphtheria epidemic is unlikely, it is necessary to prepare for it, because, when it strikes, it is often deadly.

Diphtheria is an extremely dangerous illness. It requires immediate medical care. Physicians usually prescribe Erythromycin and/or penicillin for a 14-day period. Perhaps even more important in reversing the disease is the Diphtheria Antitoxin, which is effective especially if given early in the course. The latter is given as an injection. However, this is an experimental drug and is not routinely available in emergency rooms. It must be purchased by physicians or hospitals from the CDC by calling 1-404-639-2889. Even so, wild oregano oil is superior to any drug, plus it is nontoxic.

Antibiotics alone may be insufficient to halt this disastrous infection, especially if an epidemic strikes. Antiseptic herbs, such as garlic, onion, and wild oregano, must also be relied upon. Oil of oregano can sterilize sewage, and diphtheria germs are a minor issue compared to that. The Oreganol P73 is a reliable cure for this condition. So are the OregaBiotic capsules.

Diphtheria combat kit

- oil of oregano (SuperStrength is best)—take aggressively, 2 or more drops under the tongue every half hour or as often as necessary. Also, take 5 to 10 drops three times daily in juice or water.
- bromelain/papain mixture (anti-inflammatory agent i.e. Infla-eez)— take three or more capsules three times daily on an empty stomach.
- Purely-C—take 3 capsules four times daily.
- OregaBiotic capsules—take 3 capsules three times daily.
- oil of wild lavender—rub on soles of feet, forehead, and chest.

Foods that help

- papaya plus the seeds
- meat-based broths with garlic and onion

Things to avoid

- all types of pop and milk products
- refined sugar in any form (it is immunosuppressive)

Diverticulitis (see also Constipation)

This is an inflammatory disorder of the colon, largely due to damage to the colon wall from straining at the stool. It can cause considerable pain and discomfort. Occasionally, it develops into a medical emergency, because the colon wall becomes infected with bacteria or parasites. This may lead to abscess formation. If this condition is untreated, the colon wall may rupture, causing life-threatening infections.

Diverticulitis combat kit

- wild oregano herb (OregaMax)—take 3 capsules twice daily.
- oil of oregano—take 2 drops under the tongue twice daily. Take also 5 drops in juice or water or 1 Oreganol cap 2x daily.
- oil of rosemary (for relaxing the intestinal walls)—take 5 drops in juice or water twice daily.
- Nutri-Sense protein/B vitamin drink mix—take 3 tablespoons in juice or water. Add a tablespoon of carob molasses and mix in a blender with frozen fruit. Very nourishing for the bowel, yet gentle.
- Infla-eez—take 2 or more capsules twice daily on an empty stomach.
- wild greens drops (i.e. GreensFlush)—2 droppersful twice daily

Things to avoid

- peanuts and other legumes
- nuts and seeds
- refined sugar, colas, pastries, and cookies
- white flour and foods made with flour—these must be strictly avoided.
- raw wild honey, i. e. oregano honey, 3 T. daily.

Dog bites

As incredible as it may seem over a million Americans are bitten by dogs every year. Some estimates place the number as high as 4.5 million, because many of the bites are never reported. The point is virtually anyone is likely to be bitten by a dog.

The Postal Service is well aware of the scope of this dilemma, as thousands of mail carriers are included among the victims. However, children are the most common victims. Weiss and colleagues noted in *JAMA* that nearly one half of all children, that is tens of millions of individuals, suffer at least one dog bite during their lifetimes. Unfortunately, a high percentage of these bites are on the face, neck, and head. Thus, dog bites are an enormous health issue in the United States, costing tens of millions of dollars yearly. The extent of this dilemma is so vast that bites by other animals, including cats, must be considered relatively rare in comparison. In fact, human bites are possibly the second most common "animal" bite.

Any animal bite can become infected. Bites are a type of puncture wound, where contaminated secretions are injected deep into the tissues. The deeper a puncture is into the muscle, the greater is the risk for infection. Deep wounds receive less oxygen than superficial ones. Blood flow is greatest in the skin and least in the deep muscles. This reduced blood flow largely contributes to the high risk for infection in puncture wounds.

Dog bites notoriously become infected. Any dog bite which breaks the skin, no matter how superficial, can become infected. When the teeth puncture the skin, dog saliva is driven deep into the tissues. This saliva is contaminated with billions of germs. Dog owners might find this difficult to believe, but it is true. The fact is, the saliva of dogs can readily infect humans.

In the emergency rooms physicians advise patients to leave dog bites open and rarely suture them. Experience has proven that closing (suturing) the wound traps the infections within the tissues. Not only will the wound heal poorly if it is closed, but also potentially severe or even life-threatening infections may result. This is where antiseptic spice oils are so valuable. Applied repeatedly they sterilize the wound.

Dog bite combat kit
- flush the wound liberally with clean water, hopefully clean saline water.

- oil of wild oregano (i.e. Oreganol P73)—drizzle copious amounts throughout the wound several times daily.
- oil of lavender—add to wound and rub around the wound site; speeds healing.
- oil of propolis (i. e. PropaHeal)—vastly important to sterilize wounds while speeding tissue healing, apply on wound several times daily.
- Royal Power premium-grade royal jelly—take to combat stress and strengthen the adrenal glands, 2 to 4 capsules every morning.
- bromelain/papain mixture (i.e. Infla-eez)—to reduce trauma and swelling, take 3 or more capsules several times daily on an empty stomach.
- Oreganol cream—anti-pain; also speeds healing.
- wild oregano honey—add to oregano oil and cover wound, an important step.

Drug overdose

Drugs are cellular poisons. During crises this makes them extremely dangerous to use. Drugs should only be dispensed under a doctor's direction. Yet, even under a doctor's direction they are dangerous. In April 1998 the *JAMA* reported that over 100,000 individuals are killed and another 2.2 million harmed yearly by reactions from drugs, which are properly dispensed. This fails to include the damage inflicted by improperly dispensed medications, which accounts for additional thousands of deaths and injuries. In fact, the research was skewed, because only deaths due to properly prescribed medications were reviewed and this was primarily in relation to hospitalized patients. The number would likely triple if other drug-induced disasters were included, including the dispensing of drugs or samples in doctor's offices or via mail order. What's more, millions of other individuals, perhaps as many as 5 million, suffer adverse reactions to nonprescription drugs every year.

As reported in 2005 one drug alone, Vioxx, caused some 75,000 deaths, largely due to strokes and heart attacks. Thus, the use of prescription drugs by the public in an attempt to self-medicate is dangerous. It is particularly ill-advised during disaster circumstances, when access to emergency medical care may be compromised. The point is it is likely to cause more harm than good. For instance, let's assume you develop a cough or sore throat, and you have leftover antibiotics from a previous prescription. You take those antibiotics on your own. Yet, if the problem is due to a herpes viral infection, mono, fungus, or a respiratory virus, the illness will likely be aggravated and prolonged. What's more, you may create drug-resistant germs that could cause long term illness and perhaps spread dangerously to the internal organs.

Children are highly vulnerable to the toxic effects of drugs. Nonprescription drugs and over-the-counter tablets are the primary causes of childhood poisoning. Incredibly, first on the list are multiple vitamins, which cause iron poisoning. However, perhaps even more insidious are antibiotics, which are the primary cause of prescription drug toxicity in children/infants. According to S. Knowles, reviewing data from Health Canada, fully 75% of all drug reactions in children under 16 were caused by antibiotics: over 20% were serious, that is they were capable of causing permanent damage and/or death. The reactions include severe rash, hives, diarrhea, swelling, and shock.

The liver is the organ responsible for detoxifying and removing harmful chemicals and thus bears the brunt of drug toxicity. Specifically, drugs damage the liver by depleting it of critical components, particularly vitamins and certain enzymes. The enzymes which are severely depleted are primarily glutathione and to a lesser degree superoxide dismutase. Glutathione depletion alone accounts for much of the drug-induced damage. Therefore, agents which replenish glutathione do much to repair liver damage or prevent it from occurring. Top glutathione-replenishing agents include N-acetyl cysteine (NAC), glutathione tablets, organic selenium, rosemary oil, cumin oil, oregano oil, and cilantro oil. Use only the edible oils emulsified in olive oil. Do not use aromatherapy grade essential oils, since they have not been screened for edibility. Do not use sodium selenite or selenious acid. These synthetic types of selenium may accentuate the chemical poisoning. A completely organic form of selenium is available from NutritionTest.com by calling 1-800-243-5242.

Another advantage of edible plant essential oils is that they may aid in restoring bile synthesis as well as stimulating the flow of bile. Drugs are stored in the bile-producing portion of the liver and the ideal means to eliminate them is through the bile. Top bile stimulants include oils of fennel, lavender, cumin, rosemary, and oregano, with cumin being perhaps the most effective of these. All these are available in a product called LivaClenz.

Certain herbs, such as milk thistle, beet extract, artichoke, and, particularly, GreensFlush wild dandelion/burdock formula, are well respected liver detoxifying agents. However, they are far less potent than the edible essential oils in purging the liver of poisonous compounds. What's more, the crude wild greens are also invaluable, that is a combination of wild dandelion leaf, nettles, and burdock leaf extracts, i.e. the GreensFlush drops.

Drug detoxification kit

- oil of cumin—take 10 to 20 drops three times daily.
- LivaClenz—take one dropperful twice daily.
- oil of oregano—take 10 drops twice daily.
- oil of cilantro/coriander—take 10 or more drops twice daily.
- NukeProtect—take 3 capsules every few hours until the toxicity is resolved (no more than one week on this dose). As a maintenance, take 400 mg daily.

- GreensFlush wild greens drops (only available by mail-order, 1-800-243-5242. Take 2 droppersful several times daily.
- activated charcoal—actually absorbs the drug so it can be removed through the bowels.
- crude ascorbic acid/bioflavonoids (Purely-C)—take 2 capsules every few hours until the toxicity is abated. Also, use regular vitamin C, about 1000 mg twice daily.

Foods that help

- artichokes, black radish, garlic, and onion
- beets and beet tops
- pure extra virgin olive oil plus vinegar (as a liver flush)—add the LivaClenz and wild greens drops

Note: anyone taking prescription drugs must see his/her physician before taking new items or altering the prescription.

Dry or irritated eyes

Dryness of the eyes is a classic symptom of nutritional deficiency. Vitamin A, zinc, and essential fatty acids are the missing nutrients, although vitamin B_2 deficiency may play a role. Essential fatty acids are a must for correcting this condition. Excellent sources include primrose and borage oils plus to a lesser degree flaxseed oil. Vitamin A eye drops would be curative in the event of its deficiency, which is manifested by dry and/or inflamed eyes. Also, consume foods rich in vitamin A such as organic liver, fatty fish, and whole milk products. Be sure to take essential fatty acid supplements as well as cod liver oil, because in many cases the condition is too severe to rely on food sources alone. About nine capsules of primrose oil and a teaspoon of cod liver oil daily should suffice. Also, dry eyes may be a sign of fungal infection. In this case a few drops of oil of wild oregano under the tongue would be indicated.

E. coli

This bacteria is a normal inhabitant of the bowel. It only causes problems if it overgrows or if it enters other regions such as the bladder, kidneys, and/or prostate. It was only rarely a problem prior to modern time. However, now it is a killer. This is because a number of mutant strains have been created by antibiotics. These mutant strains are highly aggressive and are capable of rapidly destroying human tissue. They essentially liquefy certain organs unless they can be quickly eliminated from the body.

No one can afford to have mutant E. coli in the body for long. It must be promptly destroyed. Unfortunately, no synthetic antibiotic is 100% capable of that. I have made it evident that natural substances, specifically oil of oregano and the multiple spice (garlic, onion, allspice, oregano), OregaBiotic, are capable of filling the void by killing noxious germs outright. A recent study performed by the University of Tennessee in concert with the FDA attempted to dispute these findings. However, unexpectedly, it was determined that a variety of natural compounds, particularly oil of oregano, killed the type of E. coli that contaminates food. Thus, natural antiseptics are lifesaving for this condition.

> **CASE HISTORY**
> A 27-year-old girl contracted severe diarrhea from mutant E. coli. The diarrhea was unstoppable; in fact, according to her mother the hospital sent her home to die. Her mother gave her one dose of oil of oregano, and the diarrhea stopped completely. This beautiful young lady is now totally healthy, but, just in case, she takes a drop or two of oil of oregano every day.

E. coli combat kit

- oil of oregano SuperStrength—take this aggressively, 2 to 5 drops under the tongue frequently; take also 10 to 20 drops internally, as often as every hour. Reduce this amount to a maintenance level of 2 drops twice daily once the infestation is destroyed.

- wild oregano capsules (i.e. OregaMax)—take 3 capsules three times daily.
- LivaClenz—take 20 drops twice daily.
- oil of cilantro/coriander—take 10 drops twice daily.
- Lactobacillus supplement (take also as a daily preventive)
- OregaBiotic—1 or more capsules three times daily.
- Garlex oil of cold-pressed garlic–10 drops several times daily.

Foods that help
- raw garlic and onion (add to foods frequently)
- onion juice—one or more cups daily
- papaya and kiwi fruit
- ginger root in food or in hot water (as a tea)

Earache and/or infection

Ear infections are one of the most difficult dilemmas faced by parents today. The incidence of this condition has risen in children dramatically over the last fifty years. Adults rarely develop them.

Nearly 50% of the incidents where parents think their child has an ear infection, he/she doesn't. This is according to the latest research by Dr. Weiss and colleagues from Phoenix's Children's Hospital. Perhaps even more astounding is the fact that these orthodox M.D.s categorically state that a large percentage of earaches completely resolve without treatment. What's more, when a true ear infection does occur, as many as 40% of them may be due to organisms other than bacteria such as viruses and fungi, both of which are immune to antibiotics.

When parents are confronted with earaches or infections in their children, they often become concerned that the infection will spread from the inner ear to the brain, which is in close proximity. This does rarely occur. Yet, what parents fail to realize is that a huge percentage of earaches are caused by toxic reactions to foods, not germs. However, bacteria often invade the ear canal secondarily as a result of the allergic reaction. In a crisis it may be cumbersome to avoid potentially allergenic foods. Combine this with stress, exposure to the elements, and communicable diseases, and earaches can become a significant dilemma.

The inner and middle ear cavities are in close proximity to the brain. So are the sinuses, roots of the teeth, and eye sockets. Infections in any of these regions could theoretically spread to the brain. Infection of the brain in children is relatively rare, but when it occurs, it is frequently fatal. These infections include meningitis, encephalitis, and brain abscess. However, an incredibly small percentage of cases of ear infections lead to brain or spinal cord infection. The vast majority of cases of meningitis, encephalitis, and brain abscesses are caused as a consequence of other factors, including poor hygiene, blood poisoning, animal bites, insect bites, pneumonia, and surgery (and its complications). People should be equally if not more concerned about these factors as they are about ear infections.

The current approach is to aggressively treat ear infections with prescription medicines. Frequently, doctors prescribe repeated doses of potent drugs, like broad spectrum antibiotics, cortisone, and codeine. Antibiotics are overprescribed by pediatricians for virtually all childhood illnesses. This is largely because doctors are afraid of being sued. Children, particularly infants, are easily overdosed by such medicines, and numerous side effects may result. Antibiotics are far from innocuous. In fact, they may occasionally cause life-threatening reactions.

Antibiotic therapy creates its own group of illnesses. These illnesses include chronic candidiasis, vaginitis, cystitis, chronic serous otitis media, pseudomembranous colitis, irritable bowel syndrome, and food intolerance.

Children are also overmedicated with anti-fever agents like aspirin and Tylenol. Other drugs are given for pain such as opium derivatives, i.e. codeine. Drugs containing codeine should never be given to children without medical supervision.

The ill effects of such drugs upon respiration are of particular concern. If lung function is depressed, less oxygen will be available for the tissues, and the results may be catastrophic. Impaired function of the immune system will result, and the function of the brain, the body's number one oxygen consumer, may be seriously impaired. If this respiratory depression occurs for a prolonged period, seizures and/or coma may result. Additionally, the systemic physiological depression induced by codeine increases the tendency for infections to spread. As a result, a self-limiting disease can be turned into a fatal one.

Antibiotics are highly destructive to bowel bacteria, particularly the friendly bacteria. They are less able to develop resistance to antibiotics than pathogens, and, thus, they are routinely destroyed in vast numbers as a result of even modest dosages. The destruction of the friendly bacteria encourages the growth of pathogenic organisms. Yeasts grow prolifically as a consequence of destruction of the normal flora, since the latter secrete a variety of substances which inhibit the growth of fungi. Thus, antibiotics both cause and aggravate yeast infections.

Antibiotics negatively affect immunity. They impair white blood cell function. Evidence exists that they cause a significant reduction in the *phagocytic index*, a measurement of the ability of white blood cells to destroy microbes. The reduction in the immune potential encourages the development of opportunistic infections, the very thing that doctors are attempting to cure.

Prolonged use of potent medicines increases patients' risks for developing a variety of ailments. Infants and children are significantly more vulnerable to these ill effects than are adults. Do not overmedicate your children.

Ear infection combat kit

- Kid-e-Kare Ear-eez (oil of warming garlic)—a few drops in the ear as needed. This is highly safe, since it is a whole food extract.
- oil of oregano (use the edible type, Oreganol P73)—this may be all you need; rub on the outer ear or the skin behind the ear. Also, internally under the tongue, several drops daily or as Oreganol gelcaps a few capsules daily until condition resolves.
- Kid-e-Kare rubbing oil—rub on face, chest, soles of feet, and outer ear
- Kid-e-Kare multiple spice gelcaps—one or more capsules twice daily.
- OregaMax capsules—take as many capsules as possible, up to 6 per day. If the child is too small to swallow, open and add to bottle or food.

Things to avoid

- milk products
- white sugar, chocolate, and candy
- apple and orange juice
- food dye-laced foods
- nitrated meats
- white bread and/or pasta

Ebola

Ebola has developed in the United States. This is what inspired the book *Hot Zone* and the resulting movie *Outbreak*. Indeed, like the book and movie the USA outbreak was monkey-induced. However, none of the individuals who were infected died. This is because the monkey virus was a weakened mutant of the more severe human type.

The human type rapidly devastates anyone in its path. As described in *Hippocrates Magazine* during the largest outbreak of Ebola yet in Africa nine out of ten individuals died. The death is gruesome but not always quick. There may be up to two weeks of intense suffering before the ultimate demise. Death is usually via organ liquefaction. If Ebola strikes, don't give up hope. Use the Ebola combat kit as aggressively as possible to save your life and the lives of others.

Ebola combat kit

- oil of oregano (SuperStrength is best)—take massive amounts, like 5 drops under the tongue every 15 minutes and 20 drops internally every hour. Rub on soles of feet and chest.
- OregaBiotic multiple spice capsule—3 or more capsules as often as necessary with juice or food.
- Purely-C—take as much as possible to impede blood vessel destruction; consume an entire bottle a day, if necessary.
- red grape powder (Resvital)—the bulk form is ideal; take up to a heaping teaspoon every hour.
- Garlex oil of cold-pressed garlic–ten or more drops under the tongue as often as needed.
- Infla-eez—take 2 or more capsules several times daily.

Foods that help

- onion juice (yellow onions are best)—drink as much as can be consumed
- raw honey—eat it by the cupful
- carob molasses—well digested and an ideal source of nourishment for fighting the infection, 1 or 2 teaspoons daily

Eczema

This condition is a type of chronic inflammation of the skin. For years no one was sure what caused it. Many presumed it was due to allergies or sensitivity to chemicals in soap, etc.

The medical profession has erred greatly in its approach to this illness. All manner of creams and ointments have been dispensed, largely to no avail. This failure is due to the fact that eczema is primarily an internal disorder, i.e. the cause is systemic. It was Rosenberg and colleagues at the University of Tennessee who first made the determination: germs are the cause of eczema. They found that the eczematous lesions and psoriatic blotches contained a fungus as well as staph and/or strep. Apparently, the germs arise from inside the body, that is from within the bowel, and infect the skin secondarily. Thus, the only way to resolve this disorder is to eradicate the infection *internally*. In other words, killing the fungus and/or bacteria is the objective. The same is true of psoriasis.

Certain substances, notably pure essential oils in a carrier base, may be helpful rubbed externally. For this purpose use a 6% essential oil cream.

Eczema combat kit

- Oreganol oil of wild oregano—take 5 drops under the tongue twice daily. Also, take 5 or more drops twice daily internally in juice or water. For tough cases the SuperStrength may be necessary—at the same or greater doses.
- Oreganol cream—rub externally on irritated skin or eczema lesions to tolerance.
- OregaMax capsules—take 3 or more capsules twice daily.
- Oreganol P73 Juice—take an ounce or more daily with meals.
- Pumpkinol oil of cold-pressed pumpkin seed—for damaged skin, 2 or more tablespoons daily.

Things to avoid

- caffeine, soda pop, and chocolate
- refined sugar and corn syrup

Emotionally distressed child

This covers a wide range of conditions wherein a toddler or child is distressed, that is out of control. No one can afford to deal with this nerve-wracking situation, whether in everyday life or a disaster. The answers are found in nutrients, herbs, spices, and aromatic plant oils.

Emotional distress combat kit

- oil of sage in olive oil—highly calming, rub on face, chest, and especially soles of feet and mid-lower back (adrenal reflex).
- Royal Power (premium quality royal jelly)—2 or more capsules in the morning.
- Royal Oil—1/2 to one teaspoon twice daily.
- Nutri-Sense—a superior, natural source of B vitamins and fatty acids, take 2 tablespoons twice daily in juice, milk, or water.
- Essence of Neroli Orange or white coffee—add a tablespoon or more to juice or hot tea; drink once or twice daily.
- Kid-e-Kare Attention drops (for psychologically damaged children)—rub on chest, spine, and feet; also, take five drops twice daily internally. Also useful for calming children.
- Kid-e-Kare Mighty Kids (fortified royal jelly formula)—to give children strength and patience, 1/2 teaspoon under the tongue as needed.
- primrose oil—take as directed or 6 capsules daily.

Foods that help

- salted roasted nuts (MSG-free)
- peanut butter with salt (high in B vitamins and protein)
- sliced turkey meat (high in tryptophan)
- fatty fish, especially salmon

Things to avoid

- candy, sugar, cookies, or sweets of any kind
- pop and other caffeinated/sugary drinks
- synthetic food dyes or flavorings

Emphysema

If there is a disease of torment, it is emphysema. In this condition the individual is literally suffocating to death in his/her own secretions. Life with emphysema is miserable and death by it even worse.

Emphysema is largely due to toxic chemical damage to the lungs. Thus, it is particularly common in industrial workers and cigarette smokers. Yet, it is also prolific in non-smokers who live in highly polluted regions like Los Angeles, New York City, and Chicago.

While the medical profession regards emphysema as incurable, the lungs have an immense capacity to regenerate. Nutrients needed for lung cell regeneration include beta carotene, vitamins C and E, flavonoids, zinc, and selenium. Essential oils also assist cellular repair.

Emphysema may also be caused by chronic infection. Molds and bacteria readily infect the lungs, causing tissue damage. If the infection is eradicated, the breathing improves significantly. Destruction of infection is key to remission of this disorder.

Nutritional deficiency is another major factor. The key deficient nutrients are vitamins A, C, and E as well as pantothenic acid, essential fatty acids, and phospholipids.

Emphysema combat kit

- oil of oregano (SuperStrength may be required)—take 2 drops under the tongue two or more times daily.
- oil of rosemary—take 2 to 5 drops twice daily in juice or water. Also, rub on chest and under nose.

- Purely-C—take 2 or more capsules twice daily.
- OregaMax capsules—take 3 capsules or more twice daily (an excellent lung tonic). **Note:** essential oils and wild herbs are more aggressive in aiding the lung function than vitamins. Crude sources of flavonoids, such as Purely-C, are also highly useful.
- OregaBiotic multiple spice capsules—take 2 to 3 capsules twice daily.
- Infla-eez potent antiinflammatory enzymes—take 3 capsules on an empty stomach twice daily.
- Oreganol P73 Juice—a potent remedy for this condition, 1/2 ounce twice daily.

Foods that help
- squash, pumpkin, sweet potatoes

Things to avoid
- any contact with smoke as well as moldy or damp rooms

Encephalitis

This is defined simply as inflammation of the brain and the surrounding linings. It is nearly always virally induced. It is life threatening.

Usually, this condition develops as a consequence of insect bites, mostly mosquitoes, however, ticks can also cause it. Worldwide, mosquitoes cause millions of cases of encephalitis, which these insects contract from the blood of rodents and other wild animals (as well as humans). Encephalitis may also develop in the aftermath of common viral illnesses; measles, chicken pox, mumps, and viral pneumonia may all result in it. It frequently develops after natural catastrophes, like floods.

In September 1999 a bizarre virus began attacking individuals throughout America. It was claimed to be carried by birds, which proved fallacious. Called the West Nile virus, it is infecting hundreds of individuals throughout the country. This virus is now causing a national encephalitis epidemic. The most likely source: an accidental release from the military-industrial complex.

Over a period of decades this contaminant will cause hundreds, perhaps thousands, of deaths. Plus, there will be countless cases of permanent brain damage. There is a need for protection from mosquito bites, which can be achieved naturally by using an herbal insect repellent such as Herbal Bug-X. This is a completely nontoxic insect repellent and may even be used on babies. The repellency lasts for two hours. Antiviral edible essential oils should be used, mainly internally. For instance, one study showed that oil of wild oregano disintegrated viruses, a power not found in drugs. However, oil of oregano itself, whether taken internally or applied topically, is a repellent.

Encephalitis combat kit

- oil of oregano—take 2 to 5 drops under the tongue every hour.
- oil of lavender—rub on face, under nose, on scalp, buttocks, and soles of feet. Or, use Kid-e-Kare rubbing oil.
- Purely-C—take 3 capsules three times daily.
- OregaMax capsules—take 9 or more capsules daily.
- Oreganol P73 Juice—highly important for neurological damage, take one ounce several times daily.
- Essence of Rosemary—take 2 or more ounces daily.
- Black Seed-plus—take 3 capsules twice daily.
- Nutri-Sense (crude rice fractions for providing much needed natural vitamins for regenerating brain tissue)
- Neuroloft aromatic antiseptic essence—1/2 or more ounces twice daily.

Foods that help

- squash (especially butternut), pumpkin, and sweet potatoes
- watercress, arugula, spinach, and parsley

- garlic/onion meat-based broths
- yolk of organic eggs (for regenerating neurons)

Endometriosis

This is an inflammatory condition of the female organs. It can afflict any of the pelvic female organs or glands, especially the ovaries, uterus, and fallopian tubes. It can even attack abdominal organs, such as the bowel.

Endometriosis occurs when fluids from the uterus regurgitate into aberrant areas, like the abdominal cavity, causing massive inflammation. The conduit for this is the fallopian tubes, the same ones that transport the eggs. Infection is the most likely cause for this condition. However, hormonal insufficiency is another major cause, that is poor output of natural steroids such as progesterone, estrogen, and cortisol.

Endometriosis combat kit

- oil of oregano (Oreganol P73)—take 2 drops under the tongue twice daily.
- premium-grade royal jelly (Royal Power, very important)—take 4 to 6 capsules in the a.m.
- oil of myrtle—rub on the vaginal walls twice daily.
- oil of rosemary—take 5 to 10 drops twice daily.
- Thyroset—take 4 capsules twice daily.
- Nutri-Sense drink mix—take 3 T. daily in juice or water.
- Resvital—take 2 capsules twice daily.
- Infla-eez—invaluable for halting pain and inflammation, 3 capsules twice daily.

Foods that help

- raw sunflower seeds
- fatty fish, especially salmon
- hard kiwi and green papaya plus the seeds.

Things to avoid

- refined sugar, candy, cookies, etc.
- chocolate, tea, iced tea, and coffee
- hydrogenated and partially hydrogenated oils
- sex during menses

Exhaustion

Exhaustion is something virtually everyone has experienced. It is usually caused by severe stress, physical exertion, or disease. Nutritional deficiency also results in fatigue/exhaustion. To survive in today's rather hostile world it is required to have a full bank of energy. Exhaustion negatively affects the individual in every aspect of life, in relationships, work, and enjoyment. There is no need to be exhausted. By taking strength-producing remedies it is possible to have plenty of energy, perhaps an excess of it, quickly.

Exhaustion combat kit

- Royal Power (premium-grade royal jelly)—take 4 to 6 capsules every morning. If necessary, take another 2 to 4 at noon.
- Oreganol P73 Juice (a strength tonic)—take an ounce twice daily.
- Hercules Strength—take 3 capsules twice daily.
- OregaMax capsules—take 2 or more twice daily.
- sage tea—make a tea by adding a tablespoon of Essence of Sage to a cup of hot water; drink once or twice daily.
- Nutri-Sense drink mix—take 3 tablespoons every morning in milk, juice, or water. Add to shakes, smoothies, cereals, or soups.

Foods that help

- salted roasted nuts
- roasted beef, turkey, or chicken (rich in carnitine, an energizing nutrient)

Exposure to the elements (see also Frostbite; Cold exposure)

Inevitably, this will develop as a consequence of a major disaster. Body temperature fluctuations, either too hot (heat intolerance) or too cold (hypothermia), are among the primary problems associated with exposure. Exposure can rapidly lead to physical damage, particularly in the elderly or very young.

Hypothermia, that is abnormally low body temperature, is the most life-threatening consequence of exposure. Every year, tens of thousands of individuals, mostly the poor and homeless, suffer from it.

Exposure means the individual is exposed to potentially dangerous elements, that is to poor weather, excessive heat, and, particularly, to excessive cold and wet. Cold wet weather is particularly dangerous, especially if the individual has no shelter. Such exposure can rapidly lead to respiratory distress and/or infection, which may prove fatal.

Cold exposure combat kit

- oil of oregano—rub on face, hands, and feet to produce heat. Take 2 drops under the tongue twice or more daily.
- Royal Power—to strengthen the adrenal glands, take 4 to 6 capsules every morning. For severe cold exposure take extra doses.
- Purely-C—take 2 to 4 capsules twice daily.
- Resvital capsules—take 2 or more capsules twice daily with juice or food.
- oil of sage and/or Essence of Sage—add to hot water and drink as a highly invigorating tea; a tremendous tonic for improving cold tolerance and reversing cold injury, including frostbite.
- wild strawberry leaf tea (Wild Power Tea)—drink one or two cups daily.

- Black Seed-plus—take 2 capsules twice daily to speed metabolism.
- Thyroset (for stimulating the thyroid gland)—take 4 to 6 capsules every morning.

Foods that help against cold
- salmon, albacore tuna, sardines, herring plus the juice
- meat broths rich in fat, onion, and garlic
- sea salt and salted foods
- hot spicy soups and sauces
- seaweed or miso soup

Heat exposure combat kit
- Royal Power—good for too hot or too cold, this strengthens adrenal action; take 4 capsules twice daily or more often during extreme exposure.
- Purely-C—crude vitamin C plus flavonoids greatly enhances heat tolerance; take 2 or more capsules several times daily.
- Resvital capsules—2 to 3 capsules twice daily.
- Garlex oil of mountain-grown garlic—5 to 10 drops twice daily (provides natural sulfur compounds, which help dissipate heat).

Foods that help against heat
- watermelon and cantaloupe, salted
- parsley and cilantro
- radishes and turnips, salted
- salted dried meat, fish, or poultry
- meat-based broths (garlic and onion added)
- salted toasted nuts (especially dry roasted)

Note: interestingly, salt and salted (healthy) foods are helpful in building strength both in cold and heat exposure.

Fainting

Few people realize that smelling salts were originally based on using essential oils as the active ingredients. This is because certain essential oils are such profound sensory activating agents that they will wake up just about anyone.

Fainting may be caused by a number of diseases. However, usually the cause is innocuous such as sudden bouts of fear or anxiety or low blood sugar. Regarding the latter it is largely the adrenal glands which control blood sugar as well as blood flow to the brain. Regardless of the cause "essential oil smelling salts" should be administered.

Fainting combat kit

- oil of bay leaf—rub on face and under nose as well as on the chest.
- oil of rosemary—rub on face and adrenal reflex in the mid lower back. Rub also on soles of feet. Give 2 or 3 drops under the tongue.
- oil of lavender—rub on face, under nose, on buttocks, and soles of the feet. Apply near or around nostrils.
- oil of myrtle—rub on the face and spine or around the nostrils.
- Royal Power—important for normalizing blood pressure, 2 to 3 capsules twice daily.

Fever

Parents, don't lose your minds over fevers. This is a natural process by which the body destroys germs. Everyone knows that heat kills germs. Fever by itself will only rarely harm or kill a human. In other words, it is not the fever that does so. It is the consequence of fever: dehydration and/or internal toxicity. As long as there is plenty of fluid in the body to buffer or insulate against high temperatures and to aid the body in the removal of toxins, fever is harmless.

In the event of high fever be sure to constantly consume the fluids. Use cool compresses on the face and forehead. Avoid using anti-fever drugs. They are the primary cause of organ damage. Such drugs should only be consumed as a last resort, when all else fails. Instead, utilize substances which help naturally break fevers. The most effective of these are the essential oils.

Fever Combat Kit

- oil of oregano—usually, rapidly breaks fever. Take internally and rub topically. Also, take the Oreganol gelcaps, up to 2 every hour.
- oil of lavender—a tremendous topical aid; helps cool skin and also breaks fever. Note: for infants and children use the Kid-e-kare rubbing oil, which contains wild lavender, sage, and oregano oils—rub all over the body as often as necessary until fever breaks.
- oil of sage—a natural coolant; take internally or rub topically.
- wild oregano capsules (OregaMax)—take 2 or more capsules every four hours to strengthen immunity and dissipate heat.
- ginger—slice fresh ginger and add to hot water as a tea.
- Essence of Neroli Orange—cooling, yet effective in normalizing heat transfer. Add one or more tablespoons to hot water and drink as a tea.
- Kid-e-Kare cold/flu capsules—one or more capsules as needed.
  Garlex oil of cold-pressed garlic—5 or more drops under the tongue as often as needed.

It seems ironic that hot spices actually help dissipate heat. They accomplish this by stimulating metabolism and by dissipating excess heat through the skin. This is readily apparent by anyone who eats hot spicy food. Often, the individual becomes hot and sweaty; this is the dissipation of heat through the skin. Thus, if you make chicken soup for fevers or infections, make it spicy.

Fire ants

These insects are not natural inhabitants of the United States, originating instead in South America. However, now they inhabit nearly all of the southern states. Fire ants are feared, because their bites are intensely painful. What's more, bites occurring in highly allergic individuals and/or individuals who have been bitten previously may cause life-threatening shock. Typical symptoms of the bites include pain, itching, swelling, redness, and, for allergic individuals, constricted breathing, shock, and collapse.

The editors of *USA Today* (1998) succinctly describe the fire ant epidemic, stating that these ants "kill, maim, and blind." Perhaps as much as one fifth of the land mass in the United States is contaminated by these pests, notably the entire states of South Carolina, Georgia, Florida, Alabama, Mississippi, Louisiana, and parts of Texas, North Carolina, and Tennessee. Recently, Southern California (Orange County) has become infested. What's more, the ants are expanding northward several miles each year.

The fire ant is a tropical ant, the demonic man-eating type of the movies. Unfortunately, it has efficiently adapted to our southern climate. What is perhaps more ominous is the fact that, perhaps through breeding with local ants, fire ants have adapted to cold weather, making their spread to unsuspecting northern states virtually imminent.

Fire ants are vicious. In the wild they kill newborn deer and baby birds. They may attack adult farm animals. They have no fear of large creatures, after all, they are immigrants from the land of big game (i.e. South America/Africa). They are a serious menace to small children. Dozens of Americans have been killed by these ants, some of them, as described by Richard de Shazo, a director at the University of Mississippi Medical Center, Jackson, Mississippi, being literally "eaten alive." The reason for their terror and toxicity isn't due to their bites per se: it is because of the highly poisonous venom they secrete when they bite. The venom itself usually doesn't kill humans. However, if an individual is allergic to it, shock and death may rapidly result.

Fire ants are learning to live indoors. For instance, in Florida they routinely enter homes in search of food. Different than normal ants, they will crawl on children (and adults) and bite them. Parents often have to scrape them off and then deal with a stinging itching lesion(s). If fire ants succeed at colonizing homes, they could be found in virtually every region of the United States, a disaster of unprecedented proportions.

The fire ant venom causes burning pain. This usually leads to intense itching, swelling, redness, hives, and pustule formation. In an individual with multiple bites allergic shock may develop, leading to collapse, unconsciousness, and perhaps death. The biggest problem is with Northerners. They are unaware of the crisis, and, thus, when visiting the South take no precautions. Often, they don't even realize that the ants are the culprit; they may think it is "hives" or "food allergy." Or, they rush to the emergency room, deathly ill, while having no clue that they were stung by ants.

Fire ant combat kit

- oil of oregano—apply to bites; take 2 drops under the tongue every hour until resolved.
- Infla-eez rubbing oil—apply to any bite region as often as needed.
- Garlex oil of raw garlic—apply to bites.
- raw onion—crush and apply to bites.

- Infla-eez—take 2 to 3 capsules every hour until resolved.
- Germ-a-CLENZ ant killing and repelling spice spray—routinely spray about home as preventative. Spray any outdoor mounds. Spray directly at invading ants. Also, use the Herbal Bug-X as a repellent and killer.

Note: when attacked by a horde of ants it is difficult to react or think. However, if possible, attack them back with the Germ-a-CLENZ and Herbal Bug-X. If unavailable make an oregano oil concoction. Grab a spray bottle and add a few ounces of hot water. Add a bottle or whatever amount is available of oil of oregano. Pump-spray in a fine or medium mist directly at the ants. If no oil of oregano is available, crush a few cloves of garlic and add this to the water. These agents are so hot that they will damage the ants' sensors, and they will either fall off or die.

Fleas

No one could believe that a human could have fleas, yet, infestation by these insects afflicts thousands of Americans every year. Many individuals are unaware that fleas can't fly; they are hopping insects and infect individuals by jumping on them and burrowing into the skin.

Fleas can cause serious disease. They transport the plague, which they contract from rats. They transmit tropical diseases such as typhus. They cause a plethora of minor problems such as itching and hives. However, the major cause of fleas in humans is more rudimentary: infestation from house pets, particularly dogs, which act as intermediary hosts for these pests.

Flea combat kit

- oil of oregano—burn the fleas out of the skin by applying the oil of oregano topically.
- oil of cumin—take 20 drops twice daily internally. Also, place on flea bites; they can't tolerate it.

- oil of bay leaf—highly valuable as a fumigant.
- oil of lavender—rub on involved regions and use for fumigation.
- Germ-a-CLENZ—spray on any fleas and any contaminated surface.

Note: pump-spray the house with Germ-a-CLENZ and/or an oregano/bay leaf mixture. Use diffusers and atomizers; bomb them out with essential oils. It is curious to note that the medical treatment for flea infestation includes fumigation with mothballs (naphthalene), which is so poisonous that the house must be vacated for 48 hours. This is the beauty of using essential oils, which are actually therapeutic when burned or volatilized. Note: avoid all perfumes/colognes.

Flesh-eating bacteria

This name is somewhat of a misnomer. No bacteria can digest human flesh by itself; however, bacterial enzymes are capable of doing so. What's more, certain bacteria produce toxins, which cause a vast inflammatory reaction. This leads to the destruction of tissues. In some cases no tissue escapes this destructive power. Organs are dissoluted. Even the bone may be dissolved.

Flesh-eating disease has existed for decades. It has primarily existed since the advent of antibiotics. Such drugs create mutant strains, which cause bizarre, in fact, deadly diseases. Reports of flesh-eating disease date back some 50 years, about the time in which antibiotics were introduced. Thus, this dangerous and deadly syndrome is man-made.

Medically, flesh-eating disease is known as *necrotizing fasciitis*. The word necrotizing proves its ominous nature, because this is defined in medical dictionaries as "the mass death of human tissue (even bone)." The involved bacteria secrete potent enzymes capable of digesting any type of human protein, essentially liquifying everything in its path.

The high vulnerability of this infection in children may be due to the increasing use of certain drugs which depress the immune system, making children more vulnerable to relentless infection. Researchers in Seattle found that children who consume anti-pain medication, particularly ibuprofen (Pediaprofen, etc.), are at a high risk for developing the infection. What's more, in adults the regular use of antiinflammatory drugs may precipitate the disease. Even aspirin increases the risks for the development of flesh-eating bacteria.

This level of destruction is caused by bacteria capable of secreting potent enzymes. As a result of antibiotic therapy the bacteria mutate, and this mutant form produces abnormal amounts of such enzymes. If produced in a sufficient amount, these enzymes can digest protein, including the protein of human skin, tissue, muscle, and bone. The key is to destroy the germ and, thus, totally halt enzyme production. Another objective is to neutralize the existing bacterial enzymes and/or toxins responsible for the damage. Strep and staph, especially the drug-resistant varieties, are the major progenitors of this disease. These germs are notoriously resistant to antibiotics, but they succumb to the powers of essential oils. What's more, natural plant enzymes, such as those found in Infla-eez, help neutralize the bacterial enzymes. These plant enzyme formulas contain key enzymes, which help denature, that is inactivate, the destructive bacterial enzymes. Furthermore, according to Turkish research spice oils readily neutralize bacterial toxins.

Recently, an evaluation was done on the power of spices against such bacteria. The flesh-eating MRSA was placed in petri dishes. The SuperStrength oil of wild oregano was added. The result was major destruction of the bacteria. When the antiseptic spray Germ-a-CLENZ was added, there was complete destruction.

Note: recently, antiinflammatory drugs have been implicated in the cause of this disease. Such drugs interfere with the normal immune response, allowing the bacteria to overgrow. This may result in flesh-eating disease.

Flesh-eating bacteria combat kit

- raw honey (wild oregano type, filled with tissue-healing enzymes)—pack all over wounded area; also, eat 1/4 cup daily.
- oil of oregano (SuperStrength is best)—take 5 or more drops under the tongue as often as necessary, perhaps every few minutes. Also, take 5 to 10 drops in juice or water every hour or two. Important note: pour the SuperStrength liberally on wound.
- Purely-C—take 3 capsules every hour or two.
- oil of lavender (wild type)—add to wound and rub on surrounding skin, soles of feet, and buttocks.
- OregaBiotic multiple spice extract (natural antibiotic)—take 2 or 3 capsules frequently, even hourly.
- premium-grade royal jelly (Royal Power)—take 4 capsules several times daily.
- OregaMax capsules—take 3 or more capsules several times daily.
- uncoated bromelain plus papain (Infla-eez)—take 3 to 4 capsules several times daily, ideally on an empty stomach.
- Germ-a-CLENZ antiseptic spray—spray on any involved region as often as necessary.

Things to avoid

- refined sugar, soda pop, chocolate, and caffeine
- pain medications, especially aspirin and ibuprofen

Flu

Few people realize that influenza is the number one cause of death from infection in the United States. While other killers, such as Ebola, Hantavirus, and E. coli, seem to dominate the headlines, they are insignificant as a cause of disability and death in comparison. For instance, while Hantavirus killed 60 and E. coli approximately 10 in 1993 through 1994, the flu killed tens of thousands, some 60,000, in 1993 alone.

A national crisis from the flu virus is plausible. In 1999 the flu struck certain regions in the United States with exceptional ferocity, the East Coast bearing the brunt of the damage. Essentially, the entire state of Connecticut was disabled. Hospitals were overwhelmed, and admissions were halted. This was a modern-day medical catastrophe. Thus, the flu is the number one agent that must be derailed in the event of crisis.

The flu virus is a rather weak germ. It is highly vulnerable to natural antiseptics, particularly spice oils. The fact is oil of wild oregano, as well as oils of cumin, sage, garlic, and allspice, kills virtually all germs tested.

The antiviral powers of oregano were recently confirmed. A study performed by *Medical Science Research* (1996) determined that both RNA and DNA viruses were completely destroyed, that is the viruses were disintegrated, by oil of oregano. Recent research proved even more compelling. A study by Ingram and Ijaz, published in *Antiviral Research,* proved that a special combination of wild spice oils (i.e. Oregacyn) killed 100% of all cold viruses—even after the viruses infected living cells—within 20 minutes. Other studies by the researchers showed a 99 to 99.9% kill on various flu viruses, including influenza A and the Avian flu strain.

Oil of Oregano, as well as the multiple spice extracts, kills the flu virus. The fact is if such extracts are aggressively used, this virus can be destroyed. There are other antiviral oils, including oils of rosemary, bay leaf, cumin, and lavender. The virus-destroying powers of raw garlic and onion are also well published. Regarding the latter the raw forms are the most effective.

Flu combat kit

- oil of oregano (Oreganol P73) use SuperStrength for tougher cases)—take 3 or more drops under the tongue as often as

possible, perhaps every few minutes. Also, take 5 to 10 drops three times daily in juice or water.
- Oregacyn respiratory capsules—take 2 or more capsules several times daily.
- OregaBiotic natural antibiotic capsules—take 2 or more capsules as often as needed.
- Oreganol P73 Juice—for strength and stamina, take a half ounce as often as needed.
- Purely-C—take 2 or more capsules every few hours.
- oil of rosemary—rub on face, neck, chest, and soles of feet.
- Kid-e-Kare rubbing oil—rub all over the body as often as needed, especially the forehead, spine, and soles of the feet.
- Kid-e-Kare cold/flu gelcaps—use this form for children, 1 or more gelcaps as often as needed.
- Kid-e-Kare wild cherry throat spray—ideal for infants and children, spray on the back of the throat as often as possible.
- Garlex oil of cold-pressed garlic—10 or more drops under the tongue as often as necessary.

Foods that help
- hot meat-based broths with onion and garlic
- tangerine, grapefruit, and/or tomato juice
- anything high in vitamin A, like organic liver, salmon, sardines, etc.

Things to avoid
- chocolate and refined sugar (impede the immune response)
- soda pop and other sugary drinks as well as milk products

Food poisoning (see also individual illnesses)

Food poisoning develops when the individual consumes food or beverages which are either infected with or contaminated by microbes. It is the most common cause of sudden illness globally. Every day, hundreds of thousands of Americans contract food poisoning, largely from eating outside the home. In other words, restaurant, catered, institutional, and picnic food is the source of the majority of cases of food-related illness. The individual may become ill in the home, but this is much less common as a source of severe food-borne illness, that is compared to eating out.

According to the *Associated Press* when food poisoning outbreaks occur on a large scale, there is no way to warn everyone. In one instance it was discovered early in the crisis that commercial ice cream was heavily contaminated with Salmonella. Despite the warnings on national TV several thousand individuals became ill. Thus, the government cannot completely protect the public in the event of an epidemic. Yet, protection can be found in wild spices, like oil of oregano, oil of edible cinnamon, and oil of cilantro/coriander, which pack enormous antiseptic powers. Such protection can be achieved by taking a multiple spice capsule such as OregaBiotic (or Oregacyn). The OregaBiotic is a general natural antibiotic, while the Oregacyn is geared more for respiratory disorders.

No one is immune from this epidemic. Even healthy eaters and vegetarians are vulnerable. *Family Practice News* reported that organic vegetables which were not carefully washed caused an E. coli epidemic, which lead to the death of a child. A similar epidemic involving commercial red lettuce lead to the death of 25 people in Illinois. According to the CDC in 1996 alone some 20,000 Americans were sickened from Salmonella/E. coli-tainted alfalfa/radish sprouts.

Bacteria are only one component of this crisis. The role played by parasites may be even greater. Parasites are larger organisms than bacteria, and include worms, flukes, amoebas, and protozoa. In the United States a wide range of parasites may be contracted from food, causing diarrheal diseases. Incredibly, one researcher described a rate of parasitic infections in U.S.

citizens as high as 74%. The majority of these germs were likely contracted by eating contaminated food or drink. Foods commonly infested with parasites include raw meat, raw fish (sushi), vegetables, and fruit.

To minimize the risks, be sure to carefully wash and/or peel all fruits and vegetables and avoid the consumption of raw meat. Use also antiseptic sprays for preparing food. Made from edible spice oils such sprays may be misted directly on suspect food.

Food poisoning combat kit

- oil of oregano—2 or more drops under the tongue repeatedly until symptoms abate. Also, take 5 to 10 drops (or more) twice daily in juice or water.
- HerbSorb crushed Eastern herbal formula; take 2 capsules several times daily.
- OregaBiotic capsules—take 2 or more capsules several times daily or as much as is needed to halt the symptoms.
- raw honey—1/4 cup two or three times daily.
- Lactobacillus acidophilus and bifidus (i. e. Health Bac)—take 1/2 teaspoon as often as needed.
- oil of cilantro/coriander—add to food freely as needed.
- Germ-a-CLENZ antiseptic spray—as a preventive spray on all food; use as a food soak, a teaspoonful in a half gallon of water.
- Garlex oil of cold-pressed garlic—five or more drops as needed.

Foods that help

- vinegar
- horseradish
- raw garlic
- cilantro/coriander (or Oil of Cilantro-plus)

Fractures

Little can be done by the lay person for this condition. It requires immediate medical care. Only rarely would the general public be called upon to assist in care. However, in the event that medical care is not accessible, utilize the following home remedies:

Fracture combat kit

- bromelain/papain combination (i. e. Infla-eez)—take 3 capsules three or more times daily on an empty stomach.
- oil of oregano—anti-pain, anti-inflammation. Take 10 drops three times daily. Rub topically as needed. The SuperStrength is ideal.
- OregaMax wild oregano capsules—rich in naturally occurring calcium, magnesium, zinc, and phosphorus, it provides nutrients for bone healing. Large amounts must be taken such as 12 capsules daily. Works well as a calcium supplement.
- Royal Power—high grade royal jelly helps combat stress and speed healing.
- zinc—this nutrient speeds the healing of any wound; take at least 75 mg daily.
- silica—organically bound silica speeds the healing of bone injuries.

Note: Individuals with severe fractures must be kept still. If the individual must be moved, make a splint to immobilize the involved region as much as possible to prevent further damage.

Things to avoid

- caffeine and refined sugar, both of which deplete trace minerals
- diuretic drugs (also cause the urinary loss of minerals)

Frostbite

This is one of the most dangerous of all tissue injuries. It is caused by a sudden collapse of the small blood vessels, which supply the skin and soft tissues. When the tissues are frozen by exposure to extreme cold, blood flow is curtailed. Thus, there is no oxygen delivery to the tissues. This leads to death of the involved tissues, known as gangrene.

Frostbite is largely preventable. Proper clothing is essential. The individual must realize that metal is the coldest substance, because it retains cold energy. Thus, touching cold metal with bare skin is one of the easiest ways to get frostbite.

Hot, tangy herbs/spices are highly protective against the cold, because they help the body produce and dissipate heat. Thus, the key to preventing and treating this condition is to accelerate the heat index of the blood. This is a novel concept, wherein the metabolic rate and blood flow are increased so that the body and the blood are highly resistant to cold. Certain trace minerals are particularly effective in accelerating metabolism, notably magnesium and potassium. Spices are top sources of these minerals. Plus, hot spices contain substances, notably the flavonoids and phenols, that accelerate blood flow. To protect yourself against the cold eat hot, spicy food.

Frostbite combat kit

- aloe vera—apply to the frostbite region; use it straight from the plant.
- oil of oregano—apply liberally as often as possible; also, take a few drops under the tongue often.
- oil of rosemary—apply to the frostbite region, and take 10 drops twice daily in juice or water.
- pantothenic acid—take 500 mg every few hours to help induce healing.
- raw honey—apply to the frostbite region.

- cayenne pepper—for prevention, add to shoes or inside gloves (the same can be accomplished with oil of oregano).
- Oreganol cream—rub as needed to speed healing.
- salt; add a half teaspoon in 12 ounces of water and sip (helps improve the pumping power of the heart, aiding blood flow).
- bromelain and papain (as Infla-eez)—take 4 capsules three or more times daily on an empty stomach.
- Essence of Sage and/or Essence of Neroli Orange—add to hot water and drink as a tea; drink several cups daily.

Foods that help

- *Taber's Medical Dictionary* advises to drink beef broth instead of pop or juice.
- plenty of hot herbal teas (sage tea is the best)

Things to avoid

- candy, sweets, and sugary drinks
- caffeine, chocolate, soda pop (caffeine and cocoa's theobromines impair circulation to the extremities)

Gallbladder attack

No one can imagine the dilemma of suffering a gallbladder attack without medical help. Yet, not every attack needs to result in gallbladder surgery.

Individuals with gallbladder problems are making a grave error by avoiding the consumption of fat. The gallbladder thrives on it. Without it, the organ degenerates. As reported in *Medical Tribune,* March 1993, low fat diets place individuals at "substantial risk of developing gallstones." The authors note that fat causes the gallbladder to "fully contract", in other words, it totally empties, which is the main way to prevent gallstones.

How to combat gallstones and gallbladder attacks:

- extra virgin olive oil—drink a quarter cup with a few tablespoons of vinegar two or three times daily; this should purge the gallbladder of stones and, thus, halt the attacks.
- LivaClenz—take 10 or more drops added into each olive oil purge (stimulates bile formation and aids in stone dissolution). Then, take 10 to 20 drops daily on a regular basis.
- GreensFlush—causes the flushing of bile through the liver and gallbladder, 20 or more drops twice daily (this may also be added to the olive oil purge or can be taken separately).
- HerbSorb—take 2 or more capsules with each meal.
- Nutri-Sense protein/lecithin drink mix (contains fatty acids and lecithin, which help dissolve stones)—take 3 heaping tablespoons in the morning in juice or water.

Foods that help

- avocados, Greek-style olives, and extra virgin olive oil
- vinegar
- fresh beef and/or lamb, fat included
- fresh calves' or lamb's liver, organic

Things to avoid

- eggs (in allergic individuals yolk may incite a gallbladder attack)
- white bread, white rice, refined sugar, sweets, soda pop
- fried food and/or margarine
- bakery items, sweet rolls, and/or cookies
- apples and apple juice

Genital herpes

It is estimated that a minimum of one fifth of all Americans suffer from this infection. In individuals under 30 years of age perhaps one in three have it. This may account for the recent estimation that as many as 56 million Americans harbor the germ. Thus, this viral infection is an epidemic of enormous proportions.

The herpes virus has a predilection for infecting the genitals, largely because of the rich supply of blood and nerves in this region. The virus may reside in blood vessels, within human cells, and in the nerves, while failing to cause obvious symptoms. The fact is the virus preferentially lives in the nerves, specifically the tiny condensations of nerve bodies known as *ganglia*. There are dozens of ganglia in the nerves of the pelvis buried deep in the low back, buttocks, sacral region, and inner pelvis. The virus hides there, only to resurface after traveling down the nerves to the skin and mucous membranes of the genitals as well as on the buttocks. It may also erupt on the sacrum. The infection is incited by stress, cortisone intake, high amounts of chocolate/sugar, and vitamin deficiency. However, the most common cause is merely exposure: contracting the infection from an infected individual through sexual intercourse.

Genital herpes combat kit

- oil of oregano (P73)—dilute as follows: add 5 drops into a tablespoon of olive oil and apply directly to involved regions. Also, fill gelatin capsules and take 2 or 3 capsules twice daily.
- oil of myrtle—apply to involved region as often as necessary.
- OregaMax capsules—take 3 capsules twice daily.
- Infla-eez (to eliminate inflammation and improve blood flow)—take 3 capsules twice daily on an empty stomach.
- oil of propolis (i. e. PropaHeal)—take 10 drops twice daily in juice or water. Also, apply to any suspect lesion. Note: the PropaHeal is highly effective in eliminating pain and swelling. Propolis is a potent antiviral agent, and the PropaHeal is significantly more powerful than commercial propolis extracts.

Things to avoid
- chocolate especially (the high arginine content of this food stimulates the growth of herpes viruses)
- nuts, especially peanuts (high in arginine)
- infected humans

Giardia and/or Cryptosporidium infection

This is already an epidemic. According to *American Family Physician*, February 1998, in 1984 there were just six proven outbreaks of Giardia infection, i. e. giardiasis. In 1993-94 there were 34 outbreaks. In 1998 there were over 100. The infection usually occurs in the summer, but in children attending day care centers it may occur continuously.

Giardiasis is caused by a parasite, an organism larger and more difficult to kill than a bacteria. Contaminated water or contact with animal/human feces is the usual instigator. Campers and outdoors buffs frequently contract it from drinking untreated "natural" water from lakes and/or streams.

Giardia has a predilection for infecting the intestines, specifically the upper part of the duodenum. Thus, it may produce symptoms typical of a stomach ulcer. Symptoms of Giardia infection include:

- foul smelling sloppy stools
- diarrhea
- bloating
- flatulence, which is foul smelling (like rotten eggs)
- constant belching, especially in the morning
- nausea
- weight loss and lack of appetite

Giardia readily infests the gut, preferring the upper part of the small intestine and lower stomach. It may also infect the colon.

The organism causes massive damage, leading to poor digestion and absorption. This is why weight loss, exhaustion, abnormal stools, and malabsorption of nutrients is so common in chronic Giardia infection.

A recent study demonstrated the powers of spice oils, particularly oil of wild oregano, in the destruction of parasites. Through culture a number of parasites were found in the bowels of test subjects. The oil of oregano was administered. Then, the bowel was re-cultured. All parasites were killed. What's more, Mexican investigators determined that wild oregano in small concentrates killed giardia.

Cryptosporidium, another water-based protozoan, causes a similar infection. The ultimate source is apparently sewage runoff from farm animals. This germ may aggressively attack the sick, weak, or immune compromised and may cause death.

Giardia/Cryptosporidium combat kit

- oil of oregano—take 10 or more drops three times daily in juice or water.
- OregaMax—take 3 capsules twice daily.
- raw garlic—eat 2 or more cloves daily.
- Black Seed-plus—take 3 or more capsules three times daily.
- Infla-eez—take 2 or more capsules twice daily on an empty stomach. This enzyme will help kill the parasites. Combine with a handful of raw pumpkin seeds.
- Intesti-Clenz—a special combination of spice oils for killing parasites, 10 drops twice daily.

Headaches

There are hundreds of causes for headaches. However, the major factors are food intolerance and hormonal disturbances. These subjects are covered in great detail in my book, *Natural Cures for Headaches.* The book helps the individual discover the cause of his/her headaches. Then, it describes precisely how to eliminate them. The critical role of food allergies, structural defects, and hormonal disturbances in migraines is emphasized and explained.

Headache combat kit
- ginger root—slice the fresh root and immerse in hot water as a tea.
- Migraten capsules—special spice extract and herbal capsules, which help reverse migraines and other headaches. Take 2 capsules every hour to halt the attack. Also, take 2 capsules daily as a preventive.
- oil of oregano—rub on painful regions, forehead, temples, and/or sinus region. Take 1 or 2 drops under the tongue twice daily.
- oil of lavender—rub on forehead, chest, and soles of feet; take 2 drops under the tongue 3 or more times daily.
- Royal Power premium royal jelly plus herbs—to regenerate adrenal gland function, take 4 to 6 capsules every morning.
- Thyroset—to boost or normalize thyroid function take 2 or more capsules twice daily.
- *Neuroloft (with* wild St. John's wort wild rosemary)—take 2 or more caps at onset; continue taking 1 or more every hour or so until resolved.
- GreensFlush wild greens drops—one of the most potent migraine-reversing remedies, a few drops under the tongue as often as needed.

Things to avoid
- candy, chocolate, soda, sweet rolls, donuts, and cookies
- wine and beer
- wheat, corn, malt, and citrus fruit

Heart attack

A heart attack in the field is very difficult to combat for the lay person. First, how does the individual who is observing the event know for sure it is a heart attack? True, there are instances where it is completely obvious. Yet, often even doctors may be confused by the symptoms and may misdiagnose it as "indigestion" or "stress." Since stress is perhaps the main cause of heart attacks, remedies which combat stress, such as royal jelly and wild rosemary, are ideal.

There are certain telltale signs of heart attacks that hold true in 90% of the instances. An individual may have one or, usually, several of these signs. These signs/symptoms include:

- sudden episode of severe chest pain over heart on the left chest
- sudden severe pain in the jaw
- left-sided chest pain which runs down the left arm
- nausea
- vague indigestion sensations, usually in the upper abdomen, that can't be relieved
- left shoulder pain
- occasionally, right-sided chest pain
- pale complexion and cold sweat (clammy)

Obviously, if such symptoms develop, seek medical care immediately. If such care is unavailable, combat it with the following home remedies:

Heart attack combat kit

- Resvital—1/2 teaspoon under the tongue as often as possible, or two capsules several times daily.
- fresh onion juice (from yellow onions)—take only a Tbls at a time. Give every hour, if tolerated. Rub onion juice on the chest. Onion juice contains substances that help dissolve blood clots.

- oil of rosemary—take 10 to 20 drops twice daily.
- oil of oregano (P73)—take 5 drops under the tongue twice daily. Rub on chest and over heart reflexes as an aromatic rejuvenator.
- OregaMax capsules—take 3 or more capsules twice daily.
- Thyroset—take 3 or more capsules twice daily.
- Royal Power premium royal jelly—take 2 to 4 capsules several times daily.
- Oreganol P73 Juice—a critical agent, take 1/2 oz. or more twice daily. For those in critical condition sip on small amounts as often as possible: helps strengthen the heart muscle.
- Infla-eez—antiinflammatory enzymes, take 2 capsules on an empty stomach as often as possible.

Things to avoid
- Fear: heart attack victims are tense and scared. Attempt to soothe them. Don't add to their fears.
- caffeine, colas, iced tea, and sugary juices
- wine or other alcoholic beverages

Heart failure

In this condition the heart is unable to pump blood fast enough to prevent it from backing up into the venous system. First the lungs fill up with fluid. Then, the fluids overflow into the remaining tissues. The individual becomes essentially waterlogged.

Heart failure combat kit
- raw honey—take as much as 1/2 cup three times daily.
- oil of cilantro plus coriander—take 10 to 20 drops twice daily.
- coenzyme Q-10—take 200 mg daily.
- Infla-eez—take 2 capsules several times daily.

- magnesium chelate—take 800 to 1000 mg daily.
- vitamin E—crude natural source only, i. e. the Pumpkinol, four tablespoons daily.
- HerbSorb—take 4 or more capsules three times daily.
- oil of oregano—take 5 or more drops under the tongue 3x daily.
- Oreganol P73 Juice—one ounce twice or more daily.
- Resvital powder—1/2 teaspoon as often as possible.
- CranFlush natural diuretic—20 drops three times daily.

Foods that help
- cooked beef hearts
- avocados, olives, extra virgin olive oil

Things to avoid
- caffeine, chocolate, refined sugar, and soda pop
- processed meats (i.e. those containing nitrates)

Heat exhaustion/stroke

Heat can destroy anyone. The young and old, healthy and strong all can be decimated by it.

Being exposed to an excess of summer heat can lead to a variety of illnesses. Usually, heat causes relatively minor discomforts such as dizziness, fainting, muscle cramps, swelling, sunburn, and exhaustion. However, in certain individuals the excess heat can kill.

Heat exhaustion is largely the result of heat-induced sweating, which depletes the body of water and electrolytes. The loss of fluid and/or its evaporation from the skin disrupts the body's normal cooling mechanism, which is entirely dependent upon the volume of the body fluids. As a result, the body core temperature may rise suddenly. Fortunately, most individuals become noticeably sick and attempt to shelter themselves from the heat. Typical symptoms include dizziness, weakness, malaise, nausea, vomiting, rapid heart rate, and headache.

Some individuals don't sweat much even when exposed to extreme heat. In fact, the hotter their bodies become the less they sweat. This is a dangerous circumstance, because, without sweating, there is no way to dissipate heat. The heat becomes trapped within the body, leading to physical collapse and, in the extreme, heat exhaustion or stroke. Such heat vulnerable individuals suffer from a bizarre but common condition known as adrenal insufficiency. The fact is lack of sweating is a warning of adrenal failure.

Heatstroke is the more extreme version of heat exhaustion. It is always a medical emergency. The elderly and individuals with chronic disease are at the highest risk. When the body loses its ability to dissipate heat, the body temperature rises suddenly. Sweating virtually stops. Literally, the individuals boil to death. Often, such individuals collapse and nothing can seemingly be done to revive them.

If heatstroke develops, medical help must be summoned immediately. The objective is to reduce the body temperature through any means possible. If such help is unavailable, the following steps may prove lifesaving:

- get the individual out of the sun.
- fan the body aggressively.
- apply cool water, ice packs, wet sheets, etc. Cool water and the application of water cooled cloths is preferable to ice.
- if a shower can be accessed, spray the shower water in the finest mist possible over the individual at a temperature of about 60 degrees Fahrenheit.

Note: be aware that aggressive attempts to cool the individual may lead to further shock. To avoid this massage the body vigorously with essential oils, particularly the spine, legs, buttocks, and feet. However, remember, this is a medical emergency, so seek professional help urgently. Do not attempt to treat this condition on your own unless there is no other option.

Heat exhaustion combat kit

- Royal Power premium-grade royal jelly—take 4 capsules every hour or as necessary until the condition improves.
- red grape powder (Resvital)—take 4 capsules two or more times daily. Or, place the powder in the mouth and melt with saliva, which releases the nourishment from the extract.
- Purely-C—3 to 4 capsules immediately, then 1 or 2 capsules every hour with mineral water.
- oil of lavender—rub on face, spine, and chest.
- oil of sage or rosemary—rub on feet and spine.
- Royal Oil premium-grade liquid royal jelly—take a teaspoon or more daily.

Heatstroke combat kit

- oil of lavender—rub on spine, face, under nose, and chest.
- oil of sage—rub on soles of the feet and spine.
- oil of rosemary—rub over spine and adrenal reflex (mid lower back).
- Royal Power (if the individual can swallow)—2 or more capsules every hour with mineral water.
- red grape powder (Resvital)—2 or more capsules every hour with mineral water. Or, place the powder in the mouth and allow to melt.
- Purely-C—4 capsules immediately, then 2 or more capsules every hour with mineral water.
- Hercules Strength caps—take 3 or more caps three times daily.
- Royal Oil premium-grade liquid royal jelly—take a teaspoon or more daily.

Foods that help

- sea salt (add a teaspoon of salt to 12 ounces of water and sip)
- watermelon, salted with sea salt
- cucumbers, salted with sea salt
- radishes and turnips, salted with sea salt

Things to avoid

- completely avoid all sugar-sweetened drinks and caffeinated beverages.
- strictly avoid artificially sweetened foods or beverages.
- avoid all alcoholic beverages.

Hemorrhoids

This is due to pressure on the delicate veins of the lower rectum. It is frequently caused by constipation, although infection and nutritional deficiency are often involved. Vitamin C, bioflavonoids, vitamin K, folic acid, and vitamin E are usually lacking. However, a lack of fiber is the greatest nutritional deficit. Remember, hemorrhoids are veins. Thus, substances which nourish the venous tissues are invaluable for preventing, as well as eradicating, this condition.

Hemorrhoid combat kit

- Nutri-Sense (as a source of soluble fiber and bowel softening lignins)—take 3 heaping tablespoons daily.
- Purely-C (as a source of crude vitamin C and flavonoids)—take 3 capsules three times daily.
- Infla-eez—take 3 capsules on an empty stomach twice daily.
- oil of bay berry—apply topically for shrinkage.
- oil of myrtle—apply this flavonoid-rich oil directly on the hemorrhoids.
- OregaMax capsules—take 2 or 3 capsules three times daily.

Foods that help

- water; be sure to drink at least 6 large glasses daily
- papaya and kiwi
- tangerines, apricots, and blueberries

Things to avoid

- refined sugar, soda pop, and candy
- white flour, bread, and white rice

Hepatitis

This is defined as inflammation of the liver. It is a destructive inflammation, leading to the death of liver cells. If untreated, the liver tissues become scarred. This is known as cirrhosis.

There are dozens of causes for the inflammation. The main ones include alcohol excess, drug abuse, prescription drugs, nonprescription drugs, as well as a wide range of germs. Primarily, viruses are the causative germs, but a variety of parasites, as well as fungi and bacteria, may cause it.

Hepatitis, particularly the viral type, is currently an American, as well as global, epidemic. As many as a half million Americans are newly infected every year. It's virtually like a viral flu of the liver in terms of incidence as well as severity. Public health officials seem puzzled as to why so many Americans are developing hepatitis. It is not so complex. The hepatitis viruses and parasites are contracted through contamination, whether through blood, filth, secretions, or sexual contact. In other words, close contact with human fluids, excretions, or secretions is virtually a prerequisite for the development of this disease. Another possibility is if human waste contaminates food or water. This is an indirect means of contracting this dreaded disease. Yet, ultimately, it is human waste that is causing it. Blood transfusions, as well as contact with blood, are a major source for contracting this disease.

Hundreds of outbreaks of hepatitis occur in the United States every year. Yet, frequently, the source is never determined.

There are perhaps a dozen or more strains of hepatitis, with new ones seemingly discovered yearly. Hepatitis A is perhaps the most commonly occurring type globally. Recently, in the United States outbreaks have been traced to imported frozen fruit, particularly strawberries from Mexico.

Hepatitis C has recently become the most dominating type, accounting for the majority of new cases. The fact is the infection is an epidemic in America. It is a hidden infection, presenting initially with relatively mild symptoms and then smoldering within the body, causing prolonged infection and, therefore, tissue damage. The infection may have existed 5 to 10 years or longer before it is diagnosed. This may explain why there are as many as 5 million Americans infected with this virus. However, evidence of it may be discovered early, especially if it develops after blood transfusions, a major source for the infection. Yet, blood transfusions are not the only source. Recent evidence indicates that it is readily transmitted sexually and if an individual has the virus, there is a least a 15% chance of contracting it from such an individual. Yet, contact with blood products or secretions remains a major risk factor. It may also be eventually proven that contaminated food and water may spread the infection.

A clinical trial by North American Herb & Spice Co. has been completed for this disease, strictly using natural substances. In this case three main formulas, the Oreganol, Oregacyn Liver, and GreensFlush wild greens, were used. The results were highly positive, with improvement in 18 of 20 patients and a virtual complete cure in the majority. In the majority viral titers declined by some 90%—and in some instances virtually 100%—while liver function largely returned to normal. There were no toxic effects of such medications.

Hepatitis combat kit

- oil of oregano (SuperStrength may be necessary) — 5 to 10 drops under the tongue several times daily. Also, take 5 to 10 drops in juice or water twice daily.
- LivaClenz—take 20 drops twice daily in juice or water.
- GreensFlush wild greens formula—take 40 drops under the tongue twice daily.
- oil of cilantro plus coriander—take 10 or more drops daily.
- Oregacyn Liver—take 3 or more capsules with every meal.
- Infla-eez (to aid in digestion and reduce inflammation)—take 2 or 3 capsules with meals.

Foods that help

- sardines and salmon
- artichokes and beets
- radishes and turnips (black or Russian radish is best)

Things to avoid

- alcohol and all drugs, herbal preparations, etc. containing it
- refined sugar, white flour, white rice, corn sweeteners
- prescription and nonprescription drugs of all types (except interferon)

Herbicide poisoning (see Pesticide/herbicide poisoning)

Herpes (see Cold sores, Genital herpes, Shingles)

High blood pressure attack

High blood pressure, known medically as hypertension, is a common disease, but only in Westernized countries. Diet is a major factor in the cause of this disease. In other words, what an individual eats and drinks is directly related to creating high blood pressure. While the role of diet is immense, the primary cause is a mere beverage: alcohol. In my clinic fully 40% of all high blood pressure patients were social, or, more rarely, heavy drinkers. Complete removal of the alcohol caused the blood pressure to normalize rapidly. Dietary causes, as well as stress, were the major factors in the remaining patients. In this regard the major cause was the excessive consumption of caffeinated soft drinks. Yet, contrary to popular belief, fat is not the major culprit in the diet: it is sugar. Greater details of the role of diet, toxins, and infections in the cause of high blood pressure are found in Dr. Ingram's new book, *Natural Cures for High Blood Pressure*.

High blood pressure combat kit

- oil of rosemary—take 10 to 20 drops twice daily. For extremely high blood pressure, take 20 drops three times daily or take 5 drops under the tongue every hour.
- CranFlush—take 20 drops twice daily.
- oil of lavender—rub on face and chest at night for relaxation. Add to atomizer or diffuser. Take 2 drops under the tongue twice daily.
- red grape powder (Resvital)—take 4 capsules three times daily or more often if necessary. Resvital is entirely safe to take in large quantities.
- oil of wild oregano (Oreganol P73)—take 2 or more drops under the tongue twice daily.

Note: oil of oregano is a strong tonic for the heart. If under doctor's care for high blood pressure, especially in extreme cases, seek a doctor's advice before using. Even so, the oil helps cleanse the blood of pathogens, and so is invaluable for reversing this disorder. This is a safe spice, and, thus, it cannot cause any harm. The fact is in many individuals the regular intake of the Oreganol causes a decline in blood pressure, in fact its eradication.

- Sesam-E—a potent substance to normalize blood pressure, take 1 tablespoon twice daily.

Foods that help
- sardines, salmon, halibut, and/or herring

Things to avoid
- alcohol: absolutely none should be consumed
- refined sugar and all sweets, particularly soda pop

Hip pain

Sudden hip pain in women over 50 may be an ominous sign. It may signal a fracture of the hip.

Hip pain usually results from injury. In women it may be caused by bone loss, that is osteoporosis. Hip pain may be caused by strain in the lower back, which leads to a type of referred pain to the hip. In this instance the lower back must also be treated. A strained knee may also induce hip pain.

Sudden severe hip, knee, or back pain may all warn of fractures, particularly in women over 40. Such fractures may occur without trauma. In other words, the bones simply crack.

Hip pain/fracture combat kit
- oil of oregano (i. e. Oreganol P73)—take 5 to 10 drops two or three times daily in juice or water and take 2 or 3 drops under the tongue several times daily or to tolerance. Rub the oil on the involved region twice or more daily.
- Infla-eez antiinflammatory formula—2 or more capsules as often as needed on an empty stomach.
- vitamin D (as cod liver or halibut oil caps) — 6,000 I.U. daily
- OregaMax (as a source of crude natural calcium and magnesium) —take 9 or more capsules daily; works as well as calcium pills.

- red grape powder (i. e. Resvital)—take one teaspoon three times daily.

Things to avoid

- large amounts of aspirin, ibuprofen, or acetaminophen
- Don't sleep on the stomach or back; sleep on the side instead

Other ideas: an expert in structural therapy might help ease the pain, that is a well trained D.O., chiropractor, acupuncturist, or body worker.

Histoplasmosis

This is a fungal infection primarily of the lungs. However, the germ often attacks the entire body.

Histoplasmosis is the epidemic of river country. It should be called "River Fever." That is because the mold/fungus which causes this disease thrives in areas of constant moisture and is exceptionally prolific in the Ohio and Mississippi River valleys, where moderate temperatures encourage its growth. It is also common in the middle South and Appalachian regions in areas like Pennsylvania, Kentucky, Virginia, West Virginia, and Tennessee. This is a soil fungus that thrives in moderate climates with lots of moisture. Regions wherein there are large congregations of birds and, therefore, large amounts of bird droppings are to be treated warily. This is because bird droppings greatly accelerate the fungus's growth.

The primary signs and symptoms of histoplasmosis include fever of unknown cause (this fever may last for months), fatigue, low blood count, low white count, intestinal or stomach ulcers, and asthmatic symptoms. The fact is an individual in any of the aforementioned regions who develops persistent lung systems such as cough and wheezing should be considered infected by this disease until proven otherwise.

Histoplasmosis combat kit

- oil of oregano (P73)—take 5 or 10 drops under the tongue several times daily. Also, take 5 to 10 drops in juice or water twice daily.
- Oregacyn respiratory, three capsules twice daily and for extreme cases, three capsules three or four times daily.
- wild oregano herb (OregaMax capsules)—take 3 or more capsules twice daily.
- oil of rosemary—take 2 or 3 drops under the tongue twice daily; rub on chest or add to diffuser. Also, take 5 to 10 drops twice daily in juice/water.
- Oreganol P73 Juice—take 1/2 oz. twice daily; add to diffuser and volatilize.

Foods that help

- raw garlic and onion as well as green onions
- hot, tangy spicy soups

Things to avoid

- humidifiers and damp rooms
- refined sugar, sweets, chocolate
- wheat or other common grains (they are often mold contaminated)

Hives

This reddish skin lesion is far from an illness of the skin. Allergic toxicity is the primary cause of hives. Foods, chemicals, drugs, food additives, and perfumes all may induce hives. They may also be caused by infections. Here, the primary culprits are parasites. Yet, even in this instance the parasites produce noxious chemicals, which provoke the hives.

Hives are usually signified by bright red blotches occurring virtually anywhere on the body. They represent an abrupt inflammation in the small blood vessels that supply the skin.

The redness represents the extensive degree of inflammation and irritation which develops. It is obviously a toxic reaction to some substance, and this substance is usually something which is ingested, in other words, what we eat, breathe, and drink causes the majority of cases of hives. Infection represents the second major cause, and parasites, as well as fungi, are the primary players. Insect bites may also result in hives. However, drug reactions are the number one cause; this is even more important as a cause than food.

Hives combat kit

- oil of oregano (Oreganol 73)—use topically and internally, take liberally under the tongue and/or internally until lesions clear.
- wild oregano herb—either as OregaMax or Hercules Strength (the latter is useful in the event of allergy to onion or garlic); take 3 capsules three times daily.
- Royal Power premium-grade royal jelly (unless allergic to bee stings)—take 4 capsules every hour or two until condition clears.
- Oreganol Cream—rub on involved region, as often as possible
- Infla-eez antiinflammatory capsules—an ideal topical rub take 4 capsules twice daily.

Things to avoid

- citrus fruit, particularly oranges, lemons, and limes
- wheat, rye, corn, and barley
- chocolate
- apple juice

Hookworm

According to Peters and Gilles, authors of *A Colour Atlas of Tropical Medicine and Parasitology*, fully a quarter of the world's population, billions of individuals, are infected with hookworms. This is astonishing, since this parasite can only thrive in hot climates. However, much of the global population is concentrated in tropical and subtropical regions, where hookworm infestation is endemic. Likely countries/regions in which the infection is contracted include India, southern China, Malaysia, Indonesia, northeastern Australia, Japan, Southeast Asia, Italy, Sicily, northern Turkey, Egypt/North Africa, and Burma. Regarding the recent (2004) Indian Ocean tsunami hookworm infection will become pandemic; few physicians will make the diagnosis, since the symptoms are often vague. Individuals who must walk barefoot will readily develop the infection, particularly if there openings or wounds on the feet.

In the Americas the parasite is found in the soil of virtually all of South America (except Chili and Argentina) and most of Central America. However, travelers to these regions are also vulnerable. They may contract the infection, which leads to chronic health problems, such as digestive disorders, fatigue, heart disease, weight loss, and skin diseases. In the United States hookworm infests primarily the Southeast, notably Florida, the Carolinas, Georgia, Louisiana, Alabama, Mississippi, Tennessee, Arkansas, Missouri, and parts of Texas. However, there is a complicating factor that has led to more widespread infestation in the United States: dog hookworm. This worm is disseminated primarily by dog feces. It may or may not cause systemic disease. Often, infection is represented by localized creeping tracts usually on the feet. Symptoms of systemic hookworm infection include:

- exhaustion
- weak muscles
- shortness of breath
- swelling in the extremities
- swollen abdomen
- vague digestive problems

Hookworm destruction/combat kit

- Oreganol oil of wild oregano—take 10 or more drops three times daily in juice or water or if using Oreganol gelcaps, 3 or more caps twice daily.
- Intesti-Clenz—take 1 or more droppersful twice daily in juice or water.
- GreensFlush wild greens formula—to purge the bowel and liver in a natural way take 20 or more drops twice daily in juice or water.
- oil of fennel—the top anti-hookworm oil, take 2 or more droppersful twice daily.
- Garlex raw cold-pressed garlic oil—20 or more drops twice daily.

Foods that help

- spinach and watercress (wash well)
- papaya and kiwi (always eat the papaya seeds)
- fresh organic or grass-fed red meat (cooked no more than medium to replenish parasite-depleted blood)

Things to avoid

- raw meat or fish
- dog feces

Hot flashes

Hot flashes are regarded exclusively as a female problem. Now men are also suffering from them. The causes in men are unknown, although, like women, it is probably hormonal. In women the flashes are induced by an imbalance in hormone production. Specifically, it is believed that as women age they fail to produce sufficient amounts of estrogens, or the proper balance of hormones, resulting in a wide range of symptoms, including hot flashes, fatigue, mood swings, loss of libido, and depression.

Hot flashes combat kit

- Royal Power—4 capsules every morning or Royal Oil, 1-2 tsp.
- sage tea or oil of sage (edible type in olive oil)—drink the tea twice daily. Rub the oil on the mid-lower back (adrenal reflex).
- oil of fennel—10 drops twice daily in juice or water.
- Essence of Neroli Orange (or white coffee)—add one or two tablespoons in hot water as a tea, preferably at night after supper. Also, add to cold drinks if desired.
- Thyroset—to strengthen thyroid function, take 3 to 4 capsules twice daily.
- oil of myrtle (for improving sex drive and reversing vaginal dryness)—rub on vaginal tissue twice daily.
- EstroNorm multiple herbal formula—for balancing female hormones two capsules twice daily. This is a purely herbal and wild spice formula (plus kelp and royal jelly).

Things to avoid

- chocolate and refined sugar
- synthetic estrogens

Hypothermia (see Cold exposure)

Impetigo

This is perhaps the most contagious of all childhood bacterial infections. It is usually caused by staph or strep; in some instances, both of these germs are involved.

Usually, impetigo strikes the face, notably the cheeks and especially around the mouth and nose. When it develops about the mouth and nose, it is often confused with cold sores i.e. Herpes virus. It may also occur on the arms or legs. Typically, lesions form a pustule, which breaks, dumping germs. The germs readily spread and the contagion may strike anywhere on the body. It may also infect other individuals.

To avoid the rampant spread of this infection do not touch the skin or pustules with bare hands. If any lesions are touched, wash hands thoroughly with soap and hot water; add a few drops of oil of oregano to pump or bar soaps to aid in antisepsis.

Impetigo combat kit

- oil of oregano (the most important herbal therapy)—apply topically and take internally.
- raw honey—apply topically.
- OregaMax capsules—take 2 capsules every four hours.
- Oreganol cream—highly effective in healing any lesions. Apply topically to speed healing and minimize scarring, apply as needed.

Things to avoid

- don't allow children to keep long fingernails. The impetigo germs may be housed underneath them. Keep the fingernails clipped.
- raw honey, applied topically and taken internally

Influenza (see Flu)

Ingrown toenail

This seems like a minor problem. Yet, an ingrown toenail can become extremely painful and can also result in secondary infection. It is usually caused when the individual is too aggressive with clipping of the toenail. Always clip the nail in a straight line. Don't clip the corners aggressively, because, if you do, the nail may grow into the skin, causing severe pain, inflammation, and infection.

Ingrown toenail combat kit

- oil of oregano (SuperStrength is best)—apply vigorously into nail bed or surrounding area twice daily. Also take 5 to 10 drops under the tongue twice daily.

Insecticide poisoning (see pesticide/herbicide poisoning)

Insomnia

During a crisis it is essential for the individual to rest. Lack of sleep quickly devastates human health during adversity. A rested body and mind provide the strength necessary to survive.

Insomnia is frequently related to blood sugar disorders. When the blood sugar drops, the brain misfires, leading to an irritated state. High protein snacks eaten late at night balance the blood sugar mechanism. To help relax the nervous system use sedative essential oils such as oils of sage, oregano, and lavender.

Insomnia combat kit

- oil of oregano—rub on chest and neck at bedtime.
- Essence of Sage—add two tablespoons in hot water and drink as a late night tea.
- Oreganol P73 Juice—a natural sedative take 1/2 oz. twice daily; take right before bedtime. This is particularly effective if there is restlessness or spastic muscles.
- oil of lavender—rub on chest and neck at bedtime. Add to a diffuser or atomizer.
- oil of sage—take a few drops in hot water or rub on feet or back.
- wild strawberry leaves and borage flowers (a natural sedative) —drink a cup of hot Wild Power Tea before bedtime. Add whole milk and wild oregano honey, if desired.
- Royal Oil emulsified/fortified fresh royal jelly—a half teaspoon twice daily.

Foods that help

- salted roasted nuts, especially if eaten at bedtime

- salted turkey meat (sugar free), eat at bedtime
- full fat cheese, eat at bedtime
- sweets, especially late at night

Itchy skin/scalp (see also Hives)

There are four common causes of itchy skin: contact with poisonous plants, allergic reactions to drugs or other chemicals, allergic reactions to foods, and fungal infections. Thus, the cause should be relatively easy to determine. Fungal infections may result in itchy skin, because fungi secrete poisons, which cause inflammation and, therefore, itching.

Itchy skin/scalp combat kit

- oil of oregano—this is the mainstay; rub on any itchy region. Also, take 2 drops under the tongue as often as necessary.

Note: fungal organisms, like *Candida albicans* and tinea, can cause itchy skin by secreting poisons, which cause inflammation and therefore itching. Oil of oregano is antifungal.

- tea tree oil—use as needed, topically only.
- Scalp Clenz (a tremendous cleanser for sensitive or itchy skin)—rub into the scalp and add liberally to shampoos.
- oil of myrtle—soothing for topical application; especially useful for itchy vaginitis.

Foods that help

- beets and beet juice (include beet tops, if possible)
- radishes, especially Russian or black radishes
- olive oil and vinegar (stimulates the flow of bile)

Things to avoid

- all drugs, including antihistamines and antibiotics

- alcohol of all types, including the use of alcohol as a base material
- lye-based soaps and perfumes
- refined sugar (increases the growth of fungi)
- jewelry containing nickel

Jaundice

This is caused by liver damage. The damage is induced primarily by toxic chemicals and/or germs. Major causes of jaundice include alcohol abuse, drug abuse, prescription drug reactions, and viral hepatitis. The condition is manifested by the accumulation of bile pigments, i.e. bilirubin, in the skin as well as the whites of the eyes. Severe jaundice is an indication of massive liver damage. This is usually due to a virus, although parasitic infections may also cause it. Of course, alcohol is the major cause of jaundice.

Jaundice combat kit

- oil of cumin (a potent antioxidant for the liver)–take 20 drops twice daily in juice or water.
- oil of rosemary (purges the liver of poisons and bile)—take the same as above.
- LivaClenz (a multi-edible essential oil formula for regenerating liver function and increasing glutathione synthesis)—take 10 or more drops three times daily.
- beet juice tablets or powder—take several tablets or a teaspoon three times daily.
- oil of oregano (especially valuable in the event of infection)—take 5 drops twice daily.

Foods that help

- beets and beet tops, ideally gently cooked
- radishes of all types, especially black/Russian radish

Jock itch (see Athlete's foot)

Joint pain

Joint pain may be a manifestation of a severe disease, or it may be due to injury. It may also warn of infection. This is especially true when it afflicts one joint only. Bacterial infection often causes pain in an isolated joint. However, parasitic infestation, particularly by amoebas, may cause pain in multiple joints. For instance, rheumatoid arthritis is believed to be due to a systemic amoebic infection. Single joint pain, like knee pain, may also warn of Lyme disease.

Joint pain combat kit

- oil of oregano—rub on involved region; take 2 or more drops under the tongue twice daily. Also, take 5 to 10 drops in juice or water twice daily.
- Infla-eez oil—rub several drops twice daily on the involved region.
- Infla-eez capsules—take 2 or more capsules twice daily on an empty stomach.
- Purely-C all natural vitamin C—take 4 capsules twice daily.

Kidney infection

This is usually caused by bacterial infection, although yeast and parasitic infections are increasingly involved. These infections are particularly common in young children, especially girls. The elderly are also highly vulnerable. Kidney infections frequently develop as a consequence of prolonged surgeries, which require the placement of urinary catheters. The yeast Candida albicans is the most notorious culprit in post-surgical kidney infections. Kidney infections which fail to improve despite repeated antibiotic therapy are likely due to yeast infestation. The yeasts thrive in the kidneys and may provoke repeated bladder infections; they may also cause bladder and vaginal yeast infections. The health dramatically improves when the kidneys are sterilized of all invaders.

Kidney infection combat kit
- oil of oregano—take 3 drops under the tongue three times daily. Also, take 10 to 20 drops in juice or water three times daily.
- red grape powder (Resvital)—take 4 capsules three times daily. For severe infections double this amount (for bulk consumption, take three or more heaping teaspoons daily. This is safe to take in large amounts, because it is a food-like substance).
- CranFlush wild cranberry extract—20 or more drops twice daily.
- Wild Power Tea (natural diuretic for aiding stronger urination)—drink 2 or more cups daily.
- OregaBiotic—2 or more capsules twice daily.

Foods that help
- cranberry, as a juice or extract—take often, as much as desired.
- Pomegranate Syrup—add a tablespoon to ice water and drink twice daily.

Kidney stones

This is a disaster of major significance regardless of the circumstances. The pain of kidney stones is one of the most gruesome of all types of organ pain.

Repeated kidney stones are a sign of chronic infection. When germs infect the kidneys, they cause inflammation, and this leads to stone formation. The usual culprits are bacteria and fungi. Nutritional deficiency is another major factor. A lack of magnesium, potassium, pyridoxine, vitamin C, and even calcium may play a role. Vitamin D deficiency is also a factor, since this substance controls calcium metabolism and most stones are made of calcium. However, vitamin A deficiency is the primary factor inducing kidney stones. Chronic kidney stone formation nearly always warns of a severe vitamin A deficiency.

Kidney stones combat kit
- red grape powder (Resvital)—take 4 capsules three times daily and if using the powder, one or two teaspoons twice daily.
- oil of fennel—take 20 drops three times daily.
- OregaMax capsules—take 6 or more capsules daily.
- CranFlush wild cranberry extract—take one or two droppersful three times daily.
- Purely-C—take 6 or more capsules daily.
- oil of wild oregano—5 drops twice daily.

Foods that help
- Pomegranate Syrup—mix a tablespoon in ice or sparkling water, and drink twice daily.
- organic calves' or lamb's liver (as a source of vitamin A)—eat a pound per week.
- cranberry (either concentrate or extract)—use as much as possible.
- parsley—chew on a bunch daily; or, make parsley juice and drink a cup daily.

Things to avoid
- caffeine, alcohol, chocolate
- refined sugar and all sweets
- calcium supplements made from oyster shell, calcium carbonate, dolomite, or bone meal

Killer bees (see also Bee stings)

A laboratory freak, killer bees are the scientist's worst

nightmare. Now they have become a public menace of enormous proportions.

Killer bees are a product of genetic experiments in Brazil gone awry, an attempt by scientists to increase the productivity of local bees. They mated the placid local honey bees with aggressive African honey bees. The bees escaped from the lab and mated with Brazilian bees in the wild, corrupting their gene pool. These "synthetic" bees retained their aggressive nature and have become international monsters.

In only a few years the bees have hewn a path from Brazil all the way to the southern United States. They are now found in virtually all southern states. In the process the bees have attacked hundreds of thousands of mammals, including humans, killing and maiming thousands. In fact, thousands of humans have been viciously attacked by killer bees, many fatally. Deaths from killer bees occur daily. The number of the human victims, and the death and devastation they wreak is mounting. For those who proclaim that genetic engineering is for the benefit of humankind, here is merely one example of the devastation resulting from such human bungling and arrogance.

Killer bee combat kit

- oil of oregano (SuperStrength may be necessary)—rub this on any sting immediately. Also, drip it on the bees if they are attached. During the attack attempt to give several drops under the tongue frequently. Or, just get it into the mouth. If possible, find a pump spray bottle; add hot water and oil of oregano; spray the bees. Also, spray at any attacking bees. This will drive them off and/or kill them. The oil destroys their sensitive scent glands. Other anti-bee oils include oil of cumin, bay leaf, and, perhaps, tea tree oil.
- OregaMax capsules—give as many as possible.
- red grape powder (Resvital)—take as much as possible.

- pantothenic acid (500 mg capsules)—take 2 every hours to block circulatory shock.
- Herbal Bug-X—spray on body as an insect repellent. Also may be sprayed at bees to neutralize them. This is completely non-toxic.

Special Note: the key is to take the anti-toxic essential oils under the tongue for quick absorption into the blood. This is a lifesaving maneuver. Give 2 or more drops of oil of oregano under the tongue repeatedly to halt or prevent shock-related death. It is the shock, that is the collapse of the circulatory system, that kills, not the bites themselves.

Foods that help
- vinegar—pour full strength on bees and stings
- sea salt—drink a solution of salt water to block circulatory shock

Things to avoid
- perfumes

Laryngitis

Extreme hoarseness is the well known symptom of this condition; people who have laryngitis commonly are reduced to a whisper or perhaps no voice at all. It is usually due to a virus, which directly infects the vocal cords. The nerves to the vocal cords may also be attacked. Laryngitis is usually induced by stress. It may also develop as a consequence of sinus infection, in other words, the infection begins in the sinuses and eventually leads to laryngitis. It is important to note that hoarseness may also be a warning of vocal cord cancer.

Loud speech, stress, or arguing may precipitate this condition. Constant consumption of allergenic foods also increases the risks.

Laryngitis combat kit

- oil of oregano—take 2 drops under the tongue every few hours or more often if necessary.
- oil of rosemary—take 10 drops twice or more daily.
- oil of sage—take 5 drops twice daily.
- Essence of Orange Blossom—highly soothing; add one or two tablespoons in warm water as a tea, adding raw honey if desired.
- raw crude honey—add to hot herbal tea or Essence of Neroli Orange, and drink several times daily.
- Kid-e-Kare wild cherry or berry throat spray—mist on the back of the throat as often as necessary.
- OregaSpray wild oregano, bay leaf, lavender spray—mist on back of throat as needed.

Foods that help

- Pomegranate Syrup—add a tablespoon to hot water and drink several times daily.
- raw honey or carob molasses—soothing and easy to consume

Things to avoid

- arguments
- chocolate (stimulates the growth of viruses)
- corn, wheat, and rye

Lead poisoning

Lead poisoning usually develops over a prolonged period. The vast majority of cases occur in individuals who work in factories which utilize lead or in people living in older homes. Regarding the latter the source is lead paint, lead-containing dust, and lead water pipes.

Despite its well known toxic effects American industry still relies upon lead. In fact, besides iron and steel lead is the most widely used industrial metal. This puts both workers and those living near the factories at risk. At the greatest risk are those in the following industries:

- battery
- construction
- demolition
- firing range
- foundry
- gas station
- jewelry
- pipe fitters/plumbers
- pottery
- soldering
- stained glass
- welding

Lead is absorbed through the skin, but ingestion and inhalation of lead particles are the major means of contamination. What's more, once entering the body lead is highly soluble in fatty tissues, so it readily pollutes the fatty brain, nerve sheaths, and spinal cord. Also, because it dissolves so easily into the tissues, it is difficult to remove. This heavy metal is also readily absorbed by bone, which fiercely binds it. This may account for the musculoskeletal symptoms so common in lead poisoning. Because of the fact that inhalation is a major means of lead contamination, wearing a mask is a simple and effective method to prevent lead exposure in the event of a major urban disaster. Early signs of lead poisoning include:

- fatigue
- memory loss
- irritability
- vague muscle, bone, or joint pain

- headaches
- stomachaches and cramps
- numbness

As the illness progresses the following symptoms may develop:
- impotence and/or loss of sex drive
- vague digestive problems
- loss of sensation in the arms/legs
- weight loss
- constipation
- vomiting
- constant headache

Chronic lead poisoning also results in anemia. Thus, in an individual suffering from these symptoms who is also anemic, lead poisoning is virtually assured. Sudden exposure to lead exhibits certain symptoms, notably:

- abdominal tightness, cramps, and colic
- constipation
- severe fatigue
- convulsions, vomiting, seizures, and other symptoms of brain damage

Sudden overwhelming lead exposure readily occurs during disasters, especially earthquakes or toxic chemical releases. Chelation therapy is the only way to extract large amounts of lead. This is by irreversibly binding the metal so that it can be eliminated through the kidneys and gut. Medically, this requires a type of intravenous therapy. It involves the IV infusion of a drug called EDTA, which binds, that is chelates, the lead and removes it from the body through the kidneys. However, this is impractical during a crisis. The following is a protocol of natural substances which bind and remove lead from the body:

Lead poisoning detoxification kit
- LivaClenz (to purge the liver of bile and lead molecules)—take 20 or more drops of twice daily.
- GreensFlush wild greens formula—take 40 or more drops twice daily.
- calcium chelate (helps drive lead out of bone)—take 2000 mg daily.
- OregaMax capsules—a major aid for chelating heavy metals, take 4 capsules three times daily.
- red grape powder (Resvital)—rich in organic acids, which aggressively bind heavy metals, take 4 or more capsules three times daily. If using bulk, take 3 or more teaspoons daily.

Things to avoid
- all calcium supplements made from bone meal and oyster shell calcium (high in lead residues)—bone meal may also be contaminated with the Mad Cow agent.

Leg cramps

This is almost exclusively due to nutritional deficiency. Poor circulation may also play a role. Nutrients which are primarily deficient include pantothenic acid, folic acid, calcium, magnesium, sodium, potassium, and vitamin E.

Calcium deficiency may be the major factor in the cause of leg cramps in women, particularly in those who shun the typical calcium-rich foods such as fresh milk, cheese, yogurt, sardines, canned salmon, and dark greens. What's more, since calcium absorption is dependent upon vitamin D, leg cramps may also warn of a deficiency of this sunshine-dependent nutrient. This may also explain why some women have an increase in leg or foot cramps during the winter. Liver disease increases the risks for leg cramps, because the liver produces a protein required for calcium transport.

For immediate relief rely on anti-inflammatory essential oils. Rub these oils over the involved region to enhance blood flow, reduce pain, and relax the nervous system.

Leg/foot cramp combat kit
- pantothenic acid—take 500 mg twice daily.
- Pumpkinol (as a source of natural vitamin E to aid circulation)—2 tablespoons twice daily.
- OregaMax capsules—2 or more capsules twice daily (as a source of natural calcium–phosphorus).
- oil of oregano—rub on involved region and take 2 drops under the tongue repeatedly until cramps stop.
- oil of rosemary—take 5 drops under the tongue repeatedly until cramps stop.
- folic acid—take 5 to 10 mg daily.
- calcium and magnesium—take 1000 mg of calcium and 500 mg of magnesium daily.
- Royal Power (an excellent source of natural pantothenic acid; aids cortisone production)—take 4 capsules twice daily.

Foods that help
- glass of warm milk with honey (the natural sugars in the honey aid in calcium absorption)
- large handful of salted almonds, filberts, or roasted peanuts

Lice

Having lice crawling on the body or in the hair elicits all manner of emotional reactions. The thought alone can create hysteria. The most common type is the one which attacks the hair and scalp, i.e. head lice. Other types include body lice and pubic lice.

Head lice attack the scalp, because it is a warm climate, perfect for their metabolism. Obviously, bald individuals are innately protected. The lice tend to adhere close to the scalp, because they require body heat to survive. The eggs are also found close to the scalp and are attached to the hair follicles. The main site for egg attachment is the back of the head. The problem is that the infection festers without symptoms for perhaps weeks before it is discovered. By then the entire family and home may become infested.

Essential oils are the remedy of choice. Their solvent action makes them ideal for combating this condition, because the oils dissolve the eggs. Plus, the antiseptic powers of the oils kill the lice outright. To begin treatment, comb repeatedly with a metal or hard plastic comb; start combing from the base of the scalp forward. If possible, saturate the comb with an anti-lice essential oil compound such as Scalp Clenz. Scalp Clenz contains potent spice oils, which destroy all traces of lice, while dissolving the nits. Cover the entire head /scalp with the oil twice daily or simply add it to shampoo.

Lice combat kit

- oils of oregano, fennel, cumin, and bay leaf: add 1 part of each oil together (or, use Scalp Clenz, which is a mix of such oils and is specific for killing lice); rub into scalp and hair. Repeat as often as necessary until all lice and eggs are destroyed.
- oil of oregano (edible type, P73): take 5 drops under the tongue twice daily.
- diffuser or atomizer: fumigate the rooms and bedding with Germ-a-CLENZ
- Scalp Clenz—thoroughly saturate the hair and scalp with this; allow to sit for 1/2 to 1 hour, then wash. All lice will fall out as will the nits. Repeat as often as necessary although a single application usually suffices. May also be added to shampoo, about 6 to 8 droppersful per 8 ounces. Wash and let sit as long as possible, then rinse.
- metal comb

Lyme disease

Lyme disease is caused by the bite of ticks, usually deer ticks. This disease is an epidemic on the East Coast, however, cases have been reported virtually everywhere. Regions at the highest risk include New York and New Jersey.

Lyme is supposedly one of the most difficult to diagnose of all diseases. Yet, it shouldn't be. Lyme mimics the flu, that is it is represented by mild to moderate muscle aches, fever, malaise, etc. Yet, the flu rarely occurs in the spring and summer, which is when it usually strikes. A significant percentage of Lyme victims develop a rash a week or so after the tick bite. The rash is non-itching and circular. No such rash is seen in the flu.

It is a major error to misdiagnose Lyme disease as the flu. This is because a large percentage of infected individuals develop chronic disease, which may be debilitating or even life-threatening. Great effort must be made to procure a precise diagnosis. High suspicion should exist for wilderness buffs who develop sudden flu-like illnesses during the spring or summer. Dog owners are also a high risk category, especially if the dogs venture outdoors. Erroneous diagnosis and/or treatment may result in chronic Lyme, which is devastating. Symptoms of chronic Lyme include joint pain, stiff spine or neck, muscle aches, exhaustion, poor concentration, headaches, numbness, and fatigue.

Lyme is difficult to cure by any means, medical or herbal. However, recent data indicates that prolonged treatment of the individual with anti-Borrelia compounds, whether natural or synthetic, offers hope for a cure. For instance, researchers publishing in *Modern Medicine*, September 1997, determined that after a 90-day course of tetracycline over 60% of Lyme patients improved significantly. However, it is important to note that long term antibiotic therapy has numerous risks, for instance the development of fungal infections as well as drug-resistant mutants. This is why natural substances are so valuable. There is no risk with long term use of natural substances with germ-killing power such as cinnamon, oregano, garlic, cumin, onion, etc. Rather, there is often significant improvement, perhaps cure. At a minimum medicine and natural cures should be combined to provide the individual with the best odds for a cure.

Medical authorities have deluded themselves to believe that a tick bite leads to only one circumscribed infection. Ticks are fully contaminated with a wide range of germs, which they derive from the blood of rodents. Thus, usually, multiple infestations result from a single bite. This is clearly evidenced by an article published by researchers at the University of Wisconsin; these researchers discovered that a significant percentage of Lyme patients also had in their blood other tick-acquired germs. It is likely that perhaps dozens of different germs are injected by a single tick bite. Recall that Lyme smoldered in humans in this country for decades before it was discovered. This illustrates the importance of natural antiseptics, such as oil of oregano, which are capable of attacking a wide range of invaders. In order to eradicate these germs from the body every tool possible must be used. The Lyme spirochetes are difficult to kill. High and prolonged doses of spice oils often are necessary.

Tick combat kit (for destroying the tick)
- fine point straight tweezers
- oil of oregano (SuperStrength is best)—saturate a cotton ball and hold over tick until it dies. Remove the dead tick carefully with tweezers. Grab the tick as close to its attachment as possible.
- tea tree oil—also useful by saturating tick or a cotton ball held over it.
- cotton balls (saturate with the oils and suffocate the tick)

Tick disease combat kit (in case of infection)
- oil of oregano (SuperStrength is preferable)—take 10 or more drops under the tongue three times daily. Also, take 10 to 20 drops in juice or water two or more times daily. For extremely

tough conditions, double this amount. Oreganol capsules are an alternative, 3 or more twice daily.
- wild oregano herb (OregaMax capsules)—take 3 capsules three times daily.
- Oregacyn capsules (also good for Lyme-related joint pain)—2 or more capsules three times daily.
- Infla-eez—to eliminate muscular and joint inflammation and to aid in the destruction of the germs, 2 or 3 capsules twice daily on an empty stomach.
- Oregano P73 Juice—take 1 or more ounces twice daily. For severe cases increase the dose, for instance, three ounces twice daily.

Foods that help
- papaya and its seeds
- horseradish
- raw garlic and onion; also, onion/radish juice

What to do if a tick is attached
- Don't touch the tick with your hands unless no other option is available.
- Saturate the tick with oil of oregano and/or tea tree oil.
- Saturate a cotton ball with these oils and hold the ball gently over the tick. Do this until the tick suffocates (dies).
- When dead, grasp the tick as close as possible to its attachment site with the tweezers. Pull the tick out slowly but gently. If the tick is crushed and secretions pour out, saturate the involved region with tea tree or oregano oil, and wash the region, as well as the hands, thoroughly.
- If tweezers are unavailable, cover the fingers with tissue or a paper towel (or a plant leaf) and pull out the tick. Do not cut the tick open, as this will spread its dangerous secretions and blood. Rather kill it with the essential oils.

How to avoid tick bites

If you are in a tick-infested region and are exposed to the elements, here are some simple steps that may help protect you:

- Never sit directly on the ground, and avoid sitting or squatting near tall grass.
- If you must sit on the ground, place light-colored sheets or bedding underneath you. Or, place cardboard or plywood on the ground. This will make it easier to see ticks.
- Wear socks over the pants to force ticks to crawl up the legs so they can be spotted.
- Tuck shirts into pants and wear tight long sleeve shirts, if possible.
- Take the time to inspect for ticks regularly, no matter how time consuming or difficult it seems.
- DEET-containing tick repellents are potentially carcinogenic. If possible, use natural tick repellents such as Herbal Bug-X. However, it may be necessary to maintain a can or two of commercial tick repellent in case all else fails. Premethrin is a less toxic alternative to DEET. However, this is applied to the clothing rather than the skin. One application lasts about two weeks to keep the ticks away. However, the Herbal Bug-X and, particularly, the Germ-a-CLENZ can be sprayed on the clothing and allowed to sit. Since they are organic they may tend to stain, although in most cases the residues are readily washed out.

Malaria

Once exclusively a tropical disease, malaria has invaded temperate regions: through travelers. This does not mean that outbreaks will occur in Chicago or New York City. Yet, it is remotely possible that pockets of infection could develop in the southern United States.

There is an effective drug for malaria, a quinine derivative, yet, it is not without side effects. Still, the condition is highly serious and relying upon drug therapy alone may be inadequate.

The fact is this germ is difficult to kill, because it hides inside red blood cells. It does so to evade the immune system, plus it feeds upon these cells. The malaria parasite should be bombarded with every possible antiseptic/antiparasitic substance available.

Malaria combat kit

- oil of oregano (SuperStrength is best)—take 5 or more drops under the tongue several times daily. Also, take 10 to 20 drops in juice or water twice or more daily or use Oreganol caps (1 cap equals 7 drops of oil).
- wild oregano capsules (OregaMax)—take 6 or more capsules
- OregaBiotic—3 or more capsules twice daily
- Oreganol P73 Juice—2 ounces twice daily
- Intesti-Clenz antiparasitic formula—20 drops under the tongue twice daily.

Measles (regular and German)

This is highly contagious, perhaps one of the most contagious infections known. Measles begins with a cough, high fever, eye irritation, with the development of a rash within 4 to 5 days. Ear infections, as well as viral pneumonia, may develop afterwards. Rarely, if the fever is high enough and if the child becomes severely dehydrated, brain damage may occur.

German measles is also known as "3-day measles." Less contagious and harsh, it is only a threat in pregnant women, who may pass the infection to the fetus. Birth defects are believed to be a possible consequence. Symptoms are a rash, fever, fatigue, and aching limbs. The following amounts are appropriate for children.

Measles combat kit

- oil of oregano—take 2 or more drops under the tongue several times daily; also, take 2 drops in juice or water twice daily. Add to raw honey.
- OregaMax capsules—take 3 or more capsules daily.
- Oreganol cream—rub on any rash, also on the buttocks, soles of feet, and chest.
- Kid-e-Kare rubbing oil—add to diffuser and rub on the body.
- Purely-C—take 2 capsules three times daily.

Things to avoid

- soda pop; give juice instead (this at least provides vitamin C)
- chocolate, beans, nuts, and seeds

Melanoma

In California medical scientists list melanoma as an absolute epidemic. It has risen in incidence at a stupendous rate throughout the United States. In 1935 the individual had only a 1 in 2000 risk of developing it. Now the risk is nearly 1 in 75. That is an epidemic.

Melanoma may develop anywhere on the body and can even occur in the mouth and under the nails. However, it most commonly occurs on the torso, oddly enough, in areas not regularly exposed to the sun. This is supposedly a sun-induced disease. Yet, its distribution certainly gives credence to the theory that regular measured exposure to the sun is somehow protective. In fact, a study in Canada of thousands of men regularly exposed to the sun as outdoor workers showed a decreased incidence of melanoma compared to the normal workforce.

When this disease strikes, it elicits great fear. There is no need to fear. As always, medical treatment should ideally be combined with nutritional support. Certain vitamin deficiencies are associated with heightened melanoma risk, and these nutrients should be supplemented in the diet. A lack of vitamins A, C, E, D, and beta carotene all increase the risk for melanoma. These nutrients should be taken to prevent it as well as to eradicate it after it strikes. B vitamins which protect against it include pyridoxine, pantothenic acid, and riboflavin. Selenium and zinc also offer protection. As always, be sure to seek medical care if a suspicious lesion develops.

Spice oils offer the most profound actions against these lesions, often offering hope for a cure, as demonstrated by the the following example.

CASE HISTORY:
Mrs. H., a 94-year-old melanoma victim, was under the care of her daughter. The daughter saturated the large metastatic melanoma with the SuperStrength Oreganol. Within three days the melanoma tissue fell out of the skin, leaving a hole, which eventually healed.

Melanoma Combat Kit

- wear white/light-colored cotton clothing that covers most of the exposed parts
- large-brimmed hats are mandatory
- top quality sunscreen containing antioxidants
- oil of oregano (SuperStrength is best)—rub into the lesion three times daily. Also, take 5 or more drops under the tongue twice daily.
- oil of rosemary—rub on the involved region as often as desired.
- Infla-eez—take 3 capsules on an empty stomach three times daily.
- Pumpkinol crude pumpkin seed oil—as a natural source of phytosterols and vitamin E take 4 tablespoons daily. The Sesam-E, with potent anticancer compounds, may also be added, two tablespoons daily.
- BerriesFlush (wild berries extract, with rare flavonoids)—40 drops twice daily.

- GreensFlush (wild greens extract)—40 drops twice daily.
- NukeProtect with organic selenium—take 3 or more capsules twice daily.
- Oreganol P73 Juice—drink two or more ounces twice daily.•
- Essence of Rosemary—drink two or more ounces twice daily.

Things to avoid

- refined vegetable oils and hydrogenated oils
- deep-fried foods of all types
- sunbathing
- sun exposure at high noon

Meningitis

Meningitis is a life-threatening condition, which is defined as inflammation and infection of the brain. This is an extremely treacherous disease, which often fails to respond to even the most aggressive medical therapy. The fact is certain of the meningitis germs are entirely resistant to synthetic antibiotics. Thus, if this disorder breaks out during a crisis, the individual must be armed with other means besides drugs. What is really frightening is that outbreaks of meningitis are developing virtually everywhere. Plus, the germ which causes these epidemics is unusually aggressive. The bizarre bacteria, known as ET-15, is twice as deadly as the normal agent.

Meningitis has reached virtual epidemic proportions. A vaccine will only aggravate the dilemma. Only natural medicines can reverse this disease. What's more, in ancient times, incredibly, the Islaamic physician ar-Raazee found a bizarre treatment curative: bloodletting. Apparently, this procedure stimulated the immune system, cleansing the body of this germ.

The symptoms of meningitis are fairly predictable. The major symptoms include:

- high fever
- headache
- nausea and vomiting (possibly)
- stiff neck (this is of great importance, since the flu, colds, strep throat, etc. don't present with stiff neck). Doctors know that if the individual is extremely ill, the neck should be gently moved to see if it is rigid. This distinguishes meningitis from virtually any other infection.

Note: infants don't usually develop stiff necks. The usual symptoms in infants are:

- temperature instability
- listlessness
- unusually high pitched cry (feeble cry)
- no appetite
- weak sucking response
- irritability
- vomiting and/or diarrhea

Be aware that the main issue with infants is that there is a sudden change in their normal physical condition or mental state. If their behavior is highly unusual, be suspicious of significant infection. As always, if an outbreak of meningitis occurs, see your physician immediately. The following amounts are for children over 5 years of age.

Meningitis combat kit

- P73 edible oil of oregano—take a few drops under the tongue frequently, like every 15 minutes. Gently rub the neck and head with the oil of oregano (SuperStrength is preferable).
- (for children) Kid-e-Kare rubbing oil—rub on forehead and under nose several times daily. Also, rub on the soles of the feet and up and down the spinal column several times daily.

- OregaMax capsules—take as many capsules daily as possible.
- Purely-C (as a source of immune-stimulating ascorbates)—take 2 or 3 capsules as often as possible.
- Infla-eez (bromelain/papain), to improve blood flow to the brain—take 2 or more capsules on an empty stomach three or more times daily.
- OregaBiotic—2 capsules every hour or two, that is until symptoms dramatically improve. Then, take 2 twice daily for week or two.
- Resvital—take a teaspoon twice daily. In severe cases take a teaspoon several times daily.
- Garlex oil of cold-pressed garlic—20 drops under the tongue as often as possible.
- Bloodletting (under a doctor's care)—slowly remove 1/2 pint, then observe. Be sure to combine this therapy with the aforementioned natural medicines.

Foods that help
- raw honey (wild oregano or wild Mediterranean flower); consume at least three tablespoons daily
- ginger root: slice and add to hot water; drink to combat nausea or upset stomach

Menstrual bleeding (heavy)

Bleeding from the vagina usually only has one cause: a bleeding uterus. It is one of the most commonly occurring conditions in women, afflicting up to 15% of the population. Chronic excessive bleeding may lead to anemia and weakness. If unstoppable, it could result in a life-threatening crisis.

Short of a hysterectomy, medical doctors offer little successful therapy. In fact, J. Rosenfeld, M.D., writing in *American Family Physician,* January 1996, indicates that this condition hasn't been studied thoroughly in the U.S., nor have any proven drug therapies been devised. Yet, for thousands of years primitives, as well as advanced societies, have found effective therapy among herbs. While herbs may frequently be invaluable, they don't always work. This is because the uterus may be diseased beyond repair, which leads to profuse bleeding. If bleeding is continuous or unresponsive to conservative measures, surgical intervention may be necessary.

Menstrual bleeding combat kit
- oil of fennel—take 10 drops twice daily internally.
- oil of rosemary (apply to vaginal walls).
- oil of oregano—dilute with extra virgin olive oil; apply to the vaginal walls. Also, take 2 drops twice daily under the tongue.
- oil of sage (to balance the hormone system)—take 5 to 10 drops twice daily.
- essential fatty acids (primrose or borage oils)—take 4 capsules twice daily.
- uncoated bromelain (Infla-eez)—take 2 or more capsules twice daily on an empty stomach.
- Royal Power—to build up the strength of the adrenal glands, 3 capsules twice daily.

Things to avoid
- refined sugar, soda pop, corn syrup, and all sweets
- caffeine, chocolate, and iced tea

Menstrual cramps

Menstrual cramps are not an inevitable consequence of being a female. There are a number of physical causes for them. Nutritional deficiency is a major factor. Nutrients which improve the function of the uterus and help prevent cramps include pantothenic acid, magnesium, vitamin E, essential fatty acids, and vitamin B_6.

Excessive cramping may also warn of uterine and/or cervical infection. Major culprits include yeasts (Candida albicans), viruses, and bacteria, the most notorious being Chlamydia.

Menstrual cramps/difficulty combat kit
- antiinflammatory enzymes (i. e. Infla-eez)—take 2 or more capsules on an empty stomach twice daily.
- Royal Power high grade royal jelly—3 capsules twice daily.
- oil of oregano (Oreganol P73)—3 to 5 drops under the tongue twice daily.
- oil of myrtle—apply to the vaginal walls twice daily.
- oil of rosemary—apply to the vaginal walls twice daily. Also, take 5 to 10 drops twice daily in juice or water.
- Purely-C—take 2 or more capsules three times daily; with severe bleeding double the dosage.
- essential fatty acids (Pumpkinol)—take 4 tablespoons daily.

Foods that help
- fatty fish (salmon, halibut, sardines, mackerel, bluefish, trout)
- unripe raw pineapple (eat the top, that is the part closest to the stem); papaya and its seeds

Things to avoid
- totally avoid chocolate, coffee, colas, and other sources of caffeine

Mercury poisoning

Mercury poisoning can occur in several ways besides touching or swallowing globs of mercury. This highly toxic metal is a component of hundreds of industrial chemicals. Billions of pounds of mercury are found in storage tanks across the United States. The fact is mercury, in the form of solid, liquid, and/or gaseous compounds, is transported via rail and truck by the megaton throughout the United States every year.

Fungicides and insecticides are often mercury based. Thus, poisoning by these chemicals may be due to mercury components.

The most commonly occurring type of mercury poisoning is due to chronic exposure. This exposure is primarily in the mouth via mercury amalgam dental fillings. Research indicates that mercury fillings poison the kidneys, brain, adrenal glands, and liver. The best means of treatment is to remove the mercury load from the body. Existing fillings should be removed and additional ones should be avoided. Poisoning can also be acquired through vaccinations, since mercurial compounds are used as "preservatives."

All mercury compounds are aggressive poisons. They act by destroying the protein of human cells, in other words, they decimate human enzyme systems. The enzymes are absolutely critical for the existence of the body's life forces. In addition, mercury binds to cell membrane proteins, leading to the rupture of cells. Toxicity may occur via ingestion, inhalation, or direct contact with the skin. Symptoms of acute poisoning include:

- abdominal pain
- diarrhea
- nausea and vomiting
- respiratory distress
- loss of sensation
- loss of coordination
- headache
- seizures

Mercury poisoning combat kit
- Oil of Cilantro-plus—take 20 to 40 drops twice daily. For extreme conditions take 80 drops twice daily.

- LivaClenz—take 20 or more drops twice daily.
- NukeProtect—take 3 capsules three times daily. This contains organic selenium and numerous other antidotes.
- GreensFlush wild greens formula—2 droppersful under the tongue twice daily. For extreme conditions double or triple this amount.
- red grape powder (Resvital)—take 1 teaspoonful twice daily.
- Purely-C—take 3 capsules two or three times daily.
- BerriesFlush—20 to 40 drops twice daily.

Migraines (see Headaches)

Mite allergy

Dust mite allergy is a primary cause of respiratory distress, sinus problems, asthma, and other common disorders. It is not the only cause of these illnesses, however it contributes to them in a major way. As described by T. Johnson, M.D., in *American Family Physician*, fully 1 in 10 individuals and 9 of 10 asthmatics react to the residues of these pests.

The problem of mites has been aggravated by modern living: they love living along with humans. They love our homes and thrive at the temperature in which we thrive. In particular, they flourish in the moist tropics and in subtropical regions, like the southeastern United States.

One rather shocking fact is that mites don't just reside on the ground or in dust. They seek to reside as close to the human body as possible. This is why they flourish in bedding, where they have a captive source of nourishment for several hours. A pillow alone may house as many as a quarter of a million of these pests. A study published in 1995 by Australian researchers discovered that mites thrive in human's clothing. The researchers found that there are enough mites and mite secretions on virtually anyone to provoke allergic reactions or respiratory problems in susceptible individuals. Perhaps even more grotesque is the fact that other research documents how mites thrive on our bodies, that is on the skin and in the hair, despite normal hygiene. Therefore, additional tactics must be utilized to destroy these vermin.

Essential oils kill mites effectively. Top anti-mite essential oils include the oils of wild oregano, lavender, bay leaf, and rosemary. The most aggressive of these is oil of oregano. Add a combination of these oils to body shampoos or pump soap for washing to help keep mites off the body. ScalpClenz is a special combination of these oils that is ideal for killing hair/scalp mites. This may be added to shampoo to regularly kill such mites. The Germ-a-CLENZ spray may also be used for this purpose.

Mite combat kit

- oil of oregano—take 2 drops under the tongue whenever needed; add to diffuser and volatilize into air.
- oil of bay leaf—take 5 drops daily and add to diffuser; pump-spray into air and add to wash cycle.
- oil of rosemary—diffuse into air; add to wash cycle.
- ScalpClenz—rub into scalp or add to shampoo to kill hair/scalp mites.
- Germ-a-CLENZ all natural spice spray—ideal for spraying throughout the house, on carpets, or bedding, use as needed.

Other ideas

- wash all clothes and bedding in hot water. Only hot water kills mites, as they can survive cold/warm washes. Add bleach when appropriate. Better yet add a few drops of oil of oregano, per wash cycle.
- rub oil of oregano, oil of bay leaf, and/or oil of lavender on the skin before dressing. This will allow the oils to "fumigate" the clothes throughout the day. This is particularly valuable

for wool clothes, which can't be washed in hot water. Wool clothes retain the greatest numbers of mites. Spray all wool clothing with a distant mist of Germ-a-CLENZ.

Mold allergy/poisoning

This section is perhaps the most important of any in this book. Mold poisoning is a monumental cause of illness, disability, disease, and death. It is rarely diagnosed, in fact, it is almost never considered. Yet, it is pervasive and insidious and frequently causes human distress, perhaps for years or even decades before it is recognized if ever.

Did you know that it is virtually certain that molds are the most dangerous of all germs and that they have caused throughout history a greater degree of disability and death than the plague? It was M. K. Matossian, in her book *Poisons of the Past: Molds, Epidemics, and History*, who wrote that molds are wreaking havoc on the human race, causing sudden death, physical exhaustion, and mental aberrations. Regarding the latter she mentions how mold poisons, through contamination of stored food, caused massive outbreaks of psychosis, often affecting entire cities. Matossian further writes that it was ergotism, a form of mold poisoning, which caused the illnesses that led to the notorious Salem Witch Trials. These poisons are capable of completely disabling the neurological system, as well as the immune system, making the individual extremely ill.

CASE HISTORY:

A 28-year-old woman was admitted to the psychiatric ward for acute psychosis, which developed after she went on a sugar and chocolate binge. Doctors noticed she also had a rash on her feet, legs, and hands, which appeared to be a fungal infection. Her mother insisted that the doctors consider using an antifungal approach to help her daughter. All sugar and starch were eliminated from her diet. Oreganol P73, a natural antifungal agent, was administered aggressively; 20 drops three times daily. She was also given Royal

Power, 4 capsules three times daily, to rebuild her adrenal glands. Within 48 hours the patient's behavior improved to such an extent that she was released. In addition, the rash had improved significantly. Thus, a medical and social disaster was averted.

Mold-contaminated foods are not the only culprits. The molds found in the air and, particularly, inside homes and other buildings may be highly toxic. What's more, they can readily invade the body, infecting virtually any region or organ. Apparently, the toxic effects of these "household molds" are particularly dangerous for children. The CDC recently reported a high number of illnesses, as well as deaths, due to an indoor mold known as *Stachybotrus atra*. This mold produces potent chemicals which cause immune depression and internal bleeding. Children have been killed by inhaling these mold poisons. They bleed to death into their lungs. However, untold thousands more have been poisoned, many fatally, and, again, no one suspects it. The dilemma is so serious that the *American Academy of Pediatrics* issued a warning to all doctors entitled "Toxic Effects of Indoor Mold."

It doesn't take much to induce damage. Just a tiny quantity, less than the amount placed on a pinhead, is enough to decimate an individual. J. S. Marr, M.D., writing in the *JAMA*, notes that these "extremely potent...poisons...cause numerous diseases in trifling amounts." He further describes that the Tenth Plague of ancient Egypt was probably due to such mold toxins, which proliferated as a result of floods. The fact is the current outbreaks in the United States are largely due to the plethora of severe floods, which have decimated numerous regions such as south Texas, central Iowa, North Dakota, Missouri, Ohio, and parts of California. Symptoms of mold poisoning are highly variable. However, the most common manifestations include:

- unquenchable thirst
- poor appetite (or excessive appetite for sugar)

- bizarre heat sensations (hot flashes)
- cold extremities, worsened when eating certain foods
- intolerance to weather extremes, hot or cold
- tingling sensations
- joint pain and/or spinal stiffness
- itching or redness of the skin
- swelling and/or blistering of the skin
- hysterical and/or psychotic behavior
- loss of hearing
- headaches and/or sinus pain
- nosebleeds
- exhaustion
- asthma-like symptoms
- skin eruptions, eczema, and/or psoriasis
- nausea and/or vomiting
- dark-colored smelly stools
- depression
- internal bleeding
- apathy
- inability to cope

Not all of these symptoms need to necessarily be present for infestation to be proven. If you have 6 or more of these symptoms, mold toxicity is highly likely. A score of 10 or more indicates massive mold contamination.

Mold allergy/poisoning combat kit

- oil of oregano—take 5 or more drops under the tongue twice daily plus an additional 10 drops twice daily in juice or water. For severe exposure take it more often.
- wild oregano herb (OregaMax capsules)—take 3 or more capsules twice daily.
- Oregacyn respiratory—take 2 or more capsules twice daily.

- Lactobacillus complex (i.e. Health-Bac)—take several capsules daily. Take at a different time than oregano oil.
- OregaSpray natural wild spice anti-mold spray—use to cleanse the air of mold. Also, spray in mouth or on roof of mouth as an antidote.
- organic selenium, zinc, and manganese—to activate the mold detoxification systems.
- Purely-C—crude ascorbic acid plus bioflavonoids to activate white blood cells, 2 or 3 capsules twice daily.
- Fung-E-Clenz (a special formula of natural spice/herb oils for removing fungal residues and toxins from the body)—take 10 or more drops twice daily in juice or water (or under the tongue).

Note: the oils should be volatilized to cleanse the air and penetrate the lungs directly. Use a diffuser or atomizer.

Foods that help
- garlic and onions (raw)
- cloves and cinnamon

Things to avoid
- rye of all types
- wheat and corn

Mononucleosis

Mononucleosis, known commonly as mono, is caused by a virus belonging to the herpes family. The virus usually attacks adolescents and college students and is readily transmitted sexually, primarily through kissing.

The mono virus specifically attacks the lymphatic system. This is why swollen lymph glands is a major sign of this illness. The liver and spleen are a part of the lymph system and are also aggressively attacked. Antibiotics are of no use in this condition and usually aggravate it.

Mono combat kit

- OregaBiotic—take 2 or more capsules several times daily.
- oil of oregano (Oreganol P73)—take 5 or more drops under the tongue several times daily. Rub on feet, buttocks, and abdomen.
- OregaMax capsules—take 3 capsules three times daily.
- LivaClenz—take 20 drops twice daily in juice or water.
- Oregacyn Liver—2 or more capsules several times daily with food or juice.
- GreensFlush wild greens formula—take 20 drops twice daily.

Things to avoid

- alcoholic beverages
- antibiotics
- prescription painkillers, aspirin, and acetaminophen

Mosquito bites

Mosquitoes, seemingly mere pests in North America, are the number one direct transmitter of infectious disease globally. They cause a wide gamut of diseases, including yellow fever, dengue fever, malaria, worm infections, and encephalitis.

There is a simple way to prevent these infections: avoid getting bitten. This implies the use of repellents. However, the commercial repellents are themselves poisonous. According to investigations at Guelph University in Ontario, Canada, there is a natural repellent that is equally as effective as the synthetics. Called *Herbal Bug-X*, it is 98% effective. Herbal Bug-X is relatively new and may be ordered by calling 1-800-243-5242. It comes in either a spray or dropper bottle form. It is an edible repellent, meaning that in the dropper form it can be taken orally to build up internal repellency. The spray form offers at least two hours of protection. It can be applied repeatedly.

Another therapy is to detoxify the bite as soon as it occurs. This is accomplished through the application of essential oils. The oils of oregano, cumin, lavender, bay leaf, and bay berry all offer anti-toxic actions.

Mosquito combat kit
- oil of oregano—apply to bite region and take a few drops under the tongue as often as necessary. Taken internally, this acts as a repellent.
- raw garlic—crush cloves and apply small amount to bite.
- mosquito netting
- Herbal Bug-X spray—spray on exposed skin as often as necessary.
- Herbal Bug-X drops—take 10 or more drops under the tongue twice daily to build up internal repellent powers.

Things to avoid
- perfumes

Muscle soreness and weakness

This can happen to anyone. Usually, it is a symptom of overexertion or infectious disease. Certain illnesses, such as chronic fatigue and fibromyalgia, may be manifested by it. Common causes are chronic stress, infection, allergic reactions, and nutritional deficiency. Poor circulation and blood pooling add to this aggravation.

Muscle soreness/weakness combat kit
- Infla-eez antiinflammatory enzymes—take 3 or more capsules twice daily on an empty stomach.
- sea salt—consume a heaping teaspoonful daily in food.
- Infla-eez rubbing oil—rub as needed several times daily.
- oil of sage—rub on sore muscles and on soles of feet.

- Resvital (as a source of muscle-strengthening chromium)—take 3 capsules twice daily.
- Purely-C—as a source of natural vitamin C, two capsules twice daily.

Foods that help
- papaya plus the seeds
- salted roasted nuts, especially almonds and filberts

Nail bed infection

Known medically as *paronychia*, this infection is usually caused by a fungus, notably *Candida albicans*. Less commonly, bacteria are the culprits. In either case it is a painful infection, which may persist unless it is aggressively treated. It is manifested by swelling around the nail bed, redness, and extreme pain.

Nail bed infection combat kit
- oil of oregano—take 3 drops under the tongue three times daily. Soak the finger in a solution of oil of oregano and olive oil. Or, simply rub the oil twice daily on the involved region.
- oil of lavender—rub on the involved region.
- bromelain (as Infla-eez)—take 3 or 4 capsules three times daily on an empty stomach.
- Purely-C—to boost white blood cell activity take 3 capsules twice daily.

Things to avoid
- nail polish and artificial nails
- harsh soaps
- sugar and other sweets

Nasal polyps

The primary cause of nasal polyps appears to be a vitamin deficiency, that is a lack of vitamin A. Zinc deficiency may also play a role. Food allergies are an aggravating factor. However, infection, that is chronic infection, is a more likely cause. This makes sense, since both vitamin A and zinc are required for normal immune function.

Nasal polyp combat kit
- vitamin A (as cod liver oil)—teaspoon twice daily with meals.
- zinc—50 mg daily.
- Infla-eez, high potency antiinflammatory enzyme formula—take 3 capsules twice daily on an empty stomach.
- oil of oregano—5 or 10 drops under the tongue twice daily.
- Black Seed-plus—take 3 or more capsules twice daily. Also, open capsules and add contents to food or chew on the seeds.
- Oregacyn respiratory—take 2 capsules twice daily.
- Oregano oil (P73)—under the tongue take 3 or more drops twice daily.

Nausea

This is one of the most uncomfortable of all conditions. It is caused by inflammation in the gut, although head injuries also lead to nausea. The inflammation may be due to infection, stress, chemical poisoning, alcohol toxicity, drug reactions, pesticide/herbicide intoxication, or allergic reactions. Nausea of pregnancy is another consideration. In fact, nausea is one of the earliest symptoms of pregnancy. It is also the primary symptom of motion sickness.

Nausea also has an ominous component; it may be a sign of intestinal or stomach cancer. Whatever the cause, herbs and spices are effective remedies. Even in cancer they often relieve the agony.

Nausea combat kit
- ginger root, either fresh, dehydrated, or capsules: take as needed.
- oil of ginger (from the entire ginger plant emulsified in extra

virgin olive oil)—take 2 or 3 drops with each meal or as needed.
- Oregacyn Digestive capsules (or Infla-eez)—take 1 or two capsules as needed until nausea abates.
- oil of fennel—take 5 drops in warm water once or twice daily.
- Essence of Neroli Orange—delicate and soothing; add two tablespoons to hot water and drink as a tea.
- Oreganol P7 Juice—drink an ounce as often as needed.
- Black Seed-plus—take 2 capsules two or more times daily.
- pressure point wristbands

Things to avoid
- Food: rest the gut as long as possible or until the nausea abates.
- alcohol of any type
- synthetic chemicals, aspirin, and radiation

Nerve gas poisoning

This seems unlikely, yet it happened in Japan. When sarin gas was released in the subway system, thousands of individuals were overcome; some permanently. Nerve gas poisonings could just as easily occur here, whether deliberate or accidental. As reported in the *Chicago Tribune* in December 1998, some 150 gallons of the deadly nerve gas sarin, the same one that poisoned the Japanese, spilled at an Army incineration facility in Utah. Apparently, no one was hurt and the spill was contained or at least so Army officials claim. Yet, if this would have become airborne, it was enough gas to destroy all of Salt Lake City, a mere 20 miles away.

While nerve gas poisoning is unlikely, if it does occur, no one will be prepared; the government offers no curative aid. However, major incidents affecting thousands of individuals will assuredly occur, both in the Western world and developing countries. Thus, the following protocol provides the individual with the best odds for survival. What's more, a poison gas attack is far from remote. The military-industrial complex has perpetrated such attacks previously, even against its own citizens.

Nerve gas combat kit
- gas mask and protective clothing
- oil of cumin—take 10 drops every few minutes.
- oil of rosemary—10 drops every few minutes; take also under the tongue 2 drops frequently.
- oil of oregano—take 2 drops under the tongue every few minutes.
- NukeProtect antioxidant/selenium formula—the ideal antidote, take 3 capsules several times daily.
- LivaClenz (to protect the liver from toxic chemical damage)—take 10 to 20 drops twice daily.
- Oreganol P73 Juice (to maintain physical strength and prevent collapse)—drink several ounces daily.
- OxyOrega—a special antioxidant form of wild oregano, a few drops under the tongue every few minutes.
- NukeProtect—take 2 capsules several times daily.

Nervousness/Irritability

Virtually everyone has experienced a bout of nervousness. Yet, it becomes a disease when it is a daily event.

Certain individuals seem to never relax. This may not be exclusively a mental issue, as it is a sign of a damaged coping mechanism. This coping mechanism is controlled by the adrenal glands. Thus, persistent nervousness is nearly always a sign of adrenal insufficiency. Symptoms of emotional instability, which include frustration, anger, crying spells, anxiety, panic attacks, depression, and extreme sensitivity, are all indicative of weak adrenals. For further information see the tests/symptom analysis in Dr. Ingram's *Nutrition Tests for better Health* or check the self-testing web site, **NutritionTest.com**.

Nervousness/irritability combat kit
- St. John's wort (wild and unprocessed)—take 2 to 4 capsules in the a.m. (made by North American Herb & Spice Co.)
- oil of lavender (wild type in extra virgin olive oil)—2 drops under the tongue twice daily. Also, rub on the chest, neck, and soles of feet.
- Royal Power premium-grade royal jelly—take 4 to 6 capsules every morning. Use more if needed to combat stress or anxiety.
- oil of sage—add a few drops to fruit juice or hot water as a tea. If using essence of sage, add a tablespoonful or more to juice or hot water.

Foods that help
- salty healthy snacks, like salted roasted nuts or salted fresh meat

Nosebleeds

Nosebleeds occur most commonly in children and teenagers. The major cause is nutritional deficiency, although infection and trauma are also involved. Nosebleeds warn of deficiencies of calcium, copper, vitamin C, zinc, folic acid, vitamin K, and bioflavonoids. Infections that may cause it include those induced by molds, yeasts, bacteria, parasites, and viruses. Mold intolerance is particularly likely to cause nosebleeds, because mold toxins, due to their poisonous actions on the liver, are a major cause of internal bleeding.

Nosebleed combat kit
- oil of oregano—rub around the nose. Take 2 drops under the tongue every 15 minutes until bleeding halts. Also, take a few drops under the tongue as an anti-mold therapy on a daily basis.
- chelated calcium—take 500 mg every 15 minutes for at least 2 hours, then 2000 mg per day for one week. Then, take 1000

mg daily as a maintenance. For best results take calcium in divided dosages, including a dose of at least 500 mg at bed time.
- Purely-C—take 6 or more capsules daily. Also, open a capsule and place contents in mouth or under tongue; repeat as needed.
- red grape powder (Resvital)—take 6 or more capsules daily.
- Lactobacillus (to antagonize the molds)—take as directed.
- OregaMax capsules (mold antagonist and natural calcium/magnesium supplement)—take 3 capsules twice daily.
- Resvital—take 3 capsules twice daily.

Nuclear catastrophe (see also Radiation poisoning)

This is virtually impossible to prepare for. However, by utilizing the information in this section you will have the best chance for survival.

There is a high likelihood of a nuclear catastrophe in the United States. This is because of the risks of nuclear power plant accidents, not from some outside military threat. The United States has the largest number of nuclear power plants in the world, over 100, and dozens of these reactors are at a high risk for leaks and/or accidents. Other risks include accidents during the transport of nuclear wastes. Currently, all nuclear power plants leak radiation, negatively affecting at a minimum anyone living within a 20-mile radius of the plant. A study in England found a tenfold increased occurrence of leukemia in plant workers, plus there is a higher than normal risk for individuals living in close proximity.

Marketed as "clean fuel", it is far from clean, since nuclear releases permanently damage the human body as well as any portion of the earth contacted. Do not be fooled by marketing language. Nuclear power plants continuously release poisonous gases into the environment as well as the water. Plus, unless aging and friable plants are systematically and permanently closed, a nuclear release/accident of massive proportions is a virtual certainty in this country. Computer mishaps merely heighten the risks.

In the USA life-threatening contamination already exists. For instance, *U.S News & World Report*, August 30, 1999, documents the existence of radioactive parking lots and streets in Paducah, Kentucky, a contamination resulting from plutonium-containing trucks parked there.

The major way to become poisoned by nuclear ions is through the respiratory passages or the ingestion of water and food. Remember, these ions are primarily minerals, that is they are large ions (bigger molecularly than vitamins), so passage through the skin is less of a problem than inhalation and/or ingestion. Thus, one of the keys to survival is to block and/or prevent inhalation and ingestion. However, radioactive ions may exert direct toxicity to the surface of the body, causing massive skin damage, ulcerations, and radiation burns.

Radiation harms the body by destroying cells, particularly the highly friable cells of the immune system. Nutritional therapy helps protect the cells through every means possible, and antioxidant nutrients are the number one tool available.

Nuclear catastrophe survival/combat kit

- oil of cumin—take 20 or more drops (one dropperful) every few minutes.
- oil of rosemary—take 20 or more drops every few minutes both internally and under the tongue.
- Oreganol P73 Juice, Essence of Sage, Essence of Rosemary —very important; drink up to a bottle of each daily. Highly protective against radiation poisoning, Oreganol P73 Juice was used successfully to save the lives of Chernobyl victims.
- OxyOrega—take 10 or more drops every few minutes plus several drops under the tongue every few minutes.
- resveratrol-rich red grape powder (Resvital)—highly

valuable for total body protection; take as much as possible. For highest intake consume the bulk type; take a teaspoon every hour initially, then a few teaspoons daily. For quickest absorption hold the Resvital in the mouth for a few moments before swallowing. With capsules take 4 to 6 capsules every hour.
- Sesame-E (as mixed tocopherols and/or tocotrienols)—take a teaspoon or more daily.
- Black Seed-plus —take 3 or more capsules every few hours.
- Oreganol cream (for radiation burns)—apply liberally to the injured region.
- raw honey (for radiation burns)—apply as needed
- Aloe vera gel—use topically on radiation burns/wounds.
- portable gas mask with anti-nuclear ion cartridges
- water filtration straws
- NukeProtect super-protective capsules (iodine/selenium formula)—in the event of major exposure take 2 or more capsules every hour. For continued protection take 6 or more capsules daily. This protects the thyroid from nuclear radiation.

Foods that help

- anything rich in saturated fat, like whole milk, butter, beef, avocados, nut butters, etc. These heavy fats block the toxicity of radioactive ions, whereas vegetable oils accelerate them.
- fatty fish
- Brazil nuts (because of their rich supply of selenium)
- papaya and kiwi fruit
- tomato paste (lycopene, the tomato pigment, intercepts nuclear ions; be sure to add olive oil to the paste, as lycopene absorption is dependent upon dietary fats)

Things to avoid

- refined vegetable oils of any type

- iron of any type (except that naturally occurring in food)
- all contaminated foods, especially meat products and milk (animals concentrate radioactivity from contaminated soil/grass)

Pesticide/herbicide poisoning

It is estimated that a minimum of 500,000 individuals develop severe pesticide poisoning every year. This is a conservative estimate; the number is probably far higher: in the tens of millions.

Pesticides are ubiquitous, although they were unknown on this planet 100 years ago. They contaminate virtually every square inch of the earth. According to M. J. Bayer, medical toxicologist at the Connecticut Poison Control Center, these chemicals are "routinely sprayed over fields and farms", poisoning thousands of individuals, especially rural workers.

A mysterious flu has been afflicting farmers for decades. Previously attributed to molds or other germs housed in grain elevators, now the cause has been elucidated: toxic farm chemicals. Researchers publishing in *The Practitioner* (March 1993) found that when 34 people with known pesticide poisoning were analyzed, all had flu-like symptoms. These symptoms included debilitating fatigue, muscle and joint aches, and severe depression. While the farmers' ailments were usually misdiagnosed as the flu, arthritis, or psychological disorders, the cause was exclusively pesticide poisoning, either chronic or acute.

Repeated exposure to pesticides is life threatening, because these chemicals poison the brain and nervous system, disrupting their impulses to vital internal organs such as the heart, lungs, and kidneys. Yet, even a single exposure can kill. What happens is the pesticide poisons enzymes in the nervous system, which are responsible for breaking down neurotransmitters. Without these enzymes, the neurotransmitters accumulate within the brain and nerves to toxic levels, causing them to go haywire. This should be no surprise, since this poisoning of the nervous system is how these chemicals kill pests. Symptoms of sudden massive exposure include:

- massive sweating
- very slow heart rate
- twitching, often violent
- vomiting and nausea
- abdominal contractions
- convulsions and/or seizures
- severe respiratory distress

Daily exposure to pesticides is a more realistic problem than exposure from a sudden disaster, like an overturned tanker car or a chemical plant release. As reported by *Mother Jones* magazine, July/August 1998, unwittingly, virtually all individuals are being exposed without realizing it, at least this is true for those who fly. Tens of millions of individuals experience vague sensations, cold sweats, claustrophobia, head pain, earache, sinus trouble, nausea, or flu symptoms during or shortly after a flight. However, few realize that these symptoms are often due to pesticide poisoning rather than from germs. In all likelihood the plane you board was treated with pesticide spray recently, perhaps the day that you enter it. Numerous airlines confirmed to the magazine that they regularly or occasionally spray their planes with pesticides, and this includes some of the world's most prominent airlines: American, Continental, Delta, TWA, US Airways, United Airlines, and Northwest. What's more, these are domestic flights, not international. When questioned about the reason for spraying airplanes and passengers with toxic compounds, the explanation is "to kill mice."

Certainly, some of this pesticide is absorbed into the traveler's body, either via inhalation or through the skin. The skin is like a sponge, and it is unable to protect us. Becky Riley from the Northwest Coalition of Alternatives to Pesticides describes this dangerous practice thusly, "Pesticides break down slowly in the enclosed, poorly ventilated aircraft...passengers are *sealed in a chamber that has been gassed and sit there for hours* (italics mine)." According to Dr. Jack Thrasher, immunotoxicologist of Alto, New Mexico, the so-called preventive spraying of pesticides on airliners amounts to the "practice of insanity." He notes that one of the typical airline pesticides, Tralomethrin, can cause severe allergic reactions, even asthma attacks. Thrasher further proclaims that the airlines "have no business spraying pesticide" on their planes and that the practice isn't even required by law. What's more, federal agencies, such as the Department of Transportation, are on record stating that they not only fail to require spraying but have no idea why the airlines do so. However, their "sterile" attitude to this crisis is edified by Bill Mosley, public affairs specialist at the DOT, who says "there is no prohibition against (the airlines) doing as they wish." Yet, it was Dr. Donald Hopkins, former Assistant Surgeon General, who stated categorically that the practice of spraying noxious pesticides on planes was not only useless but also highly dangerous. Furthermore, he noted, it has never been proven to effectively control pest growth or prevent disease. Yet, fatalities have likely occurred on airlines due to pesticide reactions and have been "misdiagnosed" as heart attacks.

Pesticides are the most poisonous chemicals known. For instance, until 1996 Northwest Airlines used a compound known as *Bolt*, which outright poisons the nervous system: one of the consequences of such a poisoning is sudden death/heart attack. What's more, a report by the *Journal of Pesticide Reform* describes the well known birth defect-inducing action of this chemical. The pesticides currently used are far from safe and have been implicated in causing birth defects, cancer, and reduced sperm counts as well as neurological disorders. Dave Noetzel, an entomologist at the University of Minnesota, also finds the practice of poisoning the interior of airliners with pesticides abhorrent, stating that at best "it is overkill" and that, in fact, it is a "meaningless procedure." In other words, the public is put at extreme risk without cause. It was Bill Plapp who also noted that this practice should be deemed illegal, because "people should have the right to transportation without being subjected to a health hazard."

A United Airlines pilot recently reported that many of the airline's employees are against the pesticide contamination. Yet, their concerns have apparently been ignored, since this silent poisoning continues.

Pesticides are highly toxic to brain tissue, and they tend to concentrate there. An article published in *Neurology*, May 1998, describes how farm chemicals dramatically increase the risk of neurological disease. The researchers found that farmers who regularly use pesticides are over four times more likely to develop Parkinson's disease than controls. This clearly illustrates the extreme toxicity of pesticides to the human organism.

Remember that pesticides are fulminant nervous system poisons. Many of them are molecularly the same as the nerve gases synthesized during World War II. Do not use them carelessly. In fact, do not use them at all.

The symptoms produced by pesticides/herbicides depend upon the type of chemical. However, the primary symptoms include:

- spasticity of the lungs, increased bronchial secretions, suffocation on secretions, swelling in the lungs.
- radical drop in heart rate or radical rise in heart rate
- nausea, vomiting, diarrhea
- excessive sweating; cold, clammy feeling
- excessive tearing
- inability to hold urine (incontinence)
- muscle twitching/jerking, weakness, and paralysis
- headache, confusion, convulsions, and coma

Note: Pesticide/herbicide poisoning is likely if there develops a sudden sickness for no apparent reason. Pesticides fail to degrade quickly and residues may remain throughout the plane even without obvious spraying. Plus, the planes are sprayed repeatedly.

Pesticide detoxification/combat kit
- LivaClenz—take 20 or more drops several times daily.
- oil of oregano—take 2 drops under the tongue often, like 5 or more times daily. Also, take 10 drops twice daily in juice or water.
- Oreganol P73 Juice—drink as much as possible, like a bottle or half bottle daily.
- red grape powder (Resvital)—take 4 to 6 capsules three times daily or a teaspoon of the powder three times daily.
- NukeProtect—take 2 or more capsules every few hours until the poisoning is resolved. Then, take 2 to 4 capsules daily.
- GreensFlush wild greens drops (an important component which purges pesticide residue from the blood and liver)—take 2 or more droppersful several times daily.
- vinegar—drink 6 or more ounces daily added to juice or water.
- Nutri-Sense drink mix (to provide nerve regenerating natural B vitamins and phospholipids)—take 3 heaping tablespoons twice daily.
- LivaClenz—take 1 to two dropperfuls twice daily. After a week or two reduce the amount to 5 to 10 drops twice daily

Foods that help
- pure extra virgin olive oil (binds the chemicals and aids in their elimination through the liver)—drink a cup per day for a few days. Add the various oils in the olive oil, and drink as a purge. Add also vinegar, if desired.

Pinworms

In children this is one of the most common causes of intestinal pain and other gut symptoms. As many as 30% of children globally suffer from this condition. The infection occurs almost exclusively in children under 14. Early symptoms include abdominal pain, constipation, and itching of the anus. Severe itching of the anus is common, and, when children scratch this region, feces and pinworm eggs become trapped under the nails. Thus, when the child eats, he/she becomes reinfected and spreads the infection to others. The fingernails house the eggs, and if they are not kept trimmed, the child may transmit the infection to virtually anyone, including family members, friends, and other school children.

Pinworm combat kit

- oil of oregano—take 5 to 10 drops twice daily in juice or water.
- Intesti-clenz—take 5 to 10 drops twice daily (it is disguised best in tomato juice). Also, rub on the anus; wash hands thoroughly.
- Oregacyn gelcaps—powerful and easy to take, 3 capsules twice daily: especially effective if taken before bedtime.
- HerbSorb—take 3 or more capsules twice daily.
- oil of fennel—take 20 drops twice daily.

Note: in the event of infection bedding must be thoroughly washed. Soap alone is not sufficient to guarantee sterility. When washing bedding or underwear, add a sterilizing agent, such as chlorine or, preferably, antiseptic essential oils such as oil of oregano, oil of bay leaf, oil of cinnamon, or oil of clove.

Plague

Odds are low for a plague outbreak in the United States. However, this dangerous illness is increasing in frequency, especially in the southwestern states. Serious outbreaks have occurred recently in India, Africa, and China.

Plague is caused by a bacteria, which is transmitted to humans via the bites of fleas. The fleas usually contract the germ from rodents. However, squirrels are the major reservoir in the western United States.

In the Third World even in the 21st century outbreaks have occurred. These outbreaks have developed primarily in Central Africa and India. Thus, a global outbreak is conceivable.

In some respects plague is one of the easiest diseases to prevent. This is because with natural antiseptics any potential bite or lesion can be effectively treated immediately. By sterilizing any suspect lesion the development of plague may be aborted.

Plague combat kit

- oil of oregano (SuperStrength may be necessary)—apply to any suspect lesion. Also, take 5 or more drops under the tongue several times daily. If needed, take 5 to 10 drops in juice or water twice daily.
- OregaMax capsules—take 3 to 4 capsules three times daily.
- Purely-C—take 2 capsules three times daily.
- OregaBiotic multiple spice capsules—(a most important defense)—2 or more capsules as often as needed.
- Oreganol cream—rub on any open wound or lesion.
- Infla-eez—to reduce tissue inflammation and swelling take 3 capsules three times daily on an empty stomach.

Foods that help

- raw garlic/onion
- crude raw honey

Pneumonia

This is a potentially fatal condition, which usually afflicts the elderly. However, increasingly it is afflicting individuals of all ages. Currently, an outbreak of pneumonia is undermining the health of middle-aged individuals as well as children. The problem is that certain individuals, many in the prime of their lives, suffer either health devastation and/or death as a result of what should be a temporary or curable illness. Pneumonia doesn't have to kill.

CASE HISTORY:
Mrs. M., the mother of my associate, was placed in a nursing home, basically to die. The-80 year-old but spry lady had just been transferred from a hospital and was in a weakened state. Complaining of a relentless cough, shortness of breath, and lack of appetite, it was obvious that she had contracted a communal germ in the nursing home and was quickly developing pneumonia; nurses discovered that her lungs were filled with fluid. It appeared she was going to die. Her daughter, with my blessings, added 2 drops of Oreganol P73 to a glass of water. Handing it to her coughing and feverish mother, she said, "Take this, doctor's orders." Grudgingly, she swallowed the concoction. By the evening the fever broke, she began eating vigorously, and slept without discomfort. By the next day the pneumonia symptoms had completely disappeared.

Pneumonia combat kit

- oil of oregano (i.e. Oreganol P73)—take 2 or more drops under the tongue several times daily. Also, take 5 or more drops twice daily in juice or water.
- Oregacyn multiple spice capsules—2 capsules as often as needed.
- oil of lavender—rub on face, chest, soles of feet, and/or spine.
- Purely-C—3 capsules three times daily (or more often, if necessary)
- OregaMax capsules—3 capsules three or more times daily.
- Infla-eez—take 3 capsules several times daily.
- Garlex oil of cold-pressed garlic—10 drops under the tongue several times daily.

Poison ivy, oak, and sumac

This condition is virtually impossible to cure with medical therapy. There simply is no effective drug for it.

This is not the case with natural remedies. A number of agents halt the itching as well as reverse the toxicity of these poisonous plants. Reliable remedies include oil of oregano, oil of lavender, tea tree oil, camomile extracts, and aloe vera. However, oil of oregano has the supremacy. It halts itching on contact, plus it dissolves the poisonous resins, which are notoriously difficult to dislodge. This is largely due to the fact that the oil is an effective natural solvent, and, thus, it dissolutes the noxious resins, neutralizing them as well as allowing their removal through washing them from the body.

Be aware that direct contact with the skin is not the only way to contract these conditions. According to *Hippocrates Magazine,* July 1998, the resins from these plants stick to footwear, clothing, and even the fur of animals. Thus, it is advisable to wash thoroughly all contaminated objects. Add oil of oregano to the wash cycle. It will help dissolve or neutralize the resin.

Oreganol Cream is also an option; it is soothing, and it also eliminates the itching. Don't use cortisone creams. According to Dr. D. Harris, a Stanford University dermatologist, they are "worthless."

Poison plant resin combat kit

- oil of oregano (Super Strength is best)—apply topically as often as needed. Take 2 drops twice daily sublingually.
- Kid-e-Kare rubbing oil—apply topically as often as necessary; for adults use the SuperStrength
- tea tree oil—apply topically only.
- Oreganol cream—apply as needed.
- OregaSpray—spray on any involved site as often as needed.

Poor appetite

Poor appetite could be caused by stress. Yet, ironically, in certain individuals stress leads to a ravenous appetite. Nutritional deficiency is another major cause. Deficiencies of certain key nutrients impair the flow of digestive juices, and this reduces the desire for wholesome food. For reasons yet to be determined the individual may have a poor appetite for healthy food, while craving instead poor quality food such as chips, pop, luncheon meats, etc.

Poor appetite is a cardinal sign of vitamin deficiency. A lack of thiamine halts stomach acid production and impairs the body's ability to process sugar. Niacin deficiency virtually aborts the body's ability to produce energy, so sorely needed for proper digestion. A lack of vitamin B_6 greatly impairs the digestion and processing of protein. A deficiency of vitamins A and D leads to a malabsorption of fat and greatly impedes calcium absorption. Thus, poor appetite represents a vicious cycle; the individual is already deficient and by failing to eat properly, he/she becomes severely deficient. The result will certainly be impaired health and, in the extreme, anorexia, which can be fatal.

Appetite stimulation kit

- HerbSorb eastern spice formula (to stimulate the flow of digestive juices)—take 2 capsules with each meal.
- Nutri-Sense natural B vitamin drink mix—take 3 tablespoons once or twice daily in juice or water.
- premium-grade royal jelly (Royal Power)—take 4 capsules in the morning.
- red grape powder (Resvital) take 2 or 3 capsules with every meal.
- OregaMax capsules—take 2 or 3 capsules with every meal.
- Royal oil—take 1/2 teaspoon twice daily.
- Oregacyn Digestive—two capsules with every meal.

Poor breast milk

Regardless of the circumstances breast-feeding women have a handy tool, that is if the milk is delivered in abundance. Milk flow can be stimulated, merely by eating certain foods and taking safe/edible herbs and/or spices. In particular, the spices appear to be the most effective for inducing milk production. Apparently, they operate by activating body metabolism.

Breast milk stimulation kit

- oil of fennel—take 5 to 10 drops twice daily or more often if needed.
- oil of cilantro/coriander—take 5 to 10 drops twice daily.
- Resvital—take 1 or more teaspoons twice daily.
- Nutri-Sense—take 3 heaping tablespoons once or, preferably, twice daily in milk or juice.
- Black Seed-plus—take 3 or more capsules twice daily.
- Pumpkinol (crude fortified Austrian pumpkin seed oil)—take 5 or more capsules twice daily.
- Royal Power—take 3 or 4 capsules twice daily.
- Nutri-Sense natural B vitamin mix—3 T. twice daily.

Foods that help

- avocados—at least 2 per day
- steak—eat the largest portions available
- fennel seed tea with raw honey
- raw honey and/or carob molasses—take two tablespoons daily; they are mild laxatives, so eat to tolerance.
- tangy or aromatic spices, notably fennel seed, anise seed, rosemary, black seed, and coriander seed
- pumpkin/squash seeds or Austrian pumpkin seed oil
- fatty fish such as salmon, halibut, and trout (must be from relatively unpolluted waters)

Postnasal drip (see Sinus attacks)

Prostatitis

This is defined as inflammation of the prostate. The inflammation may result from infection, toxicity, and/or nutritional imbalances. Nutrient deficiencies of greatest importance include a lack of vitamin D, selenium, vitamin A, vitamin C, and zinc. Prostatitis can also be caused by a host of germs. Toxicity is another cause, that is the poisoning of the tissues by various noxious chemicals. Solvents readily poison this gland, causing inflammation and swelling.

Heavy metal poisoning is another cause of prostate disorders. In particular, cadmium damages the prostate. In fact, both prostatitis and prostate cancer may be directly related to the ill effects of this metal. This is because cadmium blocks the absorption and utilization of zinc, a mineral essential for the function of this gland. Normal enzyme function in the prostate is zinc dependent, and cadmium disrupts the ability of zinc to attach to the enzymes. Taking supplemental zinc may aid in displacing cadmium from the enzymes, helping return their function to normal.

Prostatitis combat kit
- Sesam-E—take one T. twice daily.
- ProstaClenz™—a 20:1 concentrate of crude pumpkin seed oil with antioxidant essential oils; take 2 or more gelcaps daily.
- Infla-eez capsules—take 2 capsules twice daily.
- oil of oregano—take 2 or more drops under the tongue daily.
- CranFlush—take 20 drops twice daily.
- zinc chelate—75 mg daily.
- crude pumpkin seed oil (fortified with essential oils, i.e. Pumpkinol), two tablespoons twice daily.

Note: for difficult cases both ProstaClenz and the Pumpkinol must be taken. Note: Sesam-E is ideal for impotence.

Foods that help
- pumpkin/squash seeds
- sardines, salmon, herring (for the fatty acid/vitamin D content)

Puncture wounds

This is one of the most treacherous of all injuries, largely because the wound is difficult to access. In other words, it is difficult to completely cleanse the wound(s) of germs that may cause serious infection.

Puncture wounds are notoriously associated with a condition commonly known as "lock jaw," for which people now receive tetanus shots. The word tetanus derives from the name of the bacteria which causes lock jaw, *Clostridium tetani.*

The tetanus shot is of little value in a crisis. This is because puncture wounds are infected by a variety of organisms. Thus, if the germs fester in the wound, serious infections may result. Yet, all that is needed is to thoroughly cleanse any wound and use the appropriate germicides. Here are the crucial steps to take in the event of a puncture wound (or deep laceration):

1. Thoroughly flush the wound with clean water. Use pressure, such as a hose or faucet, to force debris and germs from the wound.
2. If you are helping another individual, never touch the wound with your own hands. Germs from foreign hands are a major cause of life-threatening infections in deep wounds.
3. If there is noticeable debris, such as wood or metal chips lodged in the wound, which are not dislodged with flushing, attempt the following:

a. heat a tweezers with fire until the tip turns red hot (be sure to simultaneously protect your hands); let cool. Then, without allowing the tweezers to touch any thing else, attempt to remove the foreign body (this applies to minor wounds only). Or, if no heat is avail able, spray the tweezers with OregaSpray or Germ-a-Clenz and wipe.
b. saturate the area after such cleansing attempts with Oreganol P73.

Puncture wounds are not hopeless. This is because natural antiseptics can usually salvage the dilemma. After cleansing the wound, use the following antiseptics to halt infection.

Puncture wound combat kit

- oil of oregano (i.e. Oreganol P73)—saturate puncture wound site; take 5 or more drops under the tongue twice daily.
- oil of bay leaf—saturate puncture wound site.
- PropaHeal—apply and cover, repeating every 12 hours. May be mixed with raw honey.
- raw honey—apply as needed.
- Infla-eez—for eradicating any swelling or inflammation, 3 capsules 3 times daily on an empty stomach.
- OregaBiotic—take 2 capsules several times daily.

Note: an antiseptic pack can be made by combining the oil of wild oregano, oil of propolis, and raw honey. for every three ounces of honey add 3 droppersful each of oreganol and oil of propolis. This is the ideal salve for destroying any wound infections. The wild oregano honey and the Mediterranean wildflower honey are rich in healing enzymes plus antiseptics, and, thus, they are the ideal types to use.

Radiation poisoning (see also Nuclear catastrophe)

Currently, largely as a result of global governmental instability and aging infrastructure, there is a greater risk than ever before of a massive nuclear catastrophe. Yet, besides a nuclear catastrophe or exposure from a nuclear plant there are other more pervasive ways to develop radiation toxicity. It can happen right in the individual's home: radon. This gas is found in the bedrock of every state in this country. This is a type of natural gassing, where the earth releases radon gases, which are produced as a result of chemical reactions in the earth's greatest nuclear reactor: its molten core.

The only way to determine if you are being exposed to excessive levels is to be tested, that is to have your home tested. Check the local yellow pages for companies offering this service. You may also purchase self-administered test kits.

X-rays are another type of radiation. This is the most common type of human poisoning. Most individuals are poisoned as a result of medical x-rays, which, when performed repeatedly, result in significant tissue damage. X-ray technicians, radiologists, orthopedists, chiropractors, chiropractic assistants, cardiologists, dentists, and dental assistants are highly vulnerable to developing radiation poisoning.

High tension power lines are another type of poisoning. In this case the individual is being poisoned by electromagnetic radiation. Radiation may also emanate from broadcasting centers. Microwave dishes and, particularly, powerful radio towers emit microwaves and radio waves, both of which may enter the body and disrupt the cellular machinery. These forms of radiation are highly significant and may cause a toxicity similar to radiation poisoning. Transformer stations for utilities are perhaps the greatest culprit in this category and their emissions have been directly linked to a heightened incidence of brain cancer.

Cellular phones are perhaps the most prolific and direct source of electromagnetic wave exposure. Many phones produce potent electromagnetic waves capable of inducing "cellular" damage. The electromagnetic power source is a radio transmitter that produces powerful rays, which are capable of penetrating deep into human tissue, including the brain. There, they will incite the formation of free radicals, which may potentially lead to cancer initiation. Regular use of cell phones is linked to a heightened incidence of brain cancer. A recent study indicates that frequent cellular phone users are up to four times more likely to develop certain rare brain cancers than non-users. Antioxidants particularly active in protecting brain tissue from cellular phone damage include sage, oregano, rosemary, cumin, beta carotene, selenium, vitamin C, and vitamin E. For those who must use a cell phone, daily consumption of these antioxidants is advisable. In particular the regular use of Oreganol P73 Juice, as well as the Oxy Orega, is a must for individuals who constantly use cell phones.

Computer terminals emit a significant amount of radiation. All manner of gadgets have been invented to block the radiation. Yet, there is little that can be done about it, and because the radiation must be released, a certain amount of it will be absorbed into the body. However, one significant means of protection is to take natural antioxidants on a daily basis.

Patients undergoing repeated radiation treatments and/or who are subjected to frequent X-rays are being poisoned. X-rays cause tissue damage. They do so by bursting apart human genetic material. Recent studies have determined that radiation therapy offers no significant advantage for decreasing disability or increasing life span. Yet, millions of Americans undergo radiation therapy yearly. For those undergoing this treatment it is crucial to protect the body from the X-rays' toxic effects plus repair any tissue damage that occurs.

During the 21st century radiation accidents/exposure will occur at increasing frequency. Human error, as well as computer glitches, will cause catastrophic radiation releases. As this book was going to press humanity suffered a nuclear disaster. On September 30th, 1999, as described in the *Chicago Tribune,* an "unbelievable mistake" occurred at a Japanese plutonium plant. Strictly due to human error, the fatal blunder resulted in a monstrous release of radiation. Hundreds, perhaps thousands, were sickened. As a result, in this region cancer incidence will skyrocket. Reports in the U.S. that this is a minor accident are bogus. As plutonium dust is being "washed off" buildings and streets, the press would have us believe that only minor damage was done.

The press tells lies. The fact is, plutonium is so toxic that even a millionth of a gram can kill. The Japanese press is more "consumer friendly" than the U.S. press. If the same type of accident were to occur in the United States, there would surely be an extensive coverup. Unfortunately, the 21st century will be fraught with such incredibly dangerous disasters. The greatest of these is the use of so-called depleted plutonium or uranium. Known as DU this term was invented as a propaganda ploy, that is to minimize in peoples' minds the toxicity of this substance. The fact is this substance aggressively destroys human cells, causing irreparable genetic damage. There are hundreds of thousand of victims as a result of the use of this substance. Tens of thousands of children have developed birth defects as a result of it. What's more, by the thousands U.S. soldiers are dying as a result of this murderous substance. The fact is the use of depleted uranium against humankind is a war crime. It is crucial to determine who the perpetrators are, who imposed this substance on humanity and who, while murdering the innocent, profited. Surely, major U.S. corporations are among these profiteers. Yet, the fact is those who perpetrated it must be held responsible for harming virtually the entire human race. Incredibly, the majority of these criminals are U.S. citizens. The persistent use of depleted uranium will be the doom of the human race.

When radiation-induced catastrophes occur, protection may be achieved by taking natural substances and/or antioxidants, which protect the tissues from toxic damage. The following herbs, spices, and nutrients help protect the cells and their nuclei via their potent antioxidant actions:

Radiation poisoning combat kit

- oil of rosemary (edible type in olive oil)—to combat acute radiation toxicity take as much as possible, at least 40 drops daily. As a maintenance take 10 drops twice daily.
- oil of cumin—take as much as possible; no limit.
- oil of sage—take a few drops every hour, internally and/or sublingually. As a maintenance take 5 drops twice daily.
- Essence of Rosemary—drink as much as possible, 6 or more ounces daily. As a maintenance take 2 ounces daily.
- Oreganol P73 Juice—drink as much as possibly, 6 or more ounces daily. As a maintenance take 2 ounces daily.
- red grape powder (Resvital)—for acute poisoning take 4 capsules per hour, or take the bulk powder, 1 teaspoon every hour.
- multiple trace mineral supplement (iron-free)—iron increases the toxicity of radiation.
- Sesam-E and Pumpkinol (as a source of natural vitamin E and other key antioxidants—note, this is far more powerful than vitamin E pills)—for acute poisoning take 2 tablespoons of each I.U. every hour or two. Then, take four tablespoons of each daily.
- crude natural vitamin C and flavonoids (Purely-C)—take 3 or more capsules every hour. As a maintenance take 2 or more capsules twice daily.
- beta carotene (as natural crude mixed carotenoids)—take 25,000 I.U. every hour. As a maintenance take 50,000 I.U. daily.
- organic selenium—take 200 or more mcg every few hours for a few days. Selenium is potentially toxic, so after a week

or two reduce this amount to 1000 mcg daily. After a month reduce this to a maintenance amount of 400 to 600 mcg daily.
- iodine (as Lugol's solution or potassium iodide)—this is crucial, since radiation releases nearly always include the dis semination of radioactive iodine. This chemical rapidly destroys the thyroid gland, which, as a consequence of its normal tendency, concentrates iodine. Thus, if it concentrates radioactive iodine, it unwittingly destroys itself. The key is to load the blood with natural iodine in order to block the poisonous type.
- iodine as kelp (arsenic-free; Thyroset brand is best)—take 4 or more capsules every hour (this is the safest form of iodine).
- NukeProtect™ (a special formula containing the most essential anti-nuclear/radiation ingredients, including kelp, iodine, black seed, and selenium)—during immediate severe danger take 3 or more caps every hour; during moderate danger take 4 caps three times daily; as a maintenance take 2 caps twice daily.
- oil of edible ginger (in extra virgin olive oil)—for fighting nausea and vomiting, take a few drops as often as needed.

Foods that help

- Brazil nuts (as a source of selenium)
- cloves, whole
- raw almonds and filberts (rich source of vitamin E)
- dehydrated tomatoes and tomato paste (rich source of the anti-cancer anti-radiation substance, lycopene)
- cranberry juice concentrate (for flushing radioactive chemicals through the kidneys)
- crude sea salt (or iodized salt if the former is unavailable)
- canned salmon, sardines, and tuna (as a source of natural iodine)
- canned shrimp or squid (a top source of iodine)
- raw oregano honey (to prevent radiation-induced intestinal damage)

Note: the rule with radiation poisoning is to be aggressive. The amount of antioxidants required to protect the body is dependent upon the degree of exposure. If a massive radiation release occurs, be equally massive in the treatment. Double or triple the suggested amounts if necessary. Err in excess, because, without massive protection, the tissues will be destroyed. Barring the remote possibility of allergic intolerance the mentioned items are safe edible substances and can be consumed in huge amounts. The juices are the ideal agents, because they are quickly absorbed, and the individual will need quick antioxidant power to combat radiation. Protect yourself in every means possible. Radiation poisoning is the most gruesome of all illnesses.

Ringworm

This is caused by a fungus, which attacks the skin and other superficial tissues. The fungus feeds on skin cells. It also feeds on hair and nails. The reason it is called ringworm is that when the organism spreads it makes a ring. However, despite its name there are no worms in this ring, just fungus. Ringworm is another name for athlete's foot and jock itch.

Ringworm is contagious. Humans get it from other humans, and even pets can transmit it. However, the latter can also contract it from humans.

If you develop a lesion which is ring-shaped and which is itchy and/or red, it is probably ringworm. The only way to know for sure is to procure a culture. However, in most instances this is unnecessary. The following amounts are ideal for children as well as adults.

Ringworm combat kit
- oil of wild oregano (Oreganol P73)—rub vigorously on involved region twice daily. Also, take 2 or 3 drops twice daily under the tongue.

- oil of myrtle—rub vigorously on involved regions twice daily.
- Oregacyn multiple spice formula—take 2 or more capsules daily.
- Oreganol cream (very soothing)—rub on the involved region as needed.

Things to avoid
- refined sugar, corn syrup, sweets of all types, pop, etc.
- public gyms and locker rooms
- when walking in public places or using showers in places other than the home, never go barefoot. Wear thongs or shoes.
- don't allow the feet to remain wet (outside of water) for prolonged periods. Whenever the feet become wet, attempt to dry them thoroughly as soon as possible.
- never use another individual's sneakers
- thoroughly dry feet & between toes after every shower/bath

Salmonella

This is perhaps the most feared of all food-borne infections. Currently, it is the number one cause of food poisoning outbreaks. The commercial food supply is infested with this dangerous germ. What's more, this pervasive, aggressive germ is resistant to the majority of antibiotics.

Typically, humans contract salmonella through the gut, that is through eating contaminated food. Once ingested the organism usually causes diarrhea, which can be violent. Salmonella is an exceptionally destructive bacteria and may infect virtually any organ in the body. However, it has a predilection for infecting the liver and gallbladder, where it causes extensive damage. Apparently, it hides in these regions in order to evade the immune system.

Outbreaks of salmonella food and beverage poisoning are out of control. Incredibly, according to the CDC there are some 2000 different types of Salmonella that can infect humans. At least 5 million cases of salmonella food/beverage poisoning occur in North America every year, clearly signifying this as one of the most dangerous epidemics of the modern era. That means one of every 60 or so individuals contracts this infection yearly, definitively proving this is a vast epidemic.

No one is impervious, nor is seemingly any food. Normally, scientists regard this infection as a poultry or raw egg problem. However, there are numerous other foods which act as reservoirs. In May 1998, Malt-O-Meal cereal was recalled from dozens of states after it sickened hundreds: the cause was a bizarre sub-type of salmonella known appropriately as "Agona." Also in 1998 the FDA issued a warning that alfalfa sprouts, as well as radish sprouts, were contaminated with both Salmonella and E. coli. The CDC determined that tens of thousands of individuals have been sickened by the germ-contaminated shoots. What is most disconcerting is that the CDC's research proved that despite thorough washing the germs remained, apparently because they are lodged inside the cores of the shoots.

Salmonella combat kit

- oil of oregano (may require the SuperStrength variety)—take a few drops under the tongue several times daily. Take 10 to 20 drops in juice or water several times daily.
- wild oregano and/or thistle honey as an anti-diarrheal (use wild Mediterranean honeys if possible)—take 1/4 cup two or three times daily.
- LivaClenz (to drive the germ out of the liver and gallbladder)—take 20 drops twice daily.
- OregaBiotic multiple spice capsules (to kill the germs outright)—take two or more capsules three times daily.
- GreensFlush wild greens drops—20 or more drops twice daily.

Foods that help
- ginger root
- raw onion, garlic, and green onions
- daikon and black radish

Foods to avoid
- raw eggs and poultry of any kind
- commercial milk products
- processed meats

Scabies

Scabies is caused by a mite, known medically as *Sarcoptes scabei*. The mite is from the same family as dust mites, but it is bigger and specifically infects humans. About the size of a pinhead, it aggressively invades the skin, causing severe itching and inflammation. Usually, outbreaks occur in individuals with weakened immune systems but, increasingly, they are striking the healthy population.

Scabies combat kit

- SkinClenz—rub on any involved region as often as needed.
- oil of oregano (SuperStrength variety may be required)—rub on involved region—highly aggressive mite killer. Or, for children use the Kid-e-Kare rubbing oil.
- cloves of raw garlic—crush and place on the bottoms of the feet. Also, crush garlic and apply maceration to scabies region. If irritation occurs, discontinue use.
- OregaSpray—spray on any contaminated region, bedding, clothing, etc., to prevent further mite contamination.
- Oreganol SuperStrength—for tough conditions rub as needed and also take internally, five drops under the tongue twice daily.
- Garlex oil of cold-pressed garlic—rub topically as needed.

Foods that help

- Eat as much raw garlic and onions as possible. The stench of the garlic permeates the skin, aiding in the mites' destruction.

Sciatica

This painful and debilitating condition is caused by pressure on the huge sciatic nerve, either from disrupted lower lumbar vertebrae or muscular impingement in the pelvis. Sciatica may also be induced by toxic chemical exposure, that is exposure to heavy metals and/or solvents, or alcohol abuse. However, it usually results from sudden injury to the spine, lower back, or hip.

Sciatica combat kit

- oil of oregano (Oreganol P73, Super Strength variety is ideal)—rub the oil over the pain distribution. Also, rub it over the lower back, since this is where the nerve arises. Take 5 to 10 drops twice daily with meals until pain subsides. Take 2 to 4 drops daily in juice or under the tongue as a maintenance.
- red grape powder (Resvital)—take 4 capsules three times daily.
- Infla-eez rubbing oil—apply as needed.
- OregaMax (as a source of natural herbal minerals)—take 3 capsules twice daily.
- Infla-eez (high potency antiinflammatory enzymes)—between meals, take 2 to 3 capsules twice or more daily.

Foods that help

- fatty fish (salmon and albacore tuna), almonds (high in salycilates), and dried papaya or kiwi (high in enzymes)

Things to avoid

Don't use a heating pad, wet or dry. This will greatly inflame the nerve. If medical care is unavailable, don't use prescription antiinflammatory drugs during a disaster due to potentially life-threatening side effects such as internal bleeding. Don't sleep on the back and beware of sleeping on the stomach; this is disastrous for sciatica.

Other ideas
- Keep moving, i.e. stay mobile, but don't jog. Instead, perform brisk walking. Do high step walking, if possible.

Scorpion bites

This is a limited problem for the general population, largely because of geography. Scorpions only inhabit the tropics, Mediterranean, and small tracts of the United States, notably Arizona, Texas, and Southern California. However, if hundreds or thousands of individuals are exposed to the elements in these states, scorpion bites become a significant possibility. In Mexico scorpion bites are a major disaster, causing some 1500 deaths yearly. Not all bites cause death. In fact, bites only rarely cause deaths. Usually, they cause pain—extreme pain. Yet, the type of scorpion found in the southwestern United States is unusually dangerous, offering a potentially lethal strike.

Scorpion bite combat kit
- crushed garlic cloves—apply juice or maceration to the site repeatedly until relief is achieved.
- Garlex oil of cold-pressed garlic—a ready-made option, apply liberally to any wound; take also 10 or more drops under the tongue as needed.
- oil of oregano (Oreganol P73)—apply repeatedly; take 5 to 10 drops under the tongue every few minutes.
  Note: The Super Strength variety is preferred.
- Super-high potency bromelain/papain, that is the Infla-eez—take 3 or more caps twice daily.

Foods that help
- vinegar—pour it on the bite repeatedly

Seizures

Only medical personnel can properly deal with seizures. Thus, the objective is to prevent them from occurring. This is accomplished by properly nourishing the brain and the glands which support brain function, like the adrenal, thyroid, and pituitary glands.

Essential oils are the most effective of all natural anti-seizure remedies. They have direct action upon the brain, because they are transferred to it directly. This is because the oils are volatile, and they gain quick entrance to the human body through inhalation as well as skin absorption. The highly volatile nature of essential oils allows for ready access to the brain, because there is a membrane in the roof of the nose directly connected to it. This membrane, known as the *cribiform plate*, is very thin, and the essential oil vapors pass directly through it. This is why essential oils are so famous for their relaxing actions and their rapid ability to alter mental state. However, skin absorption is also valuable, because once the oils are absorbed through the skin they are quickly trapped by the blood, which transports them to every organ in the body, including the brain.

Seizure combat kit
- oil of lavender—rub on face, buttocks, and soles of feet.
- Kid-e-Kare rubbing oil—rub on forehead, back, spinal column, and bottom of feet as needed.
- oil of Oreganol P73—take 2 drops under the tongue once or twice daily. Also, rub on chest, spine, buttocks, and soles of feet.
- Royal Power—take 4 capsules once or more daily.
- Royal Oil—sublingual royal jelly paste, ideal for children, take 1/2 teaspoon sublingually twice daily.

- Nutri-Sense drink mix/food fortifier (as a source of crude natural B vitamins for nourishing the nervous system)—take 3 to 6 tablespoons daily in juice or water.
- Neuroloft aromatic essence of wild spices—an invaluable natural substance with brain-soothing actions, 2 to 3 tablespoons daily added to hot water.
- Oreganol P73 Juice—1 ounce twice daily, helps eradicate any hidden infections in brain tissue.
- Neuroloft capsules (cross the blood-brain barrier)—one or two capsules twice daily.

Foods that help

- avocados (rich in natural B_6 and fatty acids)
- fresh red meat (rich in carnitine and electrolytes)
- sardines, salmon, albacore tuna (rich in fish oils and B_6)
- high fat foods which are rich in natural fats

Things to avoid

- food dyes and artificial flavorings
- white sugar and chocolate
- MSG and sulfites
- synthetic perfumes
- clothes that require dry cleaning (dry cleaning chemicals cause brain cell damage)
- processed meats

Shigellosis

Shigellosis is a diarrheal illness caused by the bacteria *Shigella sonnei*. As a cause of diarrheal outbreaks it is becoming increasingly common. What's more, now there are drug-resistant forms which are exceedingly virulent. The diarrhea can be severe, bloody, and life-threatening. The most common source is contaminated water, although food may be poisoned by this germ. The germ may contaminate various sites such as public water pipes, reservoirs, ice machines, private wells, and ice cubes. If you are concerned about a facility's water quality, avoid consuming the water as well as the ice.

The CDC notes that, globally, Shigella is the most common cause of bacterial dysentery. Typical symptoms include diarrhea, fever, chills, night sweats, abdominal pain/cramping as well as blood and mucous in the stool. According to research by the U.S. government oil of oregano destroys this germ.

Shigellosis combat kit

- oil of oregano (Oreganol P73, SuperStrength may be required)—take 5 or more drops under the tongue several times daily. Also, take 10 or more drops in juice or water as needed.
- LivaClenz—take 20 drops or more twice daily.
- onion juice—1/4 cup twice daily.
- ginger juice—1/4 cup twice daily. Or, use oil of edible ginger, 10 to 20 drops twice daily in juice or water.
- wild oregano or thistle honey—1/4 cup several times daily.
- Black Seed-plus—take 3 or more capsules every few hours.

Foods that help

- clear meat broths with garlic and onion

Shingles

As many as 150,000 Americans are afflicted with this disastrous disease every year. The elderly account for the majority of its victims. They are vulnerable, because shingles usually attacks individuals with sluggish or weakened immune systems. Often, it is provoked by severe stress, grief, and the intake of certain drugs, notably cortisone and arthritis medications.

Shingles is caused by a virus of the herpes family. This is the same virus that causes chicken pox. This herpes virus lives in the body, hiding within the nerves. In other words, it is not possible to "catch" shingles. It is not a skin disorder but, rather, is an internal disease which only surfaces in the skin. It is an extremely painful illness, in fact, according to Dr. S. K. Typing of the University of Texas at Galveston, it is "a medical emergency." When it attacks the nerves, it greatly damages them, often permanently, unless the germ is quickly destroyed.

Usually, shingles develops in the chest around the rib cage. It may also develop in the neck and face, behind the eye (which can lead to blindness), and in the lower back. The pain of shingles is usually excruciating. Often, none of the medical therapies are successful. The individual is left to writhe in agony, often for weeks, perhaps months or years. Natural remedies are part of the answer and often the only answer.

CASE HISTORY:
Mr. C., a young man suffering from a sluggish immune system, saw me during my professorship at the University of Osteopathic Medicine, Des Moines, Iowa. He had facial shingles, but this was only the beginning. The virus had infected his optic nerve, the nerve that supplies the eye. Aggressive treatment with natural remedies, which included intravenous doses of vitamin C and pantothenic acid, saved the eye and within two weeks all of the facial lesions were completely healed.

Shingles combat kit

- oil of oregano SuperStrength (P73)—apply directly to lesions or pain area. Take 2 drops under the tongue several times daily. Take also 5 to 10 drops twice daily in juice or water.
- OregaMax capsules—take 6 or more capsules daily.
- Oreganol cream—rub on involved region several times daily.
- pantothenic acid (use capsules, not pressed tablets)—take 500 mg three times daily.

- premium-grade royal jelly (Royal Power)—take 4 capsules three times daily.
- bromelain/papain high potency formula (i.e. Infla-eez)—take 3 capsules three or more times daily on an empty stomach.
- I.V. vitamin therapy; see if your doctor can administer this.

Foods that help

- fatty fish (salmon, sardines, tuna, mackerel, etc.)
- beef, lamb, and turkey
- papaya plus the seeds

Things to avoid

- chocolate, definitely and absolutely
- refined sugar and hydrogenated oil
- corn, wheat, rye
- all nuts and seeds, particularly peanuts

Sinus attacks

In modern medicine effective medical treatment for sinus disorders is lacking. Despite medication the attacks seemingly continue without mercy. Major causes of this disorder include infection, air pollutants, and food allergy.

Regarding infection it has largely been presumed that bacteria are the cause. A recent study (1999) by Mayo Clinic dispels this. In particular in cases of chronic sinusitis some 100% of all victims suffered from primarily fungal, that is mold, infections. Bacterial infections played little if any role.

Recently, it was discovered that certain essential oil-bearing plants, such as oregano, thyme, myrtle, eucalyptus, savory, cumin, and sage, may be useful in reversing respiratory disorders, including sinusitis. The fact is such oils are antifungal. The highly orthodox journal *The Female Patient* recommends using spices in the kitchen, as well as therapeutically, "to clear out the sinuses." These researchers suggest that the active ingredient in these herbs and spices is a group of compounds found within the essential oils known as phenol. Carvacrol, the active ingredient of wild oregano, is the most biologically active and aggressive of these phenols. Oil of oregano is the richest naturally occurring source of carvacrol and is highly useful as a tonic for the sinuses and respiratory tract. Other herbs useful for sinus disorders include fenugreek, coriander, black seed, bay leaf, horseradish, and cumin. However, wild oregano is the premier herb for the sinuses. In fact, in regards to sinusitis its utility overshadows the need for other herbs, spices, or tonics.

Essential oils readily destroy molds. It is the premise of this book that the majority of chronic respiratory disorders are caused by mold. To treat such disorders there must be a heavy emphasis on the use of spice oil extracts, particularly oil of wild oregano and the multiple spice respiratory formula, Oregacyn.

Sinus attack combat kit

- oil of oregano (Oreganol P73)—for best results take it under the tongue. Also, massage the oil over the sinuses; apply a small amount under the nose. Or, saturate a Q-Tip with the oil and pass into the sinuses once or twice daily.
- Oregacyn respiratory multiple spice capsules—take 2 or 3 capsules three times daily; this is the top remedy for this condition.
- Black Seed-plus—take 2 or more capsules twice daily.
- Oreganol P73 Juice—take 2 tablespoons twice daily.

Foods that help

- cayenne and curry powder
- horseradish
- onions, especially green onions
- radishes and turnips

Things to avoid
- milk products, especially butter
- antihistamines, especially nasal sprays
- NutraSweet and sulfites

Skin cancer

This is a current epidemic afflicting primarily fair-skinned individuals. The greatest concentration of skin cancers occurs in the United States, Canada, Europe, and Australia. Interestingly, these are also the regions where the greatest amounts of processed foods are consumed. It seems that for fair-skinned people persistent exposure to sunlight combined with the heavy intake of processed foods is the recipe for disaster.

Prolonged exposure to the sun is the primary cause of skin cancer. The fact is skin cancer, long thought to only develop over a prolonged period, can become instigated suddenly as a result of severe stress and/or extreme sun exposure. However, dietary factors play a significant role, although this issue has never been emphasized sufficiently. Certain civilizations, despite extensive exposure to the sun, have a lower incidence of skin cancer than Americans. These are cultures in which refined foods, particularly the highly refined sugars and vegetable oils, are unknown. In all likelihood it will be eventually proven that a diet high in refined vegetable oils greatly increases the risk for skin cancer.

Skin cancer combat kit
- oil of oregano—apply directly to region, and take 5 to 10 drops twice daily (SuperStrength is best)
- oil of cumin—apply directly to region, and take 10 drops or more twice daily.
- Oreganol cream—apply directly to region and surrounding skin. Also, apply to facial skin and other exposed regions preventively.

- oil of rosemary—take 10 to 20 drops twice daily in juice or water.
- red grape powder (rich in the anti-cancer resveratrol)—take 4 capsules three times daily.
- Infla-eez proteolytic enzyme—two or more capsules on an empty stomach twice daily.
- Oreganol P73 Juice—1 oz twice daily.

Foods that help

Austrian pumpkin seed oil (as an excellent source of natural zinc, beta carotene, and vitamin A)

Things to avoid

- constant direct exposure to sunlight. Wear a hat. Don't totally avoid sunlight, but be sure to protect yourself. Clothing is the best protection.
- refined vegetable oils
- hydrogenated oil and nitrated meats

Smoke inhalation (see also Carbon monoxide poisoning)

During disasters this is one of the most common causes of human injury. It is the number one cause of fire-related deaths. The inhalation of smoke always causes tissue damage. Massive inhalation may lead to permanent damage and/or death. The agents responsible for this are various hydrocarbons liberated in smoke, which are highly caustic to human cells.

During a fire involving synthetic building materials (or even natural wood) numerous highly toxic compounds are liberated in the smoke, including acetaldehyde, formaldehyde, and cyanide. All these substances are potent cellular poisons. In the event of smoke inhalation protect your lungs and the rest of your body with agents capable of assisting in the detoxification of these compounds. In other words, take large amounts of antioxidants.

Smoke inhalation combat kit

- oil of rosemary—take 10 drops every few hours or as necessary.
- oil of oregano—take 5 to 10 drops under the tongue as needed.
- Oreganol P73 Juice—drink an ounce or more as often as needed.
- Essence of Rosemary—drink two or more ounces daily.
- NukeProtect (cellular protection system)—take 3 capsules several times daily.
- vitamin E (as crude pumpkin seed oil and Sesam-E)—total of 4 tablespoons daily.
- folic acid—take 10 mg daily.
- beta carotene (natural source)—25,000 I.U. to 50,000 I.U. daily until condition is resolved.

Foods that help

- squash, pumpkin, sweet potatoes, Austrian pumpkin seed oil
- fresh spinach (baby spinach is best), watercress, and parsley

Things to avoid

- cigarette or cigar smoke (1st or 2nd hand)

Snake bites

Compared to the other injuries addressed in this book, snake bites are relatively rare. The basic fact is that if you leave snakes alone, they will leave you alone. The vast majority of snakes are non-venomous. Even with the venomous types, the bites are rarely fatal. The fact is a greater number of individuals die because of shock or fright than from the snake bites themselves.

Even so, snake bites can be highly destructive, so it is wise to be prepared. This is certainly not a condition to treat by yourself. However, be aware that for thousands of years humanity has relied upon natural remedies for curing venomous bites. Even today these remedies are used, for instance, the application of a garlic concoction to cobra bites by East Indian snake charmers. What follows are a few of the more reliable remedies:

Snake bite combat kit

- raw garlic cloves—crush cloves and apply maceration to involved region; repeat as needed.
- oil of oregano—apply liberally. Repeat every hour or two. Take 5 drops of the oil internally every hour. After a few hours, reduce this to 10 drops twice daily until the condition is resolved.
- LivaClenz—for preventing venom-induced liver damage; take 20 drops several times daily until the problem is resolved.
- juice of raw onion—squeeze as much juice into the wound as possible. Drink any remaining juice.
- bromelain/papain (i. e. Infla-eez)—take 3 capsules three or more times daily to reduce swelling and inflammation.

Things to avoid

- Obviously, avoid panic: stay calm. Panic may do more harm than the snake bite. Get medical help as soon as possible.

Sneezing attacks

This is usually caused by allergic reactions. In particular, it is a common consequence of mold sensitivity. There is one reliable remedy: P73 oil of oregano. Combat it by taking 2 or more drops under the tongue as often as necessary to halt the attack. If this doesn't suffice, dilute the oil in olive oil (5 drops in a teaspoon of oil) and drip into the nostrils. Beware: this burns temporarily; the eyes tear and turn bloodshot. However, this dissipates rapidly and there is no harm done to the tissues. Oregacyn respiratory is another highly effective medicine, which relieves this. A powerful antihistaminic Oregacyn quickly eliminates allergy-related symptoms. Thus, it is a cure for allergic attacks as well as hay fever.

Sore throat

Sore throat is primarily an epidemic afflicting children. Unfortunately, it has become an epidemic among adults as well. It is usually caused by bacterial and/or viral infection. The germs attack the epithelial, that is skin cells, which line the throat, causing inflammation as well as cellular destruction. They also invade and attack the lymph glands, causing swelling and pain.

Most individuals regard strep as the major factor when dealing with a sore throat. However, this condition may be caused by a variety of bacteria as well as viruses and fungi. Mold toxins, which are readily disseminated in the air and which may be consumed via poisoned food, may also cause sore throat. In this instance the mold toxins poison the immune system of the throat, causing severe pain and inflammation. Food allergy is yet another cause. Often, a combination of these factors is involved.

Sore throat combat kit

- P73 oil of oregano—take 2 or more drops under the tongue frequently until soreness is gone. Also, gargle with the oil added to salt water. The salt plus oregano oil are synergistic in germ-killing.
- OregaMax capsules—take 6 or more capsules daily.
- raw honey (with or without vinegar)—use as a natural antiseptic gargle. Or, eat (literally drink) the honey, 1/4 to 1/2 cup daily.
- Purely-C (crude natural vitamin C plus flavonoids)—take 3 capsules twice daily.
- Germ-a-CLENZ natural spice oil spray—spray in back of throat as often as necessary.

- Kid-e-kare natural wild cherry throat spray (for infants, toddlers, and children)—spray on back of throat as often as necessary.

Foods that help
- onion/garlic/chicken broth
- vinegar and/or salt water gargle
- ginger root tea
- Austrian pumpkin seed oil (as an excellent source of immune-boosting nutrients)

Things to avoid
- antihistamines and aspirin
- corn, popcorn, wheat, and rye
- soda pop and caffeinated beverages, including iced tea

Sour mood and/or negativity

There is nothing worse than being burdened by an individual who is constantly negative. Negativity and/or moodiness not only is harmful to the perpetrator, but it also assaults any bystander. The point is no one can afford to spend time/energy cajoling emotionally deranged adults (or teenagers) during high stress incidents. Halt this negativity with home remedies designed to strengthen the mind, boost mental acuity, erase apathy, and balance the mood. Remember, mental disturbances often originate from physical ailments such as hypoglycemia, adrenal weakness, and/or nutritional deficiency. For instance, a deficiency of thiamine results in depression and/or anxiety as well as mood swings. That is why this substance is known as the "morale vitamin." There are numerous other nutrients which could be deficient (for more information on the significant role of nutritional deficiencies in mental conditions see Dr. Cass Ingram's *Nutrition Tests for Better Health* or the web site, NutritionTest.com). Do not always assume bizarre behavior is exclusively due to a psychological problem.

Sour mood combat kit
- Neuroloft (helps balance mood and enliven spirits)—drink straight, add to citrus juice, or, preferably, pour into hot tea as an exotic and reviving beverage. Add 1 or more tablespoons per cup of beverage.
- Essence of Rose Petals—same directions as above.
- premium-grade royal jelly (Royal Power)—take 4 or more capsules every morning before breakfast.
- St. John's wort (wild high flavonoid type is best)—take 2 to 4 capsules with breakfast.
- Essence of Rosemary—add an ounce twice daily in juice or water.
- Nutri-Sense crude rice fractions/polish drink mix (as a completely natural source of thiamine and niacin)—take 3 or more heaping tablespoons in juice, water, or milk once or twice daily.

Things to avoid
- refined sugar and sweets, especially soda pop
- ice cream

Spider bites

A bite by a spider evokes a great deal of fear, but it is mostly overplayed. The only truly fatal spider bites are caused by the notorious and much feared funnel web spider of Australia and the Brazilian wandering spider, the most fatal of all. North American spiders are largely harmless, except black widows and brown recluses. Their bites are only rarely fatal. However, the bites are painful and can cause significant tissue damage. In fact, *Taber's Medical Dictionary* describes black widow bites as being "excruciatingly painful." Brown recluse bites may be less painful, but the results are equally catastrophic. Often, entire chunks of tissue die as a result of the poisonous effects of the venom.

Obviously, if a bite by a venomous creature occurs, get medical help immediately. Yet, the key to minimizing the damage is to apply natural antivenoms to the wound/bite region as soon as possible and also to take natural substances which combat the poisoning. It doesn't matter what type of spider bite there is (usually the individual fails to see the culprit). The treatment remains the same regardless.

Spider bite combat kit
- raw garlic cloves—crush cloves and place a maceration over the wound. Repeat every 4 to 6 hours.
- oil of oregano (Super Strength is best)—apply several drops directly on the region; gently massage into tissues. Take 2 or more drops under the tongue every 15 minutes initially (for up to 2 hours), then 2 to 5 drops twice daily as a maintenance. drops under the tongue every hour or two until resolved.
- raw honey—place over wound region by itself or with the garlic maceration.
- oil of propolis (PropaHeal)—powerful antiinflammatory, 5 or more drops several times daily; also may be used topically.
- Infla-eez—take 3 capsules several times daily, ideally on an empty stomach.

Note: if there is only a sluggish response, take a greater amount of oil of oregano; double or triple the dose. Antivenom is available at hospitals.

Sprained joints

Sprains and strains are widespread in athletically active individuals. Such injuries are a major dilemma in adolescents, especially those involved in aggressive sports.

There are no dependable medical treatments for these injuries. However, natural remedies are a real boon, as they are astonishingly effective when nothing else seems to help. In particular, through the application of oil of oregano, swelling and pain are often eradicated within minutes. The following amounts apply to teenagers and adults. For children reduce the internal amounts by half.

Sprained joint combat kit

- oil of oregano—rub over involved region. Take 5 to 10 drops twice daily in juice or water (SuperStrength is the best for topical application).
- bromelain/papain combination (Infla-eez)—take 3 capsules on an empty stomach three times daily. In the event of a severe sprain double this amount. If the swelling is severe, increase the amount to 5 or more capsules three times daily.
- Infla-eez rubbing oil—rub on the involved region as needed.

Staph infection

Virtually everyone has suffered from some type of staph infection. This hardy bacteria causes boils, pimples, infected ducts/cysts, skin eruptions, psoriasis, sinus infections, sore throats, wound infections, cellulitis, impetigo, and bronchitis, conditions which many Americans suffer with routinely. It is also a major cause of food poisoning.

Staph is also a major perpetrator of life-threatening infections such as flesh-eating bacteria, bone infection (osteomyelitis), pneumonia, spleen infections, vaginal infections, kidney infections, and blood poisoning. In fact, the commonly feared "red streaks" in the tissues which develop from infected wounds are usually caused by staph infections.

The greatest dilemma with staph is that it has become increasingly resistant to antibiotics. Currently, a bizarre type of mutant staph has been attacking humans, which is immune to all synthetic antibiotics. Known as MRSA (methicillin resistant Staphylococcus aureus) this germ could likely prove fatal in virtually any individual. Deaths from the germ have been reported in Japan, Canada, England, and the United States. It usually attacks hospitalized patients, particularly those undergoing surgery or taking multiple medications. In Canada, where supergerms such as Staph aureus are prolific as the result of the excessive use of antibiotics, massive epidemics are inevitable. Modern medicine offers nothing to stop it.

Now there is a new strain of staph, which is even worse than MRSA. Known as VRSA, this staph is completely immune to antibiotics. The VRSA is even immune to Vancomycin, the most powerful staph-killing drug known. According to physicians in the New York region infections by this mutant staph in area hospitals have already reached epidemic proportions. Only natural substances will stop such germs from mercilessly consuming human lives. For instance, according to Cornell University (1998) staph is readily destroyed by natural compounds, including wild oregano oil, for instance, Oreganol capsules, onion, and garlic.

Staph infection combat kit

- oil of oregano (P73)—take 5 or more drops under the tongue several times daily. Take 10 drops three times daily in juice or water. For tougher conditions use the SuperStrength oil of oregano, 2 to 3 drops under the tongue several times daily plus 10 to 20 drops two or three times daily in juice or water. Rub on any suspect lesion.
- Purely-C—take 6 or more capsules daily to stimulate white blood cell activity against staph.
- OregaBiotic—take 3 or more capsules several times daily.
- Infla-eez—take 2 or 3 capsules three times daily.
- red grape powder (Resvital)—take 1 teaspoon 3 times daily.
- raw garlic—take as needed, topically or internally
- pumpkin seeds or, preferably, Austrian pumpkin seed oil (as a source of immune-boosting zinc and vitamin A)

Stomachache

Perhaps the most common ailment of children, stomachaches can afflict virtually anyone. This is one of the most uncomfortable of all illnesses and is often difficult to relieve. This is why natural therapies are so useful, because they offer the ability to quickly abate most stomachaches. The most common causes of stomachaches include infections, particularly parasitic, anxiety attacks, food allergies, and medication reactions.

Modern research proves that certain herbs aid stomach function. Ironically, many of these herbs, for instance, ginger root, are hot/spicy. This is precisely the opposite of the approach taken by the medical profession, since spicy foods are often prohibited for digestive problems. Yet, in societies where spicy foods are the norm, digestive disorders are relatively rare. What today's medicine has failed to comprehend is that hot tangy spices are tonics, that is they stimulate digestion. Plus, they are antiseptics, which means they kill harmful microbes that cause stomachache, stomach cramps, diarrhea, and other gastrointestinal ailments.

Stomachache combat kit

- Gastronex—one capsule with meals or as needed.
- oil of ginger (olive oil emulsification)—a convenient way to gain the benefits of ginger, take 3 or more drops twice daily in juice or water. If stomachache is worse after eating, take oil of ginger with each meal.
- oil of fennel—take 10 to 20 drops twice daily in juice or water.
- HerbSorb—take 2 or more capsules three times daily.
- Oregacyn Digestive—take 2 or more caps three times daily with meals.

Stomach ulcer

There is a new theory for the cause of stomach ulcers: infection. The culprit is a hideous appearing curve-shaped bacteria known as *Helicobacter pylori*. This germ invades the lining of the stomach and duodenum, causing inflammation and, ultimately, ulceration. No one is immune from it. While it is perhaps most common in the elderly, as many as 50% of all children suffering from chronic stomach disorders have the infection.

Nutritional deficiency also plays a role in ulcer formation. Critical nutrients needed to maintain a healthy stomach lining include folic acid, vitamin C, bioflavonoids, vitamin K, vitamin A, thiamine, niacin, vitamin B_{12}, and zinc.

Stomach/duodenal ulcer combat kit

- wild oregano herb (OregaMax capsules)—take 2 or 3 capsules twice daily (plus 2 Oreganol gelcaps for fighting infestation).
- Gastronex—take 2 capsules with each meal.
- oil of oregano—take 2 drops under the tongue twice daily.
- oil of ginger (olive oil emulsification)—take 2 or 3 drops with each meal. Mix in juice or add to hot water as a tea with honey.
- crude fenugreek, cumin, black seed capsules (HerbSorb caps) —take 1 or 2 capsules with meals.
- Purely-C—take 2 to 3 capsules twice daily. In the event of bleeding ulcer, triple this dosage.
- red grape powder (Resvital)—take 3 capsules two or three times daily.
- Black Seed-plus—take 2 or more capsules with meals.

Things to avoid

- apple juice, soda pop, and caffeinated beverages
- fried foods
- nitrated meats (hot dogs, bologna, salami, etc.)

Strep A

This is the infection that killed Jim Hensen of The Muppets fame. One of the most aggressive and destructive of all germs, strep A is the primary cause of flesh-eating bacteria.

Strep A is fiercely attacking Americans. Thousands of individuals are mercilessly killed and/or maimed by it yearly. Recently (March 1999) an epidemic of this infection struck some 50 individuals in the Chicago area, killing at least 10. In these instances the germ literally ate the individuals' tissues alive, killing them within 24 to 48 hours. Physicians stood by helplessly, with no cures offered. As the media disseminated the story panic developed, causing thousands of individuals to flood hospitals.

Strep can infect virtually any organ in the body. It is a major cause of drug-resistant infections in hospitals and frequently causes post-surgical infections. Strep is a primary cause of sore throats, chest infections, heart valve infections, kidney infections, skin infections, tonsillitis, and blood poisoning.

Medicine cannot halt it. Yet, strep A can be destroyed by a wide variety of natural substances, including oil of oregano, oil of lavender, oil of bay leaf, raw garlic, raw onion, raw honey, and cinnamon. Oil of oregano is particularly harmful to this germ. One study found that the oil effectively killed strep by causing its cell walls to disintegrate.

It is automatically assumed that sore throats are due to strep infections, yet, according to *Postgraduate Medicine*, January 1997, only 10% of teenagers and as few as 40% of children presenting at doctors' offices with sore throats actually have the infection. The other causes, such as viruses, yeasts, and molds, are usually missed.

Strep A combat kit

- oil of oregano (the SuperStrength may be required)—take 2 to 3 drops under the tongue several times daily. Also, take 20 drops in juice or water three or more times daily. Rub on spine and buttocks liberally. For tougher conditions follow the same amounts using the SuperStrength. Or, use Oreganol gelcaps, 1 or 2 caps twice daily.

- oil of lavender (wild mountain grown type is best)—rub on face, chest, soles of feet, and buttocks.
- OregaBiotic capsules—take a minimum of 3 capsules three times daily.
- Purely-C (to help activate white blood cells against strep)—take 6 or more capsules daily.
- oil of cinnamon (from edible cinnamon bark, food-grade)—ideal for children, take 2 or more drops twice daily.

Foods that help
- papaya plus the seeds
- raw garlic and onion
- pumpkin seeds or, preferably, Pumpkinol (as a source of immune-boosting zinc and vitamin A)

Things to avoid
- all forms of refined sugar
- coffee, tea, iced tea, NutraSweet

Sunburn (see also Burns)

Sunburn is one of the most agonizing and noxious of all burn injuries. It is a common human injury, afflicting tens of millions of Americans every year. Every summer millions of Americans develop sunburns severe enough to cause tissue damage.

With modern technology it is possible to prevent sunburns. This is largely through the combination of protective clothing along with sunscreen. While not a magic potion, sunscreen, if used properly, will prevent severe sunburn. The problem is usually that people use too little or apply the wrong type. Light-skinned individuals in particular should slather it on. Be sure the sunscreen is guaranteed to block both types of UV light, the A waves and B waves. The best sunscreens use vitamins, as well as antioxidants, as active ingredients. These natural substances are of more value in protecting the skin than merely using chemicals, because the nutrients help heal skin damage. PABA is a B vitamin which absorbs sun rays, preventing them from damaging the skin. Some people are allergic to PABA, so test a small amount before using. Vitamin E, beta carotene, pantothenic acid, and vitamin C also block ultraviolet rays, while helping repair any damage. Ideally, also use sunscreens that have an aloe vera or camomile base, as both of these herbs help induce skin healing.

Certain antioxidant-rich essential oils, particularly spice or herbal oils, act as natural skin protection. This is because such oils, like oils of sage, lavender, and rosemary, are highly potent antioxidants. I have successfully used oil of wild sage and oil of wild rosemary in the Mediterranean to halt sunburn and heal damaged tissue. Simply rub these oils on the body in the morning and at night.

Don't use sunscreens as an excuse to bake yourself. Use them to protect the skin from normal sun exposure. A recent study found that sunscreens may cause individuals to receive damaging sun exposure, because of a failure to experience the benefit of the natural warnings of being burned such as redness, peeling skin, pain, etc. As always, avoid constant direct exposure to the sun. Indirect exposure provides plenty of nourishing sunshine without the damaging effects. Remember, fair-skinned individuals have no natural protection against the sun, and they must guard themselves against it. What's more, protective covering, that is the judicious use of hats and other protective clothing, is equally as important as sunscreen in avoiding the damage.

Sunburn combat kit

- aloe vera gel or cream—helps cool skin and speeds healing.
- oil of oregano—aggressive and powerful; prevents scars and halts pain; apply as needed (stops pain and blistering).
- SkinClenz—soothing/cooling; speeds healing.
- oil of lavender—soothing/cooling; speeds healing and is a

natural anesthetic.
- Infla-eez—take 2 or more capsules several times daily.
- oil of wild sage or rosemary—rub topically on exposed parts, morning and evening.
- Kid-e-Kare rubbing oil—for children this is ideal; apply to any burn injury.
- oil of propolis (i. e. PropaHeal)—apply to the burn as needed.

Swimmer's ear (see also ear infections)

This is merely an infection or irritation of the outer ear canal. It is commonly contracted from swimming in germ- or parasite-infested water. Few people realize that the water in swimming pools, lakes, or seas is readily contaminated with pathogens. When the numbers of these pathogens in natural waters reaches certain levels, swimming is banned. However, even during "legal" swimming periods, a large enough number of pathogenic organisms remain in the water and can cause human diseases. The water-borne pathogens readily infect the outer ear canal. Viruses, bacteria, bacteria-like organisms, fungi, protozoans, amoebas, and parasitic worms can all gain entrance to the body through the ear canal.

Most outer ear infections are caused by bacteria and fungi. The skin of the outer ear offers a moist, nutrient-rich environment, which is precisely what these organisms require for growth. Candida commonly infects the outer ear canal, and usage of antibiotics and/or birth control pills increases the likelihood for the development of this infection. Symptoms depend upon whether the infection is acute or chronic. In acute infection symptoms include pain, aching, and discharge. With chronic infection the symptoms are primarily fullness in the ear, excessive wax, irritation, and itching.

Treatment is simple; application of essential oils on the outer ear and, if necessary, in the ear canal. Do not use full strength aromatherapy oils in the ear canal. Use only the emulsified oils (in olive oil), which are safe for topical application (for instance, oil of oregano, oil of myrtle, or oil of rosemary, etc.). Take olive/wild oil of oregano internally, 2 to 3 drops under the tongue twice daily.

Swimmer's ear combat kit
- oil of oregano (Oreganol P73)—apply about (but not in) the ear or ear lobe. Also, take 2 or more drops under the tongue once or twice daily.
- oil of myrtle—apply on skin behind the ear as an aromatic aid.
- oil of bay leaf—apply on skin behind the ear as an aromatic aid; this may also be put into the ear.

Swollen feet and ankles

A number of disorders can cause swelling in the lower extremities, some of which are serious and some harmless. Usually, swelling is a sign of dysfunction of the internal organs. Sluggish function of the kidneys, heart, and/or liver can lead to swelling. Other causes are obesity and food allergy. Parasitic infestation causes swollen extremities, particularly in the legs. One-sided swelling in the legs is often due to parasitic infestation, although blood clots could also cause this.

Certain nutrients aid in water mobilization and act as stimulants to normal kidney function. These nutrients include vitamin B_6, potassium, magnesium, and vitamin C. The positive effects of vitamin C are greatly aided by bioflavonoids. Yet, protein deficiency is the most common nutritional factor accounting for swelling in the extremities. This is because proteins are required for the maintenance of normal fluid balance in the body. This is why individuals with this condition often suffer from low blood levels of albumin and globulin, two important fluid-regulating proteins. These proteins are produced by the liver. Thus, liver disease may be associated with persistent swelling of the lower extremities.

Swollen feet/ankles combat kit

- oil of fennel—take 10 to 20 drops twice daily in juice or water.
- Wild Power Tea (contains natural kidney tonic herbs, wild strawberry leaves and wild borage flowers); drink two cups daily.
- oil of oregano—take 5 to 10 drops twice daily in juice or water. Also, take 2 or 3 drops under the tongue twice daily.
- CranFlush (wild cranberry extract)—20 or more drops twice daily.
- B complex—take 50 mg twice daily (to get B vitamins from totally natural sources use the Nutri-Sense and Royal Power)
- Purely-C (source of crude vitamin C combined with bioflavonoids for strengthening blood and lymph vessels to prevent leaking of fluids)—take 6 or more capsules daily.
- wild oregano or Mediterranean floral honey—two or more tablespoons twice daily.
- Resvital powder—teaspoon twice daily.

Foods that help

- anything rich in protein, specifically eggs, fresh meats, yogurt, whole milk, and fermented soy

Things to avoid

- sugar, sweets, chocolates, soda pop

Tinea capitis (ringworm of the scalp)

A disgusting appearing condition, scalp ringworm is happening in the United States in epidemic proportions. Caused by a fungus known as *Tinea*, this condition afflicts perhaps as many as 1 in 3 Americans. The fact is even simple dandruff is a form of tinea infection. Medical experts proclaim a virtual standstill in curing it. African-American individuals are particularly vulnerable to contracting this infection.

As previously stated the infection in a mild stage occurs in tens of millions and is represented by flaking of the scalp, a type of dandruff. Then, as the infection proceeds the flaking becomes more constant and the flakes larger. Next, the scalp develops a thick scaly layer of red inflamed regions, which may or may not scale. Severe infection is manifested by a ringworm lesion, a well defined round region of the scalp that is tender, swollen, and inflamed. Unless it is promptly treated, hair loss is inevitable.

Tinea capitis combat kit
- oil of oregano—rub directly on the site twice daily. Take 5 to 10 drops in juice or water twice daily. Also, add to shampoo for regular use, about 40 drops per eight ounces.
- SkinClenz—rub vigorously into scalp once or twice daily. Leave on for at least 24 hours.
- Scalp Clenz (the ideal formula for this purpose)—rub vigorously into scalp at night (to avoid staining bedding apply shower cap) twice daily. Add about 4 droppersful to 12 ounces of shampoo for regular use.

Tonsillitis

Few parents realize that tonsillitis is a normal consequence of children's lives. Children and adolescents contract a multitude of germs, and the tonsils are strategically positioned to combat them. That is why they become sore and swollen so frequently. The tonsils are attempting to prevent the germs from gaining entrance to the more significant organs, like the lungs and/or bloodstream. Tonsillitis is apparently aggravated by multiple vaccinations. The fact is such vaccinations may largely cause the illness.

Germs which commonly cause tonsillitis include strep, staph, viruses, and *Candida albicans*. It can also be provoked by food allergies as well as allergies to chemicals like sulfites, MSG, food dyes, and artificial sweeteners. The tonsils serve a critical role, since they are the first defense at the gate of entry for germs. They should only rarely be removed. Their surgical extraction greatly compromises immune function. For instance, recent studies have determined that the loss of the tonsils increases the risk for cancer.

The tonsils are under constant siege in their attempts to keep the body purified. By strengthening the immune system's ability to destroy germs, the tonsils may be relieved of a great deal of this strain. Thus, they may be retained to serve their valuable role. The following dosages are for children.

Tonsillitis combat kit

- oil of oregano—use as needed, 1 or 2 drops under the tongue or in the mouth, usually twice daily.
- wild oregano capsules (OregaMax)—during an attack take 2 capsules every hour. As a preventative take 1 or 2 capsules daily.
- raw honey in vinegar—use as a drink to sooth the throat; add water and drink.
- bromelain (as Infla-eez)—take 2 capsules three times daily on an empty stomach.
- vitamin C (as crude ascorbic acid with flavonoids)—take 2 capsules every hour until the condition resolves.
- Kid-e-kare throat spray—spray repeatedly on tonsils and back of the throat until condition resolves.
- Kid-e-kare gelcaps (natural antiseptic, small capsules)—1 to 2 every hour or every two hours until condition resolves, then preventively, one daily.

Note: the tonsils are fighting a war, trapping and destroying germs before they cause more serious damage such as pneumonia or blood poisoning. Destroying the tonsils is not the answer. Providing them with strategic support, with added weaponry; this is the most physiological means to utilize. The tonsils exist for a specific cause. Thus they should be surgically removed only as a last resort.

Things to avoid
- sweet drinks, especially soda pop
- caffeinated beverages

Toothache

Toothache is usually a sign of infection. If the infection penetrates beyond the enamel, it may enter the root of the tooth, causing severe pain and inflammation. This is known as a toothache. The pain is caused by inflammation and pressure on the nerve. This is also known as an abscessed tooth. The fact is an abscessed tooth is a sign of a deeper infection within the bone. Left untreated, the infection may enter the jaw bone, causing significant illness. Signs and symptoms of a toothache or abscessed tooth include:

- throbbing aching pain in the tooth (or teeth)
- sensitivity of the tooth to cold or hot
- swollen jaw, face, or neck lymph glands
- fever and muscle aches
- tingling sensation in the tooth
- recurrent sinus aches

Oil of oregano is the ideal agent to apply for halting toothache. It possesses monumental pain and germ-killing powers. It is also a natural anesthetic. Oil of clove, as well as cinnamon, also possesses anesthetic powers. All such oils are components of the potent gum/tooth healing formula Oregadent.

Toothache combat kit
- oil of oregano—rub the oil on the gums and teeth; saturate a piece of cotton and apply securely against the base of the

gum line of the involved tooth; for upper teeth leave overnight. Also, take 2 or more drops under the tongue as often as necessary. Another technique is to saturate a strip of cotton and then pack it around the involved site. Leave overnight, then remove. Repeat as needed.
- Oregadent multiple spice oil formula—apply to gums and tooth several times daily. Also add a few drops to toothbrush before brushing.
- OregaSpray—spray on any oral lesion or sore tissue as needed.

Foods that help
- hot clove bud tea
- wild hot oregano tea

Things to avoid
- refined sugar and sweets, especially soda pop
- chocolate

Trigeminal neuralgia

This extremely painful nerve disorder primarily affects the face. It is usually caused by a virus, which invades the facial nerve, causing extreme pain. The pain is manifested by severe jabs, which shoot like lightning throughout the distribution of the nerve. The pain may be felt all over the face, like the tip of the jaw, along the eye, over the forehead, about the lip, etc. The pain is momentary but maddening, as it may repeat itself for hours, even days. Trigeminal neuralgia is usually caused by a virus.

Trigeminal neuralgia combat kit
- oil of oregano (SuperStrength is preferable)—rub topically and take under the tongue, two or more drops three times daily. If possible, rub the oil vigorously into involved region.
- OregaBiotic—take 2 or 3 capsules twice daily with food or juice.

- Royal Power premium-grade royal jelly—take 3 capsules three or four times daily.
- oil of rosemary—rub topically as needed and take internally, 5 to 10 drops twice daily.
- Resvital (to aid in rebuilding nerve damage)—take 3 or more capsules twice daily.
- Infla-eez antiinflammatory capsules—2 or more capsules twice daily.

Tuberculosis

According to *American Family Physician* fully one third of the Earth's population is infected with tuberculosis. That makes this disease the number one global epidemic.

In the United States tuberculosis primarily strikes individuals already debilitated by other diseases. However, it is possible that outbreaks of this disease could occur in the general public. What's more, the disease can be disseminated in relatively healthy people through close contact with infected individuals. For instance, several airline attendants became infected when the organism lodged in airline air filters. Passengers are also increasingly being victimized by the potentially highly infectious recirculating air found in airliners. Unfortunately, the airliners have taken no steps to protect the public. Smokers, ex-smokers, and individuals with existing lung disease are the most vulnerable to the development of airline-induced respiratory infections. However, even relatively healthy individuals are falling victim to these infections. Be prepared just in case you are exposed to these unforgiving germs.

Tuberculosis outbreaks will likely occur in the Western world. The epidemics are cyclical, and there is a high likelihood for national or global outbreaks in the near future. Tuberculosis is highly debilitating. The fact is during the early 1900s TB was known as "consumption", because it literally consumed, that is destroyed, the individual. Ideally, the disease should be prevented via the regular application of a healthy diet, plenty of sunshine daily, and the ingestion of potent nutritional supplements. The intake of substances which destroy germs, such as antiseptic spices and herbs (wild oregano is the most powerful), is mandatory.

According to research performed at Georgetown University, published in *Molecular and Cellular Biochemistry* spice oils, notably P73 oregano oil, are even capable of destroying drug-resistant germs. The oregano oil, rather, the Oreganol P73, even destroyed TB-like germs, notably *Mycobacterium terrae*.

Tuberculosis combat kit

- SuperStrength oil of oregano—take a few drops under the tongue three times daily. Also, take 5 to 10 drops in juice or water three times daily, or take 1 to 3 Oreganol caps three times daily.
- OregaBiotic—take 2 to 3 capsules twice daily.
- Oregacyn respiratory formula—take 2 capsules three times daily and for difficult cases take 3 capsules three times daily.
- wild oregano herb capsules (OregaMax)—take 3 capsules three times daily.
- Oreganol P73 Juice—one ounce twice daily.
- Infla-eez—take 3 capsules three times daily on an empty stomach.
- Thyroset—take 3 capsules twice daily (increases metabolic rate).
- Black Seed-plus—take 3 capsules three times daily.
  Note: It is critical to stay on the doses at the recommended frequency for prolonged periods. TB takes a long time to heal.

Foods that help

- butternut or other deep yellow squash
- pumpkin soup
- fresh whole milk, particularly goat's milk
- papaya, kiwi, watercress, and chard

Typhoid fever

Now mostly a tropical disease, typhoid fever was once a major cause of epidemics in all parts of the world, including the Americas. The disease is manifested by severe fever, weakness, exhaustion, headache, and abdominal pain. In extreme cases hemorrhaging from the intestines may develop.

Typhoid fever is a bacterial disease caused by a type of salmonella that is carried by various tropical insects. It may also be caught from humans as well as infected milk, food, or water. The most common symptoms are:

- extreme fever with exhaustion
- headache
- abdominal pain
- nosebleeds
- mental confusion/disorientation
- vomiting
- intestinal bleeding (in the extreme)
- stupor, muttering, and delirium

Treatment must be aggressive, since there is a high fatality rate. Much of the treatment should be aimed at detoxification of the liver and gallbladder, since Salmonella aggressively invades these tissues. Oil of wild oregano (i.e. Oreganol P73) effectively destroys this germ,

Typhoid fever combat kit
- SuperStrength oil of oregano—take under the tongue repeatedly, 2 or 3 drops every hour. Take a few drops in water every 8 hours.
- oil of bay leaf—take 10 drops twice daily.
- OregaBiotic natural antiseptic—take 2 or more capsules several times daily.

- wild oregano herb (OregaMax capsules)—take 3 or more capsules every few hours.
- Purely-C—2 or more capsules every hour.

Foods that help
- vitamin C-rich fruit
- great quantities of pure water (add a small amount of salt)
- extra virgin olive oil—consume 1/2 cup daily for at least one week to purge the liver

Things to avoid
- caffeinated beverages
- chocolate and refined sugar

Vaginitis

This distressing condition is one of the most common causes of illness in adult females. Medical treatment for vaginitis is faulty, largely because the condition is usually misdiagnosed. Plus, the treatment, which is broad spectrum antibiotics and cortisone-containing creams, is often futile. This is because in the majority of cases the exact cause is difficult to determine. Plus, the drugs are geared to destroy specific organisms. The fact is there are dozens of germs which may cause vaginitis and most of these germs are immune to antibiotics.

Vaginitis may also be caused by chemicals, particularly synthetic dyes and bleaching agents found in clothes. Lye-based soaps may also instigate the condition. Lye is basic, while the vaginal tract is normally acidic. Thus, soaps, by altering the pH of the delicate vaginal membranes, may weaken local immunity, increasing the risks for infections, particularly yeast infections. Instead of using harsh soaps for vaginal cleansing use pure edible essential oils such as oils of myrtle, lavender, bay berry, and/or rosemary (emulsified in olive oil).

Vaginitis combat kit

- oil of oregano—take 2 to 5 drops twice daily under the tongue. Also, take 5 drops twice daily in juice or water.
- oil of myrtle—rub vaginally as often as needed.
- OregaMax capsules—take 3 capsules twice daily.
- oils of myrtle, lavender, or rosemary—for cleansing and prevention rub on vaginal walls once daily.
- natural bacterial support, that is the Health-Bac—take 1/2 teaspoon in warm water twice daily.

Foods that help

- yogurt, and kefir
- sauerkraut

Things to avoid

- refined sugar and chocolate
- synthetic underwear (retains moisture and increases the growth of yeasts, and synthetic dyes depress immunity)

Varicose veins

This often painful condition afflicts primarily women, the elderly, and the obese. Certain individuals are genetically predisposed to develop it. Varicose veins are caused by the destruction of the valves found inside the veins. The valves are needed to keep the blood moving towards the heart. Without them, the blood backs up, causing congestion, pain, and inflammation. If untreated, varicose veins can lead to potentially serious problems such as varicose ulcers, parasite infections, and blood clots.

Varicose veins combat kit

- oil of oregano (P73)—rub on the involved region; take 2 or 3 drops twice daily in juice or water.

- bromelain (uncoated, i.e. Infla-eez)—3 capsules on an empty stomach twice daily.
- Purely-C (to rebuild/strengthen the veins)—take 3 or more capsules twice daily.
- red grape powder (Resvital, rich in natural resveratrol)—take 4 capsules twice daily. Or, take 2 teaspoons daily.

Foods that help
- papaya juice and papaya fruit plus the seeds
- tangerines and grapefruit (eat the inner rind)

Venomous bites
(see also Bee stings, Fire ants, Scorpion bites, Snake bites, and Spider bites)

There are hundreds of venomous creatures capable of damaging human beings. However, insect bites are by far the most common cause, with wasps, bees, spiders, and fire ants leading the list.

In the event of a venomous bite there are two essential procedures: 1) don't panic 2) panic enough to seek medical care immediately. Use home remedies as you proceed to receive proper care. They can do no harm and will usually help immensely. The following protocol is universally applicable:

Venomous bite combat kit
- oil of oregano—apply repeatedly, every few minutes, if necessary, plus take a few drops under the tongue several times daily.
- raw garlic cloves—crush and apply juice/maceration on wound or use Garlex oil, a few drops on wound as needed and 10 or more drops under the tongue repeatedly.
- raw onion—crush and apply juice/maceration on wound.

- raw honey—cover the wound with it after applying the above remedies.
- LivaClenz (for protecting the liver against poisoning)—take 10 drops three or more times daily.
- oil of cumin (for protecting the liver cells against toxic damage)—take 10 to 20 drops twice daily.
- Purely-C—take 2 or more capsules several times daily.
- Bromelain (i.e. Infla-eez)—2 or 3 capsules every hour or as needed.

Warts

Warts are caused by a virus known as the human papillomavirus. Wart viruses are inciting epidemics, which remain largely incurable through modern medicine. The wart viruses are difficult to kill and if destroyed superficially, tend to regenerate. Amazingly, there are over 60 different wart viruses.

Wart viruses can grow virtually everywhere but they have a particular propensity for attacking the skin and genitals. They may also invade the mouth, anus, and rectum.

Warts may be a sign of nutritional deficiency, because certain nutrients are required to maintain anti-viral defenses. Nutrient deficiencies which increase the vulnerability to wart infestation include a lack of zinc, selenium, vitamin C, copper, vitamin A, vitamin D, and vitamin B_6. Be sure to take these nutrients on a regular basis.

Few people realize that warts are communicable. If an individual directly touches another person's warts, he/she can develop the infection. According to the editors of *American Family Physician* it is also possible to contract warts from towels, bedding, and other objects. However, the most common way to communicate them is through sex, largely because warts may grow deep inside the vagina, and infected women may not even know they exist. However, they may also hide within the bladder as well as the penile urethra.

Warts combat kit

- oil of oregano (SuperStrength may be required)—take several drops twice daily in juice or water. Also, take 2 or more drops twice daily under the tongue. Saturate a cotton ball or Band-Aid and apply to the involved site; leave for at least 12 hours and repeat.
- Skin Clenz—apply repeatedly to the involved site twice daily or soak a piece of cotton and tape against the region. Change dressing once or twice daily.
- OregaMax capsules—take 3 or more capsules twice daily.
- OxyOrega (supercritical form of oregano extract)—this is the type most active against warts; saturate a cotton ball and tape to the wart. Repeat until wart is dissolved.

Things to avoid

- chocolate, soda pop, and refined sugar
- nitrated meats and pork products

Water contamination

Water can either give life, or it can kill. Water-related dangers are seemingly infinite in today's civilization. In America alone tens of thousands of individuals become ill from drinking contaminated water each month. The fact is globally there are a greater number of deaths caused from drinking contaminated water than any other factor. Usually, in poor countries bacteria are the waterborne killers. In the United States also bacteria are a major player, but there are other agents of a more insidious nature. Currently, the freshwater in the United States is contaminated by a wide range of toxic chemicals. The public water supply contains thousands of noxious compounds, including heavy metals, chlorinated hydrocarbons (many of which are produced via the chlorination process), pesticides/herbicides, and radiation.

Few people realize that it is legal to dump radioactive wastes into the water channels. Nuclear power plants release untold tons of contaminated water into the sewers and rivers on a daily basis. Hospitals, as well as pharmaceutical houses, legally dispose of radioactive wastes into sewers/rivers. Ultimately, the radioactive poisons enter the public water supply and are delivered right to the tap. Without proper filtration the individual will consume a certain amount of radioactive waste, though it may be immeasurable, on a daily basis.

Humans consist mostly of water and, thus, whatever is within the water that people ingest greatly impacts health. Incredibly, the entire global water supply is polluted. The chemical companies know this, yet they continue to produce their dastardly poisons. Plus, it is getting worse daily. As described in the *Chicago Tribune* (Sept. 12, 1999) by Muhammad Omair of Ann Arbor, Michigan, there is a vitally important warning. He found that zooplankton, the smallest of all freshwater life forms, are "sprouting growths from their bellies and backs." These growths are essentially bizarre cancers, making up as much as 1/3 of the entire animal. Zooplankton are a critical link in the food chain and are a clear indicator of what the future bears for humans. According to Omair "the tumors grow incredibly fast." He has discovered them on creatures as young as two weeks. The study was performed using one of the largest bodies of freshwater in the world: Lake Michigan, which supplies water to tens of millions of people living in Illinois, Wisconsin, Indiana, and Michigan.

Why should we care about zooplankton? There should be immense concern, because these creatures are the barometer for the future of all other life forms on this planet. In fact, this event is the greatest warning signal of the potential damage caused to humans and the biosphere by toxic chemicals to date. While the Tribune infers a degree of mystery, the cause is simple; dioxin, PCBs, pesticides, herbicides, nuclear radiation, septic water, toxic metals, and similar carcinogenic poisons produced by humankind.

How is this dilemma solved? Certainly, adding a water filter to treat suspect water is perhaps the simplest solution. Currently, in municipalities chlorine and ozone are used to sterilize water. Certain essential oils render water sterile. The most potent of these include oil of oregano, cumin, lemongrass, cinnamon, lavender and bay leaf. Oil of wild oregano in the form of the Cleaning Oregano is the most effective of these, rendering septic water sterile in a dilution of 1 in 1000. Translated into common terms, this means water can be sterilized by adding 10 drops per cup (8 oz.) of water or about 20 drops per quart. If the water is boiled, much less is needed. For every cup of boiled water add 2 drops of oil of oregano. For every quart add 5 to 10 drops. The OregaSpray is also highly effective, which can be used to decontaminate any suspect region.

A special strength of oil of oregano is available for water or food decontamination as well as septic water. This formula is for topical and decontaminant use only. The Cleaning Oregano may be ordered by calling 1-800-243-5242. This resolves the septic component in a natural fashion.

For everyday protection the use of a water treatment unit may be required. These units utilize modern technological advances, which include activated carbon, to remove a wide range of impurities from the water. Some units also apply sterilization systems such as ultraviolet light. For more information about the state-of-the-art water treatment systems call LifeSource Water Co. at 1-800-992-3997. This unique system removes the vast majority of toxic chemicals. While heavy metals are removed, natural minerals are allowed to pass through. It is a high-grade system, superior to the typical type available. Ask for the factory water expert representative. Do call them; your life may depend upon it.

Water contamination combat kit
- filtration straw
- potassium iodide tablets

- oil of oregano (emulsified in extra virgin olive oil)
- pump-activated filtration device (military grade)
- chlorine pellets (if nothing else is available; bleach is too dangerous to handle)
- Super Strength oil of oregano (food grade only)

Note: Portable water filtration devices are becoming increasingly difficult to procure. This is why natural antiseptics are of such immense importance. Researchers proved that a small amount of oil of oregano, about one drop per two ounces, is sufficient to render fetid water sterile. Always boil suspect water. Then, add a drop of oil of oregano for every one or two ounces. Shake vigorously before drinking. Food grade oil of oregano (Cleaning Oregano) is available via mail order. This is primarily for food and cleansing purposes. It is also ideal for cleaning, that is decontamination of germs including mold. To order a vial of pure food grade wild oregano with proven germ-killing powers for water purification call 1-800-243-5242.

Whooping Cough

This was supposedly eradicated as a result of immunizations. Ironically, whooping cough is perhaps the most commonly occurring disease for which children are immunized. Current research indicates the organism may have at best become repressed but, in fact, is alive and infective. This is demonstrated by a recent study published in *JAMA* (August 1998) and performed in Finland, a country which fully immunizes its population against whooping cough. The researchers found that over one fourth of all individuals with paroxysmal cough have the disease. Astonishingly, virtually all of the infected individuals were immunized. The conclusion of the Finnish doctors is that whooping cough is "common in an immunized population." What an incredible conclusion it is that immunizations offer no guarantee against infection, rather, that despite immunizations the infection strikes thousands. The authors even go so far to proclaim that the value of immunizations for whooping cough (i.e. the DPT) is debatable.

In the United States, too, the majority of outbreaks of this disorder occur in immunized populations. The fact is the illness is relatively common in the United States. Researchers have determined that over one fourth of all individuals with paroxysmal (meaning sudden and spastic) cough have the disease. Thus, the individual must procure alternative means of protection besides the medical approach. The cough may be violent and persistent, scaring parents perhaps even more than the child. The key is to halt the abusive cough and destroy the organism.

Whooping cough combat kit

- oil of oregano (P73)—take 3 or more drops under the tongue repeatedly until cough stops. Also, take 1 to 3 capsules of Oreganol daily.
- oil of myrtle—rub on chest and sinuses, take 1 or 2 drops under the tongue twice daily.
- Kid-e-kare wild spice capsules (cold/flu)—take 1 to 2 capsules as often as possible.
- oil of lavender—rub on face, chest, and soles of the feet.
- Essence of Rosemary—add 1 to 3 T. in hot water and drink as a tea.
- Germ-a-CLENZ spray—mist throughout the sickroom. Spray on bedding. Add to vaporizer.
- Black Seed-plus—take 1 or 2 capsules three times daily.
- Kid-e-Kare wild cherry throat spray—mist on the back of the throat as often as possible.

Yeast/fungal infection

This is perhaps the number one health catastrophe of modern humanity. Seemingly, it afflicts virtually the entire population of the world, particularly individuals in Western countries.

The high predilection of this germ for individuals in the Western world is largely due to diet and lifestyle. The diet, high in simple sugars and refined starches, greatly enhances the growth of yeasts. Recently, researchers discovered that the consumption of even modest amounts of refined sugar leads to a rather massive overgrowth of yeasts. The use of antibiotics, which are prolific in modernized countries, readily induces yeast/fungal infections. In fact, a mere course of antibiotics leads to potentially monumental fungal overgrowth. Just think what is happening to those individuals who routinely use them. They harbor tens of billions of fungi/yeasts, a circumstance which ultimately leads to a wide range of health disorders. Illnesses associated with yeast/fungal overgrowth include chronic fatigue syndrome, fibromyalgia, arthritis, diabetes, lupus, autism, schizophrenia, eczema, psoriasis, cystitis, vaginitis, endometriosis, PMS, seborrhea, Crohn's disease, ulcerative colitis, adrenal insufficiency, hypothyroidism, obstructive lung disease, Sjogren's syndrome, and alcoholism.

In the mid 1970s researchers discovered that when certain spices were added to food, the growth of food-spoiling molds was halted. In the test tube they found that hot tangy spices were readily able to destroy fungi, even if the spices were used in small quantities. In 1998 this study was repeated by the FDA with same results: spice oils kill germs.

Many individuals regard garlic as the most powerful of all germ-killers. Yet, the researchers found that oregano, particularly the wild edible extracted oil, was the most powerful of all germ-killing spices. Commercially grown oregano exerts certain antiseptic actions. Yet, the wild high mountain varieties were determined to be even more powerful. Greek researchers, publishing in the *Journal of Agriculture and Food Chemistry* (1995), determined that the wild variety of oregano oil was 400% more powerful than any previously tested. Yet, the most monumental studies of all are being performed currently by Georgetown University (Washington, D.C.). There (2001), researchers discovered that the P73 form of wild oil of oregano completely obliterates the growth of one of the most difficult to kill of all fungi: *Candida albicans*. In a concentration of less than a half percent the oil totally decimated all fungal growth. The oil for the research is provided by North American Herb & Spice, because it is from 100% wild high mountain sources.

Nuclear contamination of the earth is causing epidemic fungal infections. The infestation of molds and fungi is caused by bizarre mutant species, which are generated as a result of radioactive exposure. In a study at the University of Iowa a notorious fungus, *Candida albicans*, was exposed to levels of radiation similar to those from a nuclear accident. Incredibly, not only did the fungus survive the exposure, but it also mutated into some 90 different forms. These mutations are extremely dangerous and can cause frank disease. Thus, the destruction of the biosphere, as well as human health, is largely the responsibility of the nuclear industry. The existence of radiation-induced mutants explains the exceptional degree of poor health found in regions near nuclear plants. For instance, it was recently determined that the high incidence of leukemia in individuals living near British nuclear plants is due to bizarre viral infections. While the supposed levels of nuclear irradiation may meet "accepted norms," the mutant germs are insidiously invading living creatures. The so-called clean fuel is destroying the world.

The use of nuclear fuel components for bombs or even for fuel generation causes devastating pollution, leading to cancer. The residues of these nuclear components create mutated fungi, which cause chronic disease. For health to be returned the fungi must be purged.

Yeast/fungal infection combat kit

- oil of wild oregano—take 5 or more drops twice daily under the tongue. Also, take 5 to 10 drops twice daily in juice or water.
- wild oregano capsules (OregaMax)—take 3 or more capsules

twice daily; so tasty you may open capsules and add to food.
- OregaBiotic capsules—take 2 or capsules twice daily.
- NukeProtect organic selenium/iodine formula—for increasing the capacity of white blood cells to destroy yeasts, take 400 mcg daily.
- chemical-free kelp (i.e. Thyroset)—kelp boosts thyroid function, which increases metabolic rate. Yeasts/molds thrive in individuals with lowered metabolic rate. Take 3 or more capsules daily.
- Fung-E-Clenz (a patented formula containing a special blend of natural spice and herb oils)—to cleanse the body of fungal toxins and residues, take 5 or more drops twice daily.

Foods that help
- garlic, leeks, shallots, onions
- cinnamon and cloves

Things to avoid
- alcoholic beverages, especially beer
- refined sugar
- cortisone and antibiotics
- estrogen and birth control pills
- antacids and H-2 blockers

Yellow fever

According to *JAMA* the occurrence of yellow fever is increasing dramatically. The increase is so frightening that experts regard worldwide epidemics as inevitable. Areas at greatest risk for outbreaks include Africa, South America, Central America, and the southern United States.

Here is the concern. Yellow fever is caused by a virus. The virus is carried by a mosquito, which normally lives in the tropics. However, now this mosquito has adapted to urban areas as a residence. In fact, it is found in numerous major American cities, including North American cities such as Miami, Houston, Baton Rouge, and New Orleans. Thus, explosive outbreaks are possible in these cities.

Like dengue and Ebola, yellow fever kills via hemorrhage as well as by destroying the immune system. It takes about 3 to 6 days for an individual to develop symptoms after being bitten. Often, the symptoms are so mild that they are mistaken for the flu, and, thus, no diagnosis is procured. However, a significant percentage become seriously ill. The illness develops over three phases, as follows:

Phase 1: sudden fever, headache, sore aching muscles, nausea, vomiting. Then, it stops for a few hours or up to 24 hours, returning cyclically.

Phase 2: a toxicity may develop, liver damage (represented by yellow jaundice), spitting of blood, dark blood in the stools.

Phase 3: severe high fever, total exhaustion, hemorrhaging, unconsciousness, coma, and death. The latter occurs in 50% or more of those who reach this phase. In children under ten years 8 out of 10 usually die.

In South America significant outbreaks have been reported in Brazil, Peru, Bolivia, Columbia, and Ecuador, with the biggest outbreak occurring in Peru. In Central America outbreaks are reported in virtually every country as well as the Caribbean. In North America there are currently no reported cases, with the last outbreak occurring in New Orleans in 1905, resulting in over a thousand deaths. Yet, the southern states are long overdue for the return of this cyclical disease. The likelihood of such an outbreak is postulated by S. E. Robertson, M.D., and colleagues, who make it clear that yellow fever-contaminated mosquitoes have "reinfested" most of the major cities in the Deep South.

Remember, yellow fever is a highly dangerous infection. The mortality rate is extremely high. It must be treated aggressively, with emphasis on antiviral herbs and plenty of fluids. As with all hemorrhagic fevers, major efforts should be applied to strengthen the internal tissues, particularly the blood and lymph vessels, from collapsing and/or degenerating. This means the intake of plenty of bioflavonoids, polyphenols, and vitamin C. The most powerful vitamin C for this purpose is the crude natural type as found in rose hips, acerola, citrus extracts, wild strawberry leaves, etc.

Yellow Fever Combat Kit
- oil of oregano SuperStrength—take 5 drops under the tongue every hour. Take 10 to 20 drops internally several times daily, perhaps as often as every hour if necessary. Imagine this: there are billions of viruses multiplying every hour; so bombard these as aggressively as possible.
- Purely-C—take 2 or 3 capsules every hour.
- Resvital—take 1 tsp. every hour or 4 to 6 capsules per hour.
- oil of lavender or bay oil—rub all over the face and head. Also, rub on soles of feet, lower back, and buttocks.
- Oreganol P73—take 1 or more ounces three times daily.
- zinc chelate—75 mg daily.
- OregaBiotic natural antibiotic capsules—take 2 capsules three times daily or more often, if necessary.

Foods that help
- Essence of Rose Petals tea (highly aromatic, soothing; helps break fever) or white coffee (i.e. orange blossom floral essence); drink as often as desired. Prepare by adding 1 or 2 T. in a cup of hot water.
- vitamin C-rich juices
- papaya plus seeds
- onions and garlic

Appendix A

Ordering Information for Nutritional/Herbal Supplements

This appendix lists all the supplements mentioned in this book. The majority of these supplements are produced by North American Herb & Spice. The remainder are manufactured by a variety of other makers. North American Herb & Spice is the elite in making the most natural unprocessed supplements possible. This company specializes in wild unprocessed natural products rich in original native ingredients. Plus, the ingredients are 100% guaranteed to be free of all chemicals, herbicides, pesticides, solvents, or other noxious substances.

The products are also unique because they are primarily from wild plants growing on original native soil. Since the herbs are wild or grown on native soils from natural seeds which are environmentally protected, there is no possibility of genetic engineering. Thus, products by this company are ideal for any health crisis. Unlike pharmaceutical drugs there is no possibility of serious side effects. These products may be ordered at finer health food stores or pharmacies or by calling 1-800-243-5242 (Oreganol.com). In England these products are available at Tigon, Ltd: 011162355020 (oliveleaf.co.uk.) and in Europe, vivanatura.nl.

Product	Qty	Ingredients
Infla-eez	90 caps	bromelain (from pineapple stems), papain (from green papayas), immature tangerine
Purely-C,	90 caps	Camu camu, rose hip powder, acerola cherry, Rhus coriaria
Essence of Orange	12 oz.	orange blossom essence from (white coffee) neroli orange blossoms

Essence of Rose Petals	12 oz.	rose petal essence from Damascene roses
Oreganol P73 Juice	12 oz.	oregano essence from high mountain wild oregano
Essence of Rosemary	12 oz.	rosemary essence from high mountain wild rosemary
Essence of Sage	12 oz.	sage essence from high mountain wild sage
Oil of Lavender	.45 oz.	extra virgin olive oil and wild lavender oil
Oil of Oregano	.45 oz.	extra virgin olive oil and wild oregano oil
Oil of Myrtle	.45 oz.	extra virgin olive oil and wild myrtle oil
Oil of Rosemary	.45 oz.	extra virgin olive oil and wild rosemary oil
Cuminol (oil of cumin)	.45 fl oz.	oil of cold-pressed black seed, oil of wild cumin, edible wild fennel oil
HerbSorb	90 caps	fenugreek, cumin, black seed, coriander, and cardamom
Hercules Strength	90 caps	wild rosemary, oregano, and sage
Nutri-Sense	400 g	crude rice bran, polish, flax, lecithin, red sour grape powder, vitamin E
Oil of Bay Berry	1 fl oz.	oils of wild bay berry, myrtle, rosemary
Oil of Cilantro/Coriander	.45 fl oz.	extra virgin olive oil, oil of cilantro, oil of coriander
Oil of fennel	.45 fl oz.	extra virgin olive oil and fennel oil
Oil of sage	.45 fl oz	extra virgin olive oil and wild sage oil
OregaMax capsules	90 caps	wild oregano, Rhus coriaria, garlic, onion

Thyroset	90 caps	wild Northern Pacific kelp and wild Mediterranean oregano
Red grape powder (Resvital)	90 caps	crude unprocessed red sour grape powder
Royal Power	90 caps	premium high 10-HDA royal jelly pantothenic acid, acerola cherry
Super Strength	1 fl oz.	extra virgin olive oil and wild oregano oil of oregano
Wild Power Tea	2 oz.	wild strawberry leaves, wild borage flowers, wild hibiscus flowers
Wild St. John's wort	90 caps	wild high flavonoid St. John's wort and wild rosemary
LivaClenz	1 fl oz.	extra virgin olive oil, oils of wild cumin, rosemary, oregano & sage
Oil of Ginger	.45 fl oz.	extra virgin olive oil and ginger oil
Oil of Cinnamon	.45 fl oz.	extra virgin olive oil and cinnamon oil
Essence of Coriander	12 oz.	coriander essence from high mountain wild coriander
Essence of Lavender	12 oz.	lavender essence from high mountain wild lavender
NukeProtect caps	90 caps	selenium, iodine, cumin, kelp & more
Fung-E-Clenz	1 fl oz	blend of essential oils
Oreganol gelcaps	60 caps	oil of oregano & extra virgin olive oil
Oregacyn Respiratory	60 caps	oregano, cumin, sage, cinnamon
Neuroloft capsules	60 caps	sage, rosemary, wild St. John's wort

Non-edible Emergency and Disaster Items Described in this Text or Recommended for Emergency Protection

portable gas masks and cartridges
protective suits (against radiation/toxic chemicals)
water filtration straws
water filtration units
iodine tablets
geiger counters
diffusers (for volatilizing essential oils)

Specialty mail order food products

crude raw wild oregano honey
crude raw orange blossom honey
crude raw wild thistle honey
crude raw wild dandelion honey
crude raw wild fir tree honey
carob molasses
grape molasses
date molasses
pomegranate syrup
bulk wild oregano bunches
salted jumbo pumpkin seeds
Austrian pumpkin seed oil or ProstaClenz (from NAHS)
bulk wild rice from northern Canada

Note: The aforementioned products are of the highest quality, and, thus, are ideal for all age groups, especially children. The quality is related both to the exceptional powers of the raw materials as well as the high standards of manufacturing.

Misc. other products

•selenium chelate (organic selenium)
• aloe vera

- zinc chelate
- bee propolis (use PropaHeal by NAHS)
- calcium chelate
- lactobacillus (use the Health-Bac by NAHS)
- pantothenic acid, 500 mg

(note: the above are available at high quality health food sores or by calling 1-800-243-5242).

Select Remedies for Specific Conditions

This list is for rapid reference in order to determine the exact remedy needed. It lists the most important remedies, yet there are other substances which may be of immense value recommended within the text. The most important supplements/foods are listed, with the first item being most critical. AIDS, anthrax, nuclear catastrophe, radiation poisoning, and carbon monoxide poisoning require additional critical substances. The following are listed in alphabetical order, like the index of a book.

Note: Oil of oregano and Oreganol are used interchangeably.

A

Abdominal pain	oil of oregano, Infla-eez, HerbSorb
Aching feet	oil of oregano, oil of wild lavender, Infla-eez
Acne	oil of oregano, oil of rosemary, Nutri-Sense
AIDS	oil of oregano, OregaMax, Oreganol P73, Oregacyn multiple spice
Allergic reactions	Royal Power, oil of oregano, Infla-eez
Angina	Infla-eez, oil of rosemary, oil of oregano
Anthrax	oil of oregano, OregaBiotic, Oreganol P73
Arsenic poisoning	selenium, Resvital, oil of cumin
Asthma	oil of oregano, Oregacyn, Black Seed-plus
Athlete's foot	oil of oregano, oil of bay berry, oil of lavender

B

Back pain	Resvital, oil of oregano, Infla-eez
Bed sores	raw honey, oil of oregano, Infla-eez
Bee stings	oil of oregano, Royal Power, Infla-eez
Bell's palsy	oil of oregano, Royal Power, pantothenic acid, Infla-eez
Bites	oil of oregano, oil of bay berry, raw honey
Bladder infection	oil of oregano, CranFlush, red grape powder
Bleeding gums	Purely-C, oil of oregano, OregaMax
Blisters	oil of oregano, oil of lavender, Infla-eez
Blood clots	Infla-eez, oil of oregano, oil of rosemary
Boils	oil of oregano, raw honey, Infla-eez
Bone infection	oil of oregano, OregaMax, Infla-eez
Bronchitis	oil of oregano, oil of wild lavender, OregaMax
Bruises	oil of oregano, Infla-eez, Purely-C
Burns	oil of oregano, raw honey, oil of lavender

C

Canker sores	oil of oregano, oil of sage, Royal Power
Carbon monoxide	Oreganol P73 Juice/Rosemary, oil of rosemary, NukeProtect, Oregacyn
Cataracts	oil of oregano, Resvital, selenium
Chicken pox	oil of oregano, Kid-e-Kare rub, raw honey
Chlorine gas/liquid	oil of rosemary, NukeProtect, Resvital
Cholera	oil of oregano, OregaMax, raw honey
Cold exposure	oil of oregano, Royal Power, Thyroset
Cold sores	oil of oregano, oil of sage, Royal Power
Colds	oil of oregano, raw honey, Purely-C
Colic	oil of fennel, oil of oregano, oregano juice,
Colitis	oil of fennel, oil of rosemary, OregaMax
Concussion	oil of wild lavender, Purely-C, wild St. John's Wort
Conjunctivitis	oil of oregano, vitamin A drops, Essence of Rose Petals
Constipation	red grape powder, Nutri-Sense, Infla-eez
Cough	oil of wild lavender, oil of oregano, OregaMax
Croup	oil of oregano, OregaMax, oil Oregacyn

Appendix A   365

Cryptosporidium	oil of oregano, OregaMax, raw garlic
Cuts/lacerations	oil of oregano, raw honey, Oreganol cream
Cyanide poisoning	Oreganol P73 Juice, Resvital, oil of rosemary

D-E

Dehydration	water, Royal Power, sea salt
Dengue fever	oil of oregano, OregaMax, raw onion juice
Dermatitis	oil of oregano, oil of bay berry, OregaMax
Diabetes	oil of cumin, Oregulin, oil of myrtle, Resvital
Diaper rash	oil of oregano, Oreganol cream, oil of bay berry
Diarrhea	oil of oregano, raw honey, OregaMax
Diphtheria	oil of oregano, Black Seed-plus, OregaMax, Oreganol gelcaps
Diverticulitis	OregaMax, Infla-eez, oil of rosemary
Dog bites	oil of oregano, Infla-eez, oil of bay berry
Drug overdose/toxicity	oil of cumin, oil of Cilantro-plus, selenium
Dry or irritated eyes	essential fatty acids, vitamin A, riboflavin
E. coli	oil of oregano, oil of cumin, Garlex
Earaches/infection	oil of oregano, oil of wild lavender, OregaMax
Ebola	oil of oregano, OregaMax, Resvital
Eczema	oil of oregano, OregaMax, oil of bay berry
Ehrlichiosis	oil of oregano, OregaMax, Black Seed-plus
Emotional distress	oil of wild lavender, oil of sage, Royal Power
Emphysema	oil of oregano, oil of rosemary, OregaMax
Encephalitis	oil of oregano, Black Seed-plus, OregaMax
Endometriosis	oil of oregano, fish oils/fatty fish, Infla-eez
Exhaustion	Oreganol P73 Juice, Royal Power, Purely-C

F-G

Fainting	oil of lavender, oil of bay berry, Royal Power, oil of wild sage, oil of wild myrtle
Fever	oil of oregano, OregaMax, Purely-C
Fire ants	oil of oregano, oil of lavender, Infla-eez, oil of bay leaf

Flea bites	oil of oregano, raw garlic, oil of lavender
Flesh-eating bacteria	oil of oregano, raw honey, raw garlic
Flu	oil of oregano, raw honey, OregaMax
Food poisoning	oil of oregano, raw honey, Black Seed-Plus
Fractures	Infla-eez, oil of oregano, MCHC
Frostbite	oil of oregano, aloe vera, Infla-eez
Gallbladder attack	oil of cumin, oil of fennel, oil of oregano
Genital Herpes	oil of oregano, oil of bay berry, Purely-C
Giardiasis	oil of cumin, oil of oregano, OregaMax
Gingivitis	oil of oregano, Purely-C, Oreganol P73 Juice

H

Head lice	oil of fennel, oil of oregano, Scalp Clenz
Headaches	oil of oregano, Royal Power,
Heart attack	Oil of Cilantro-plus, OregaMax, oil of rosemary
Heart failure	Oreganol P73 Juice, CranFlush, coenzyme Q10
Heat exhaustion	Royal Power, Purely-C, sea salt
Heat stroke	Royal Power, Purely-C, sea salt
Helicobacter pylori	oil of oregano, oil of cumin, Black Seed-plus
Hemorrhoids	Infla-eez, oil of myrtle, Purely-C
Hepatitis	Oreganol, Oregacyn Liver, GreensFlush
Herpes	oil of oregano, oil of myrtle, Purely-C
Herbicide poisoning	oil of cumin, oil of rosemary, LivaClenz
High blood pressure	oil of rosemary, oil of lavender
Hip pain	oil of oregano, Infla-eez, Resvital
Histoplasmosis	oil of oregano, oil of rosemary, Oregacyn resp.
Hives	Royal Power, oil of oregano, OregaMax
Hookworm	oil of fennel, oil of cumin, oil of oregano
Hot flashes	Royal Power, oil of fennel, EstroNorm
Hypoglycemia	Royal Power, HerbSorb, Oregulin

I

Impetigo	oil of oregano, Oreganol cream, Infla-eez
Ingrown toenail	oil of oregano, oil of wild lavender

Insecticide poisoning	oil of cumin, NukeProtect, oil of rosemary,
Insomnia	oil of lavender, oil of oregano, oil of sage
Irritable bowel syndrome	oil of fennel, oil of oregano, OregaMax
Itchy skin	oil of oregano, Oreganol cream, oil of myrtle

J-K

Jaundice	oil of cumin, LivaClenz, Oreganol P73 Juice
Jock itch	oil of oregano, oil of myrtle, OregaMax
Joint pain	Infla-eez, oil of oregano, OregaMax
Kidney infection	oil of oregano, oil of fennel, Resvital
Kidney stones	Resvital, oil of oregano, oil of fennel
Killer bees	oil of oregano, raw garlic, Infla-eez
Knee pain	oil of oregano, Infla-eez, magnesium

L-M

Laryngitis	oil of oregano, OregaMax, Black Seed-plus
Lead poisoning	Resvital, oil of cumin, Purely-C
Leg cramps	oil of rosemary, Resvital, calcium, magnesium
Lice	oil of fennel, oil of oregano, oil of cumin
Lyme disease	oil of oregano, OregaMax, Resvital
Macular degeneration	oil of rosemary, oil of oregano, Resvital
Malaria	oil of oregano, OregaMax, Black Seed-plus
Measles	oil of oregano, Purely-C, raw honey
Melanoma	oil of oregano, vitamin E, beta carotene, oil of rosemary, Oreganol P73 Juice
Meningitis	oil of oregano, Purely-C, Infla-eez
Menstrual bleeding	Purely-C, Infla-eez, Resvital
Menstrual cramps	Infla-eez, Thyroset, oil of oregano
Mercury poisoning	oil of Cilantro-plus, oil of cumin, nukeprotect
Migraines	oil of oregano, Wild St. John's wort, oil of lavender
Mite allergy	oil of oregano, OregaMax, Infla-eez
Mold allergy/reaction	oil of oregano, oil of wild lavender, oil of bay berry, Oreganol
Mononucleosis	oil of oregano, raw honey, Black Seed-plus

Mosquito bites	oil of oregano, oil of bay berry, raw garlic
Muscle soreness/weakness	oil of sage, oil of oregano, Infla-eez

N-O

Nail bed infection	oil of oregano, oil of wild lavender, Infla-eez
Nasal polyps	Infla-eez, vitamin A, oil of oregano
Nausea	oil of fennel, ginger extract, HerbSorb
Nerve gas poisoning	oil of cumin, oil of rosemary, NukeProtect
Nervousness	wild St. John's wort, oil of wild lavender, oil of rosemary
Nosebleeds	oil of oregano, Purely-C, Resvital
Nuclear catastrophe Kelp/iodine,	Oreganol P73 Juice, Essence of Rosemary, oil of cumin, oil of rosemary, Resvital, NukeProtect™, oil of bay berry, oil of sage, folic acid

P

Pesticide poisoning	LivaClenz, Oreganol P73 Juice, oil of cumin
Pinworms	oil of oregano, oil of cumin, oil of fennel
Plague	oil of oregano, OregaMax, Black Seed-plus
Pneumonia	oil of oregano, oil of lavender, Black Seed-plus
Poison ivy/oak/sumac	oil of oregano, tea tree oil (wild), aloe vera
Poor appetite	Nutri-Sense, OregaMax, beef broth
Poor breast milk	oil of fennel, HerbSorb, Nutri-Sense
Postnasal drip	oil of oregano, OregaMax, Oreganol P73 Juice
Prostatitis	oil of bay berry, saw palmetto berry, Resvital
Psoriasis	oil of oregano, oil of bay berry, OregaMax
Puncture wounds	oil of oregano, oil of lavender, raw honey

Q-R

Radiation burns	oil of oregano, oil of bay berry, NukeProtect
Radiation poisoning	oil of cumin, oil of rosemary, oil of sage, selenium, Resvital, Oreganol P73 Juice, Oregano, Essence of Rosemary, Black Seed-

	plus, OregaMax, oil of oregano, LivaClenz, NukeProtect
Ringworm	oil of oregano, oil of myrtle, oil of bay berry
Rosacea	oil of oregano, OregaMax, oil of bay berry

S-T

Salmonella	oil of oregano, raw garlic, oil of cumin
Scabies	oil of oregano, raw garlic, oil of cumin
Sciatica	Infla-eez, oil of oregano, Resvital
Scorpion bites	oil of oregano, raw garlic, Infla-eez
Seizures	oil of lavender, Oil of Cilantro-plus, Royal Power
Shigellosis	oil of oregano, raw honey, raw garlic
Shingles	oil of oregano, OregaMax capsules, pantothenic acid
Sinus attacks	oil of oregano, Oreganol P73 Juice, OregaMax
Skin cancer	oil of oregano, oil of bay berry, oil of rosemary
Smoke inhalation	oil of rosemary, Purely-C, Oreganol P73 Juice
Snake bites	oil of oregano, raw garlic, Infla-eez
Sore throat	oil of oregano, Black Seed-plus, Purely-C
Sour mood/negativity	oil of rosemary, Essence of Rosemary, Royal Power
Spider bites	oil of oregano, raw garlic, raw honey
Sprained joints	Infla-eez, oil of oregano, Purely-C
Staph infection	oil of oregano, oil of cumin, OregaMax
Stomachache	Infla-eez, Herb-Sorb, Black Seed-plus, oil of ginger (in extra virgin olive oil)
Stomach ulcer	Herb-Sorb, oil of oregano, Infla-eez
Strep infection	oil of oregano, OregaMax, oil of lavender
Sugar cravings	Resvital, HerbSorb, oil of oregano
Sunburn	oil of oregano, oil of bay berry, oil of lavender (wild type)
Swimmer's ear	oil of oregano, oil of rosemary, oil of myrtle
Swollen feet/ankles	Resvital, Infla-eez, oil of fennel
Tapeworms	oil of oregano (SuperStrength), oil of fennel, oil of cumin

Tinea capitis	oil of oregano, oil of myrtle, selenium
Tonsillitis	oil of oregano, raw honey, Purely-C
Toothache	oil of oregano, Black Seed-plus, Infla-eez
Trigeminal neuralgia	oil of oregano, Black Seed-plus, Infla-eez
Tuberculosis	Black seed-plus, oil of oregano, oil of rosemary
Typhoid fever	oil of oregano, OregaMax, oil of lavender

U-Z

Urinary incontinence	Resvital, CranFlush, oil of fennel
Vaginitis	oil of myrtle, oil of oregano, oil of bay berry
Varicose ulcers	oil of oregano, Royal Power, raw honey
Varicose veins	oil of oregano, Purely-C, Resvital
Venomous bites	oil of oregano, raw garlic, Garlex
Warts	oil of oregano, oil of bay leaf, OregaMax, Zolvex
Water contamination	oil of oregano, oil of bay leaf, iodine
Whooping cough	oil of oregano, oil of rosemary, Black Seed-plus
Yellow fever	oil of oregano, OregaMax, Resvital

A special message from NAHS, makers of oil of oregano, Oreganol, Oreganol P73 Juice, and OregaMax capsules

Oil of oregano and other wild oregano products were introduced to the United States by Dr. Cass Ingram. In 1995 he discovered the antiseptic powers of the wild herb and crude essential oil as a result of a personal illness; oil of oregano had not been in use previously. He then used it successfully to help friends and family. This led to a grass roots movement, wherein the public received immense benefits. Today, oil of oregano, Oreganol caps, and OregaMax caps are among the most sought-after dietary supplements known. Now there is the antibiotic form, that is the OregaBiotic. This is a combination of the four key antibiotic spice oils: oils of onion, garlic, oregano, and allspice. The discovery will serve humanity forever, since wild oregano is one of the most potent and safe of all natural antiseptics and since few if any natural compounds can match its efficacy. Note that any reference to oil of oregano refers to the high quality mountainous wild oregano produced by NAHS. No responsibility is taken for those who utilize inferior products. The NAHS wild oregano products are guaranteed wild. The quality is guaranteed. This is a reflection of the quality and purity of the product.

A Note by the non-profit Price Pottenger Nutrition Foundation, originated by Weston A. Price, D.D.S.

The Price-Pottenger Nutrition Foundation (PPNF) believes that the full genetic expression of every human being is one of excellent health, a keen mind, and an attractive physical appearance. This potential can only be completely expressed when populations consume a diet of nutrient-rich whole foods.

The Price-Pottenger Nutrition Foundation provides guidance for the reversal of modern "civilized" dietary trends that promote disease and physical and mental degeneration. PPNF provides accurate information on whole foods and proper preparation techniques, soil improvement, pure water, non-toxic dentistry and holistic therapies. This information can help to conquer disease, prevent birth defects, avoid personality disturbances and delinquency, enhance the environment and enable all people to achieve long life and excellent health, now and into the 21st century.

The Price-Pottenger Nutrition Foundation was established as a not-for-profit organization in 1965 to provide the public and the healing professions with historical and anthropological findings and up-to-date, accurate scientific information on nutrition and health. The Foundation is known for its integrity and accuracy in making this information available to the public.

The Foundation is completely independent of commercial interests. Because of its success through the years, it has become heir to the basic research of numbers of other pioneering researchers in the field of nutrition and health.

PPNF serves as a guardian for precious archives and provides access to modern scientific validation of ancestral wisdom on diet, agriculture, lifestyle, and health. It houses the extensive files, notes and photographs of Dr. Price and Dr. Pottenger, along with the groundbreaking research of William Albrecht, Ph.D., famous soil specialist; Dr. Royal Lee, vitamin researcher; Dr. Edward Howell, enzyme researcher; Dr. Melvin Page, specialist in the relationship between the endocrine system and diet and disease; Dr. Emmanuel Cheraskin, renowned nutrition researcher; and practicing physicians John Myers, M.D. and Henry Bieler, M.D., both known for their success in the treatment of chronic illness.

Our members enjoy reading the PPNF quarterly *Health & Healing Journal;* receiving our free catalog of reprints and pre-reviewed, modern publications; access to PPNF archived material, and our list of healthcare providers. They can rely on the knowledge that the Price-Pottenger Nutrition Foundation serves as a trustworthy source of accurate information on the principles of good nutrition.

We invite you to join us and become a PPNF member. Contact us on our web site at *www.price-pottenger.org* or call us at 1-800-366-3748. Our friendly staff will answer your questions and make sure you receive your membership packet and free catalog. We look forward to hearing from you.

A Note from Dr. Cass Ingram: To all readers, I am a member of this fine organization and am currently an honorary board member. Support this organization for your own nutritional benefit and for the benefit of your loved ones and progeny.

Dr. Cass Ingram's Web Contribution

An important, monumental web site is available. This site assists the individual in determining precisely his/her nutritional needs. Using a highly sophisticated and accurate technology, this system greatly aids in the correct determination of nutritional deficiencies. The objective is to help the individual rebuild his/her health through accurate nutritional and biochemical assessment. This is followed by extensive corrective recommendations. This is a completely individualized system. It offers two components: dietary analysis and specific tests for a wide range of nutrients. It is called:

Nutritiontest.com

Test yourself for nutritional deficiencies
Look it up on the world wide web

Bibliography

Committee on Environmental Health. American Acadamy of Pediatrics: Toxic Effects of Indoor Molds. *Pediatrics.* 101(4):712–714.

Cooper, L., et al. 1931. *Nutrition in Health and Disease for Nurses*, Lippincott.

Dogan, Y., et al. 2004. The Use of Wild Edible Plants in Western and Central Anatolia (Turkey). *Economic Botany*: 58:684–690.

Flagg, E.W., Coates, R.J., and R.S. Greenberg. 1995. Epidemiologic studies of antioxidants and cancer in humans. *Journal of the American College of Nutrition.* 5(14):419–427.

Green, A. E. 1988. Wound healing properties of honey. *British Journal of Surgery.* 75:1278.

Hardy, M. and Kirk-Smith, MD. 1995. Replacement of drug treatment for insomnia by ambient odor. *Lancet.* 346:701.

Ingram, Cass. 2005. *Natural Cures for Headaches.* Buffalo Grove, IL: Knowledge House.

Ingram, Cass. 2004. *Nutrition Tests for Better Health*, Buffalo Grove, IL: Knowledge House.

Jeongmok, K., et al. 1995. Antibacterial activity of some essential oil components against five foodborne pathogens. *J. Agric. Food Chem.* 43:2839–2845.

Lawless, J, 1995. Environmental Control of Dust Mite Allergens. *The Illustrated Encyclopedia of Essential Oils: The Complete Guide to the Use of Oils in Aromatherapy and Herbalism.* Element Books.

Loosli, A.R. and J. S. Ruud. 1998. Meatless Diets in Female Athletes: A Red Flag. *The Physician and Sports Medicine.*

Matossian, M.K. 1991. *Poisons of the Past: Molds, Epidemics and History.* New Haven, CT: Yale University Press.

Montague-Drake, B. 1997. *A Biblical Herbal: the Greatest Herbal Story Ever Told.* New South Wales, Australia: Earth Images.

Mueller-Riebau, F., et al. 1995. Chemical composition and fungitoxic properties to phytopathogenic fungi of essential oils of selected aromatic plants growing wild in turkey. *J. Agric. Food Chem.* 43:2262–2266.

Peters, W. and H. M. Gilles. 1995. *Tropical Medicine: Color Atlas of Tropical Medicine and Parasitology.* New York: Mosby-Wolfe.

Presutti, J.R. 1997. Early treatment and prophylaxis against infectious complications. *Post Graduate Sports Medicine.* April (4).

Rama, N.L. and N.P. DAS. 1993 Natural Products Inhibit Oxidative Rancidity in Salted Cooked Ground Fish. *Journal of Food Science.* 58(2):318–20.

Singer, K. (ed). 1996. Patient Care. *The Practical Journal for Primary Care Physicians.* January 15, 168 p.

Stark, A. H. and Z. Madar. 2002. Olive oil as a functional food: epidemiology and nutritional approaches. *Nutrition Reviews.* 60:170–176.

Stephenson, J. 1997. Worry grows as antibiotic-resistant bacteria continue to gain ground. *JAMA.* Dec. 278:2049–50.

Rosenfeld, J.A. 1996. Treatment of menorrhagia due to dysfunctional uterine bleeding. *American Family Physician.* January.

Thomas, M. K., et al. 1998. Hypovitaminosis D in medical in patients. *New England Journal of Medicine.* 338:777–783.

Valnet, J. and R. Tisserand (ed).1990. *The Practice of Aromatherapy*, Rochester, Vt.: Healing Arts.

Index

A

Abdominal pain, 116, 117, 126, 165, 272, 294, 316, 344, 363
Aching feet, 118, 363
Acidophilus, 47, 156, 181, 182, 219 *see also* Lactobacillus
Acne, 363
Adrenal weakness, 62-65, 158, 325
AIDS, 13, 17, 20, 22, 25, 30, 37, 49, 62, 68, 73, 77, 83, 92, 102, 112, 118, 119, 162, 179, 223, 258, 293, 363, 373
Air pollution, 128
Airlines, 290, 291, 292
Allergic dermatitis, 177
Allergic reactions, 23, 75, 87, 90, 102, 120, 121, 164, 247, 273, 280, 282, 291, 323, 363
Almond, 169, 172
Alzheimer's disease, 57
Amino acids, 86, 94, 95, 99, 100, 158
Amnesia, 162
Anemia, 256, 269
Angina, 121, 122, 363
Animal bites, 195
Anthrax, 123, 124, 363
Apricots, 74, 90, 91, 234
Arthritis, 57, 60, 115, 177, 249, 289, 316, 354
Artichokes, 180, 192, 236
Aspergillus infection, 126, 127, 128
Aspirin, 13, 57, 118, 175, 177, 181, 196, 214, 215, 239, 279, 283, 325
Asthma, 7, 30, 49, 65, 77, 128, 129, 273, 277, 291, 363
Athlete's foot, 41, 129, 130, 249, 308, 364
Athlete's foot and/or jock itch, 129
Avocados, 223, 230, 288, 299, 315

B

B vitamin, 168, 180, 187, 298, 299, 334
Back pain, 62, 130, 131, 238, 364
Bad breath, 48, 165
Bay berry, oil of, 178, 182, 233, 360, 364-370
Bed sore/open wound combat kit, 133
Bed sores, 56, 131, 132, 364
Bee propolis, 26, 27, 104, 170, 363
Bee stings, 121, 134, 135, 241, 251, 347, 364 *see also* Killer Bees
Bell's palsy, 136, 137, 364
Bible, 36, 54, 88
Bioflavonoids, 75, 78, 79, 89, 139, 147, 165, 192, 233, 278, 285, 331, 336, 337, 358
Bite wounds, 137, 138
Black Seed-plus, 29, 30, 125, 128, 129, 167, 203, 207, 226, 282, 283, 288, 299, 316, 319, 331, 343, 353, 363, 365, 366, 367, 368, 369, 370
Bladder infection, 138, 139, 364
Bleeding gums, 77, 139, 140, 364
Bleeding wounds, 140, 141
Blisters, 364
Bloating, 29, 38, 120, 161, 165, 225
Blood clot, 142
Blueberries, 90, 111, 112, 180, 234
Boils, 142, 143, 328, 364
Bone infection, 144, 328, 364
Botulism, 43
Brazil nuts, 72, 73, 87, 88, 96, 288, 307
Breast milk, 29, 38, 182, 299, 368
Bromelain, 30, 31, 131, 142, 186, 189, 215, 220, 222, 269, 270, 281, 313, 318, 323, 328, 339, 347, 348, 359
Bronchitis, 77, 145, 146, 328, 364
Bruises, 56, 147, 364
Burns, 12, 26, 41, 44, 50, 56, 64, 66, 80, 86, 92, 148, 287, 288, 323, 333, 364, 369

C

Cadmium, 84, 300
Calcium, 55, 58, 59, 88, 91, 92, 95, 99, 109, 126, 140, 220, 238, 250, 251, 257, 258, 285, 286, 298, 363, 367
Calcium chelate, 257, 363
Cancer, 23, 26, 32, 40, 45, 48, 57-60, 67, 71-74, 78, 80, 84, 97, 110, 111, 127, 161, 167, 253, 282, 291, 300, 303-307, 320, 321, 339, 355, 369
Candida albicans, 18, 49, 105, 247, 249, 271, 281, 338, 355
Canker sores, 26, 64, 149, 364
Carbon monoxide poisoning, 150, 321, 363
Carnitine, 205, 315
Carob molasses, 87-89, 166, 187, 198, 254, 299, 362
Carvacrol, 319
Cataracts, 82, 364
Cayenne pepper, 87, 131, 157, 222
Cellular phones, 304
Chapped lips, 152
Chelation therapy, 256
Chicago Tribune, 7, 283, 305, 350
Chlorine gas, 153, 154, 364
Cholera, 21, 22, 155, 156, 184, 364
Cilantro-plus, oil of, 219, 272, 365, 366, 367, 369
Cilantro/coriander, 32, 33, 191, 194, 218, 219, 299, 360
Cinnamon, 33, 34, 51, 52, 96, 104, 105, 120, 124, 155, 179, 180, 218, 260, 278, 294, 332, 333, 340, 351, 356, 361, 362
Cloves, 41, 104, 136, 140, 156, 212, 226, 278, 280, 307, 311, 313, 323, 327, 347, 356
Coenzyme Q-10, 229
Cold exposure, 9, 156, 206, 244, 364
Cold sores, 26, 28, 64, 158, 236, 244, 364
Colitis, 64, 121, 161, 162, 195, 354, 364 see also Irritable bowel
Concussion, 162, 163, 364
Conjunctivitis, 163, 164, 165, 364
Constipation, 44, 46, 121, 161, 165, 166, 175, 186, 233, 256, 294, 365
Coriander, oil of 360
Cough, 6, 49, 65, 167, 169, 190, 239, 264, 296, 352, 353, 365, 370
Cranberry, 34, 35, 139, 250, 251, 307, 337
CranFlush, 35, 139, 230, 237, 250, 251, 300, 337, 364, 366, 370
Crohn's disease, 161, 354
Croup, 169, 365
Cryptosporidium, 184, 225, 226, 365
Cumin, 34-37, 42, 51, 52, 72, 82, 87, 97, 104, 124, 125, 154, 155, 179, 180, 191, 212, 216, 248, 252, 259, 260, 280, 284, 287, 304, 306, 318-320, 331, 348, 351, 360, 361-370
Cuts, 44, 50, 64, 66, 80, 141, 170, 171, 365, see also Lacerations
Cyanide poisoning, 32, 171-173, 365
Cystitis, 138, 195, 354

D

Dandelion greens, 108, 109
Dandruff, 48, 49, 65, 337, 338
Dehydration, 155, 165, 174, 175, 183, 208, 365
Dengue fever, 21, 176, 279, 365
Depression, 62, 64-68, 70, 77, 120, 196, 243, 276, 277, 284, 289, 325
Dermatitis, 133, 177, 178, 365
Diabetes, 34, 49, 90, 112, 132, 178, 179, 180, 354, 365
Dianthrones, 67
Diaper rash, 180, 182, 365
Diarrhea, 32, 33, 44-47, 64, 93, 112, 120, 126, 155, 156, 161, 174, 177, 183, 184, 190, 193, 225, 268, 272, 292, 309, 315, 316, 330, 365
Diphtheria, 6, 169, 185, 186, 365
Diverticulitis, 186, 187, 365
DNA, 39, 40, 54, 100, 216

Dog bites, 138, 187, 188, 365
Drug overdose, 50, 189, 365
Dry eyes, 192, see also Irritated eyes

E

E. coli, 6, 18, 22, 52, 54, 105, 138, 184, 193, 215-218, 310, 365
Ear infection, 194, 195, 264, 335
Earache, 10, 194, 290
Ebola, 176, 197, 198, 215, 357, 365
Eczema, 133, 198, 199, 277, 354, 365
Electrolytes, 93, 94, 174, 175, 230, 315
Ellagic acid, 90
Emotionally distressed child, 200
Emphysema, 77, 201, 365
Encephalitis, 20, 21, 195, 202, 203, 279, 365
Encyclopedia of Essential Oils, 53
Endometriosis, 204, 354, 365
Enzymes, 30, 31, 61, 62, 89, 90, 138, 149, 156, 163, 190, 202, 213-215, 229, 271, 272, 280, 289, 300, 302, 312
Essence of rosemary, 203, 267, 287, 306, 322, 326, 353, 360, 368, 369
Essential fatty acids, 99, 109, 113, 133, 152, 192, 201, 270, 271, 365
Exhaustion, 25, 62, 70, 151, 205, 226, 230, 231, 232, 242, 260, 275, 277, 344, 357, 365, 366
Exposure to the elements, 93, 195, 206
Exposure to toxic chemicals, 37, 164

F

Fainting, 173, 208, 230, 365
Fatigue, 27, 62, 65, 77, 120, 151, 165, 205, 239, 242, 243, 255, 256, 260, 264, 280, 289, 354
Fennel, 37-39, 117, 139, 161, 162, 191, 243, 244, 251, 259, 270, 283, 294, 299, 330, 337, 360, 364, 366-370
 oil of, 38, 39, 117, 139, 161, 162, 243, 244, 251, 270, 283, 294, 299, 330, 337, 360, 364-370
Fever, 21, 22, 153, 174, 176, 185, 196, 208, 209, 239, 260, 264, 268, 279, 296, 316, 324, 340, 344, 356-358, 365, 366, 370
Filberts, 96, 97, 258, 281, 307
Fire ants, 134, 210, 211, 347, 366
Fish oils, 91, 95, 99, 100, 101, 142, 315, 365
Flavonoids, 31, 35, 55, 58, 59, 66-68, 76-79, 89, 97, 112, 147, 201, 202, 207, 221, 233, 266, 306, 324, 339 see also Bioflavonoids
Flax, 152, 180, 360
Fleas, 212, 213, 295
Flesh-eating bacteria, 213-215, 328, 331, 366, see also Strep A
Flu, 6, 10, 18, 19, 21, 22, 29, 77, 151, 209, 215-217, 234, 245, 260, 268, 289, 290, 353, 357, 366
Folic acid, 39, 40, 89, 90, 140, 149, 152, 168, 233, 257, 258, 285, 322, 331, 368
Food allergy, 128, 149, 165, 211, 318, 324, 336
Food dyes, 120, 121, 129, 159, 201, 315, 339
Food poisoning, 6, 103, 217-219, 309, 328, 366
Food preservatives, 103
Fractures, 80, 144, 220, 238, 366
fresh Pineapple, 31, 90, 142
Frostbite, 25, 26, 157, 206, 221, 366 see also Cold exposure
Fungal infection, 129, 145, 147, 192, 239, 275, 353, 355
Fungi, 18, 21, 27, 37, 41, 49, 54, 55, 122, 132, 133, 145, 147, 159, 167, 181, 182, 194, 196, 234, 241, 247-250, 324, 335, 354, 355

G

Gallbladder attack, 222, 223, 366
Gangrene, 132, 133, 221
Garlex, 41, 130, 136, 157, 194, 198, 207, 209, 211, 217, 219, 243,

269, 296, 311, 313, 347, 365, 370
Garlic, 40, 41, 51, 55, 72, 73, 114, 120, 123-125, 130, 134-136, 140, 142, 146, 155-160, 181, 184, 186, 192-194, 197, 198, 204, 207, 209, 211, 212, 216-219, 226, 240-243, 260, 262, 269, 278, 280, 295, 296, 311-313, 316, 323, 325, 327, 329, 332, 333, 347, 354, 356, 358, 361, 365-371
Gas mask, 154, 172, 284, 288
Gastritis, 115
Genetic engineering, 23, 252, 359
Genital herpes, 28, 223, 224, 236, 366
Giardia, 55, 184, 225, 226
Ginger, 117, 118, 162, 184, 194, 209, 227, 269, 282, 307, 311, 316, 325, 330, 331, 361, 368, 369
  oil of, 117, 162, 282, 330, 331, 361, 369
Gingivitis, 366
Glutathione, 36, 42, 61, 71, 72, 190, 191, 248

H

Headaches, 27, 29, 36, 61, 62, 68, 70, 120, 125, 162, 165, 226, 227, 256, 260, 273, 277, 366
Heart attack, 121, 228, 229, 291, 366
Heartburn, 48, 61, 120, *see also* Indigestion
Heat exhaustion, 25, 230, 231, 232, 366
Heat stroke, 366
Heavy metal poisoning, 71, 125, 300
Helicobacter pylori, 330, 366
Hemorrhoids, 32, 49, 161, 233, 366
Hepatitis, 6, 17, 22, 184, 234-236, 248, 366
Herbicide poisoning, 236, 246, 289, 293, 366
HerbSorb, 184, 219, 223, 230, 294, 298, 330, 331, 360, 363, 366, 368, 369
Herpes, 28, 54, 68, 75, 152, 158, 164, 190, 223-225, 236, 244, 278, 317, 366
Herring, 91, 142, 207, 238, 301
High blood pressure, 115, 236, 237, 366, *see also* Hypertension
High blood pressure attack, 236
Hip pain, 238, 366
Histoplasmosis, ("river fever"), 239, 240, 366
Hives, 26, 27, 120, 121, 135, 190, 211, 212, 240, 241, 247, 366
Honey, 43, 44, 49, 87-93, 98, 111, 118, 125, 133, 134, 139, 146, 148, 153, 155-159, 162, 166, 170, 171, 177, 181, 184, 187, 189, 198, 215, 219, 221, 229, 245, 246, 252, 254, 258, 265, 269, 288, 295, 299, 302, 307, 310, 316, 324, 327, 331, 332, 337, 339, 348, 362, 364-370
Hookworm, 241, 242, 243, 366
Horseradish, 146, 219, 262, 319
Hot flashes, 38, 65, 243, 244, 277, 366
Hypertension, 115, 236
Hypoglycemia, 325, 366
Hypothermia, 206, 244, *see also* Cold exposure

I

Immunization, 128, 169
Impetigo, 244, 245, 328, 367
Indigestion, 61, 120, 228
Infla-eez, 31, 117-121, 123, 131, 134, 142, 148, 184, 186, 187, 189, 198, 202, 204, 211-215, 220, 222, 224, 226, 229, 233, 236, 238, 241, 249, 262, 266, 269, 270, 271, 280-283, 295, 296, 300, 302, 312, 313, 318, 321, 323, 327-329, 335, 339, 342, 343, 347, 348, 359, 363-370
Influenza, 20, 21, 215, 216, 245, *see also* Flu
Ingrown toenail, 245, 367
Insect bites, 195, 202, 241, 347,

see also Bite wounds; Fire ants; Spider bites
Insomnia, 48, 65, 162, 246, 367
Iodine, 45, 55, 94, 168, 170, 288, 307, 356, 361, 362, 368, 370
Iron, 58, 88, 90, 91, 94, 103, 109, 113, 133, 190, 254, 289, 306
Irritable bowel, 40, 64, 120, 161, 195, 367
Irritated eyes, 164, 192, 365
Itchy skin, 120, 247, 367

J

Jaundice, 248, 357, 367
Jock itch, 129, 130, 249, 308, 367
Joint pain, 77, 115, 249, 255, 260, 277, 367

K

Kelp, 45, 46, 72, 157, 244, 307, 356, 361, 368
Kid-e-kare, 117, 146, 153, 160-163, 165, 169-171, 197, 200, 203, 209, 217, 254, 265, 268, 297, 311, 314, 325, 335, 339, 353, 364
Kidney infection, 249, 250, 367
Kidney stones, 35, 250, 251, 367
Killer bees, 134, 136, 251, 252, 367
Knee pain, 249, 367

L

lacerations, 41, 170, 171, 365
Lactobacillus, 46, 47, 147, 155, 156, 181, 194, 219, 278, 286, 363
Laryngitis, 65, 253, 254, 367
Lavender, 47-51, 117, 118, 132, 133, 138, 145, 146, 148, 152, 163, 165, 170, 178, 183, 186, 189, 191, 203, 208, 209, 213, 215, 216, 227, 232, 237, 246, 254, 274, 280, 281, 285, 296, 297, 314, 332-334, 345, 346, 351, 353, 358, 360, 361-370
oil of, 145, 148, 165, 183, 186, 363-368
Lead poisoning, 27, 254-257, 367
Lecithin, 98, 223, 360
Leg cramps, 257, 367
Lice, 258, 259, 366, 367
LivaClenz, 37, 42, 50, 100, 126, 156, 173, 191, 192, 194, 223, 236, 248, 257, 273, 279, 284, 293, 310, 316, 323, 348, 361, 366, 367-369
Lycopene, 73, 74, 90, 288, 307
Lyme disease, 20, 249, 260, 367, *see also* Tick bites

M

Mackerel, 95, 142, 157, 158, 271, 318
Macular degeneration, 367
Magnesium, 55, 58, 92, 94, 98, 109, 126, 140, 174, 220, 221, 230, 238, 250, 257, 258, 270, 286, 336, 367
Malaria, 21, 22, 263, 264, 279, 367
MCHC, (calcium chelate) 366
Measles, 202, 264, 265, 367
Melanoma, 265, 266, 367
Meningitis, 195, 267, 268, 367
Menstrual bleeding, 112, 269, 270, 367
Menstrual cramps, 270, 271, 367
Mercury poisoning, 271, 272, 367
Migraines, 32, 48, 227, 273, 367, *see also* Headaches
Milk products, 80, 97, 146, 149, 158, 160, 162, 168, 178, 186, 192, 197, 217, 311, 320
Mite allergy, 273, 368
Mold allergy, 128, 275, 277, 368
Molds, 21, 54, 87, 105, 128, 132, 159, 201, 275, 276, 285, 286, 289, 319, 332, 354-356
Mononucleosis (Mono), 278, 368
Mood, 60, 64, 66, 68, 120, 243, 325, 326, 369
Mood swings, 120, 243, 325
Mosquito bites, 203, 279, 368
MSG, 120, 129, 159, 200, 315, 338
Muhammad, 29, 32, 350

Mulberries, 110
Muscle soreness, 280, 368
Myrtle, 49, 50, 130-133, 143, 147, 152, 170, 179, 182, 204, 208, 224, 233, 244, 247, 271, 309, 318, 336, 345, 346, 353, 360, 365, 366, 367, 369, 370

N

NAC (N-acetyl cysteine), 50, 191
Nail bed infection, 281, 368
Nasal polyps, 281, 368
Native Americans, 93, 103, 111
Natural Preservatives, 94, 104
Necrotizing fasciitis, 213, *see also* Flesh eating bacteria; Strep A
Nerve gas poisoning, 283, 368
Nervousness, 62, 64, 284, 285, 368
Niacin, 95-99, 101, 103, 109, 168, 179, 298, 326, 331
Nigella seed, 29, 30, 37, *see also* Black seed
Nitrated meats, 121, 159, 160, 197, 321, 331, 349
Nosebleeds, 277, 285, 344, 368
Nuclear catastrophe, 286, 287, 303, 363, 368, *see also* Radiation poisoning
NukeProtect, 46, 73, 119, 126, 149, 151, 154, 172, 174, 191, 267, 273, 284, 288, 293, 322, 356, 364, 367-369
Nutri-Sense, 32, 98, 99, 166, 168, 179, 180, 187, 200-205, 223, 233, 293, 298, 299, 315, 326, 337, 360, 363, 365, 368
NutritionTest.com, 73, 191, 284, 325, 373

O

Onion, 55, 120, 125, 134, 135, 140, 142, 146, 156, 157, 160, 177, 181, 184, 186, 192-194, 198, 204, 207, 211, 216, 217, 228, 240, 241, 260, 262, 295, 311, 316, 323, 325, 329, 332, 333, 347, 361, 365, 371
OregaBiotic, 52, 130, 145, 146, 155, 184, 186, 193, 194, 198, 202, 215-219, 250, 264, 269, 279, 295, 302, 310, 329, 333, 341, 343, 344, 356, 358, 363, 371
Oregacyn, 36, 42, 72, 97, 117, 119, 124, 125, 129, 151, 154, 155, 159-162, 166, 167, 173, 216, 217, 218, 235, 236, 240, 262, 277, 279, 282, 283, 294, 296, 298, 309, 319, 323, 330, 343, 362-366
OregaMax, 55, 82, 119, 121, 127, 131, 139, 140, 145, 153, 157-160, 162, 166, 167, 177-183, 187, 194, 197, 199, 202-205, 209, 215, 220, 224, 226, 229, 233, 238, 240, 241, 245, 251, 252, 257, 258, 262-265, 269, 277, 279, 286, 295-298, 312, 317, 324, 331, 339, 343-346, 349, 355, 361-371
Oreganol P73, 26, 41, 54, 55, 97, 105, 118-122, 126, 129, 130, 134-145, 148-153, 157-161, 163, 165-169, 172, 173, 177, 180, 182, 184, 186, 189, 197, 199, 202-205, 216, 217, 229, 230, 237-240, 246, 264, 267, 271, 275, 279, 284, 287, 293, 296, 302-308, 312-316, 319-322, 336, 343, 344, 358, 360, 363-369, 371
Oxygen, 73, 121, 122, 150, 172, 173, 188, 196, 221

P

Pantothenic acid, 56, 62, 63, 97-99, 118, 121, 201, 221, 253, 257, 258, 266, 270, 317, 334, 361, 363, 364
Papain, 31, 131, 142, 156, 186, 189, 215, 220, 222, 269, 313, 318, 323, 328, 359, *see also* Bromelain
Papaya, 31, 90, 131, 142, 144, 156, 160, 166, 170, 175, 186, 194,

204, 234, 243, 262, 271, 281, 288, 312, 318, 333, 343, 347, 358
Parasites, 20, 27, 29, 36, 41, 64, 122, 133, 165, 167, 184, 187, 218, 219, 226, 234, 240, 241, 285
Peanuts, 96, 97, 149, 158, 187, 225, 258, 318
Pesticide, 93, 31, 42, 49, 109, 236, 246, 282, 289-293, 349, 350, 359, 368, *see also* Herbicide poisoning
Pink eye, 163
Pinworms, 294, 368
Plague, 22, 52, 105, 120, 212, 275, 276, 294, 295, 368
Pneumonia, 23, 152, 195, 202, 264, 295, 296, 328, 339, 368
Poison ivy, 297, 368
Pomegranate syrup, 250, 251, 254, 362
Poor appetite, 70, 276, 298, 368
Postnasal drip, 300, 368, *see also* Sinus attacks
Potassium, 45, 55, 58, 87-94, 97, 98, 108-113, 174, 184, 221, 250, 257, 307, 336, 351
Price-Pottenger Nutrition Foundation, 371, 372
Primrose oil, 192, 200
Processed meats, 123, 151, 230, 311, 315
Propolis, 26, 27, 28, 49, 104, 133, 158, 168, 170, 177, 189, 224, 302, 327, 335, 363
Prostatitis, 300, 368
Protein, 30, 31, 32, 42, 56, 83, 86, 87-103, 109, 113, 120, 130, 180, 187, 200, 213, 214, 223, 246, 257, 272, 298, 336, 337
Pseudomonas, 18, 105, 144
Psoriasis, 133, 199, 277, 328, 354, 368 *see also* Eczema
Pumpkin seed, 81, 84, 199, 266, 299, 300, 321, 322, 325, 329, 362
Puncture wounds, 188, 301, 302, 368
Purely-C, 79, 95, 129, 131, 134, 140, 141, 142, 146, 147, 153, 154, 160, 163, 165, 174, 177, 186, 192, 198, 202, 203, 206, 207, 215, 217, 232, 233, 249, 251, 265, 269, 271, 273, 278, 281, 286, 295, 296, 306, 324, 329, 331, 333, 337, 345-348, 358, 359, 364-370

Q

Qur'an, 56

R

Radiation, 9, 11, 12, 26, 31, 42, 45, 50, 61, 71-73, 80, 83, 84, 87, 283, 286-288, 303-308, 349, 350, 355, 362, 363, 369
Radiation poisoning, 12, 61, 87, 286, 287, 303, 306, 308, 363, 369, *see also* Nuclear catastrophe
Radishes, 102, 151, 175, 207, 233, 236, 247, 248, 319
Rash, 177, 180, 182, 190, 260, 264, 265, 275, 276, 365
Red grape powder, 56, 79, 105, 109, 139, 141, 166, 171, 173, 198, 232, 237, 239, 250-252, 257, 273, 286, 287, 293, 298, 306, 312, 321, 329, 331, 347, 361, 364, 365
Respiratory distress, 206, 272, 273, 290
Resveratrol, 57, 59, 97, 110, 112, 287, 321, 347
Resvital, 56-59, 95, 97, 123, 126, 128, 131, 134, 139, 140-142, 154, 166, 171, 173, 177-180, 198, 204-207, 228, 230, 232, 237, 239, 250-252, 257, 269, 273, 281, 286-288, 293, 298, 299, 306, 312, 329, 331, 337, 342, 347, 358, 361-370
Rhus coriaria (mountain sumac), 55, 181, 359, 361
Riboflavin, 42, 72, 103, 109, 152, 168, 169, 266, 365
Rice bran, 81, 98, 166, 360
Rice bran and rice polish, 98
Ringworm, 308, 337, 338, 369

Rosacea, 133, 369
Rose hips, 113, 358
Royal jelly, 56, 62, 63, 118, 121, 129, 137, 158, 168, 178, 180, 189, 200, 204, 205, 215, 220, 227-229, 232, 241, 244, 246, 271, 285, 298, 314, 318, 326, 342, 361
Royal Power, 63, 118, 121, 129, 134, 137, 149, 153, 158, 168, 175, 180, 189, 200, 204-208, 215, 220, 227, 229, 232, 241, 244, 258, 270, 271, 275, 285, 298, 299, 314, 318, 326, 337, 342, 361-370

S

Sage, 42, 51, 53, 60, 63-66, 72, 82, 87, 96, 97, 104, 117, 131, 149, 154, 157, 162, 168, 173, 175, 200, 205, 206, 209, 216, 222, 232, 244, 246, 254, 270, 280, 285, 287, 304, 306, 318, 334, 335, 360-369
Salmon, 56, 99, 100, 101, 142, 157, 158, 168, 200, 204, 207, 217, 236, 238, 257, 271, 299, 301, 307, 312, 315, 318
Salmonella, 6, 18, 52, 105, 184, 218, 309, 310, 344, 369
Salt, 45, 62, 68-70, 104, 175, 180, 200, 207, 222, 233, 253, 280, 283, 307, 324, 325, 345, 365, 366
Sardines, 100, 101, 142, 157, 158, 168, 207, 217, 236, 238, 257, 271, 301, 307, 315, 318
Scabies, 311, 369
Sciatica, 312, 313, 369
Scorpion bites, 313, 347, 369
Scurvy, 76, 111, 139, 147
Seizures, 172, 196, 256, 272, 290, 314, 369
Selenium, 42, 71, 72, 73, 82, 87, 121, 126, 133, 134, 149, 154, 191, 201, 266, 267, 273, 278, 284, 288, 300, 304-307, 348, 356, 361-365, 369, 370
Shigella, 6, 22, 184, 315, 316
Shingles, 28, 236, 316, 317, 369
Shortness of breath, 120, 172, 242, 296
Sinus attacks, 120, 300, 318, 369
Skin cancer, 26, 320, 369
Skin lesions, 124, 125
Smoke inhalation, 150, 172, 321, 322, 369
Snake bites, 322, 347, 369
Sore throat, 49, 65, 185, 190, 324, 369
Sour mood, 325, 326, 369
Spastic colon, 61, 161, *see also* Colitis
Spider bites, 326, 347, 369
Spinach, 147, 169, 203, 243, 322
Squash, 102, 123, 151, 202, 203, 299, 301, 322, 343
St. John's wort, 49, 60, 66-68, 227, 285, 326, 361, 362, 364, 367, 368
Staph infection, 328, 329, 369
Stiff neck, 7, 268
Stomach ulcer, 225, 330, 369
Stomachache, 29, 32, 115, 330, 369
Strep A, 331, 332, *see also* Flesh eating bacteria; Strep infection
Strep infection, 369
Sugar cravings, 369
Sunburn, 12, 25, 230, 333, 334, 369
Swimmer's ear, 335, 336, 370, *see also* Ear infections
Swollen feet/ankles, 336, 337, 370

T

Tapeworms, 370
Tea tree oil, 247, 252, 261, 262, 297, 368
Tetanus, 138, 301
The Lancet, 48, 69
Thiamine, 97, 179, 298, 325, 326, 331
Throat tightness, 135
Thyme, 52, 53, 55, 87, 318
Thymus capitus, 53, 55
Thymus vulgaris, 52

Thyroset, 46, 157, 166, 167, 170, 204, 207, 227, 229, 244, 307, 343, 356, 361, 364, 367
Tick bites, 263
Ticks, 6, 107, 202, 260, 261, 263
Tinea capitis, 337, 338, 370
Tomato paste, 74, 151, 288, 307
Tomatoes, 73, 74, 91, 102, 175, 307
Tonsillitis, 332, 338, 339, 370
Toothache, 340, 370
Trigeminal neuralgia, 341, 370
Tuberculosis, 105, 144, 342, 343, 370
Tuna, 101, 142, 157, 158, 207, 307, 312, 315, 318
Turnips, 102, 175, 207, 233, 236, 319
Typhoid fever, 22, 344, 370
Typhus, 212

U

Ulcerative colitis, 161, 354, *see also* Colitis
Ulcers, 56, 66, 131, 132, 239, 330, 346, 370
Urinary discomfort, 120

V

Vaginitis, 49, 195, 247, 345, 346, 354, 370
Varicose veins, 132, 346, 370
Venomous bites, 41, 322, 347, 370, *see also* Spider bites, Snake bites
Vinegar, 101, 105, 112, 156, 159, 192, 219, 223, 247, 253, 293, 314, 324, 325, 339

W, X, Y, Z

Warts, 64, 348, 349, 370
Water contamination, 349, 351, 370
Watermelon, 74, 90, 139, 175, 207, 233
Whooping cough, 6, 65, 352, 353, 370
Wild oregano, 26, 37, 41, 44, 51-55, 72, 92, 93, 96, 104, 105, 119, 124, 125, 129, 132, 134, 139, 140, 141, 145, 148, 153, 156, 157, 162, 165, 166, 170-172, 181-189, 192, 194, 199, 203, 209, 214, 215, 216, 220, 226, 237, 240-243, 246, 251, 254, 262, 264, 269, 274, 277, 284, 302, 308, 310, 316, 319, 329, 331, 337, 339, 343, 344, 351, 352, 355, 360-362, 371
Wild strawberry, 76, 111, 206, 246, 358, 361
Wild Power Tea, 111, 147, 206, 246, 250, 337, 361
Wild oregano honey, 44, 92, 125, 153, 156, 162, 166, 170, 184, 189, 246, 302
Wild St. John's wort, 67, 68, 227, 361, 362, 364, 367, 368
Wounds, 12, 25, 26, 41, 44, 48-50, 56, 64, 66, 68, 83, 92, 131-133, 137, 188, 189, 242, 288, 302, 328, 368
see also Bleeding wounds; Bite wounds; Puncture wounds
Wild raspberries, 112
Wild rice, 166, 169, 362
X-rays, 303, 304
Yeast infection, 139, 165, 167, 181, 196, 250, 345
Yellow fever, 279, 356-358, 370
Yogurt, 46, 120, 155, 169, 257, 337, 346
Zinc, 83, 84, 133, 140, 192, 201, 220, 266, 278, 281, 282, 285, 300, 321, 3329, 331, 333, 348, 358, 363